COMPUTATIONAL LINGUISTIC TEXT PROCESSING

LOGICAL FORM, SEMANTIC INTERPRETATION, DISCOURSE RELATIONS AND QUESTION ANSWERING

COMPUTATIONAL LINGUISTIC TEXT PROCESSING

LOGICAL FORM, SEMANTIC INTERPRETATION, DISCOURSE RELATIONS AND QUESTION ANSWERING

RODOLFO DELMONTE

Nova Science Publishers, Inc.
New York

For permission to use material from this book please contact us:
Telephone 631-231-7269; Fax 631-231-8175
Web Site: http://www.novapublishers.com

LIBRARY OF CONGRESS CATALOGING-IN-PUBLICATION DATA

Delmonte. Rodolfo.
Computational linguistic text processing:logical form, semantic interpretation, discourse relations and question answering / Rodolfo Delmonte.
p. cm.
ISBN 13: 978-1-60021-700-5 (hardcover)
ISBN 10: 1-60021-700-1 (hardcover)
1. Discourse analysis – Data processing. 2. Computational linguistics. I..Title.
P302.3.D444 2007
401'.410285 – dc22

Published by Nova Science Publishers, Inc. ✢ New York

CONTENTS

LSLT – Lexical Semantic Language Theory

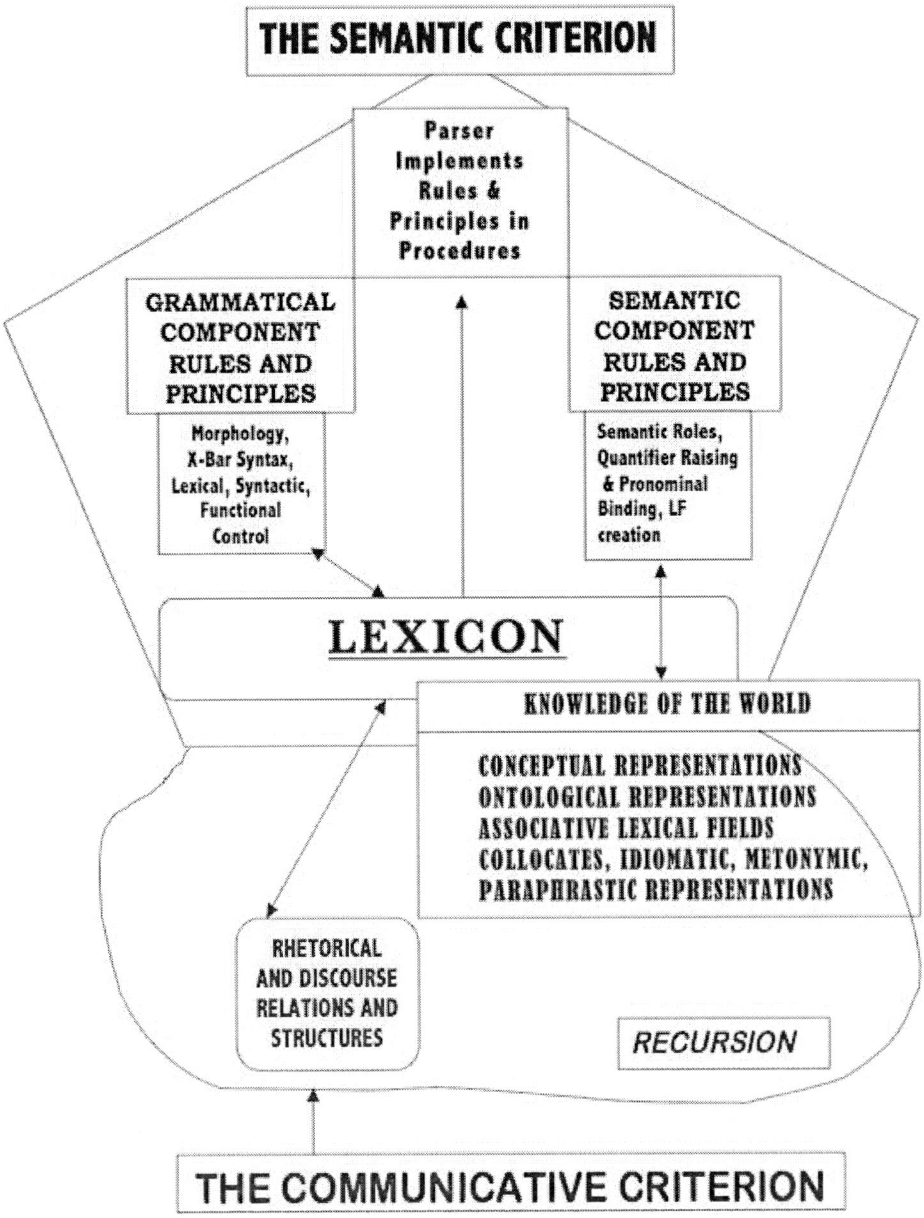

INTRODUCTION

1. THE FOUNDATIONS

The topic of this book is the theoretical foundations of a theory LSLT – Lexical Semantic Language Theory - and its implementation in a the system for text analysis and understanding called GETARUN[1], developed at the University of Venice, Laboratory of Computational Linguistics, Department of Language Sciences. LSLT encompasses a *psycholinguistic theory* of the way the language faculty works, a *grammatical theory* of the way in which sentences are analysed and generated – for this we will be using Lexical-Functional Grammar -, a *semantic theory* of the way in which meaning is encoded and expressed in utterances – for this we will be using Situation Semantics -, and a *parsing theory* of the way in which components of the theory interact in a common architecture to produce the needed language representation to be eventually spoken aloud or interpreted by the *phonetic/acoustic language interface*. LSLT will then be put to use to show how *discourse relations* are mapped automatically from text using the tools available in the 4 sub-theories, and in particular we will focus on *Causal Relations* showing how the various sub-theories contribute to address different types of causality.

We assume that the main task the child is faced with is creating an internal mental LEXICON which we further assume should contain two types of information: Grammatical – to feed the Grammatical component of the language faculty – and Semantic – to allow for meaning to be associated to each lexical entry. This activity is guided by two criteria:

Semantic Criterion

The goal of the language faculty is that of creating meaning relations between words and (mental representations of) reality, that is events, entities and their attributes

Communicative Criterion

The goal of the language faculty is that of allowing communication between humans to take place

---

[1] A complete version of the system used to produce the linguistic representations included in this book and in Book 1 will be made available with the publication of Book 1.

Both criteria are taken as primitives: the developmental evidence of communicative intentions is given in Bara(2007). That communicating implies understanding hence the need of semantic processing follows.

We start by addressing the *psycholinguistic theory* in which the basic goal is the creation of meaning relations between linguistic objects – words – and bits of reality – situations for short. To do that we set forth the strong claim that in order to have Analysis and Generation become two facets of the same coin, Semantics needs to be called in and Lexical information be specified in such a way as to have the Parser/Generator work properly. In this respect, syntax only represents a subcomponent of the Grammatical theory and as such contributes to the definition of the primitives of the LSLT. We assume that some type of X-bar syntax is inherited and innate together with innate knowledge of basic syntactic principles and parameters – or Universal Grammar (UG). As is usually assumed by all linguistic theories, language acquisition activates both universal grammar and some peripheral grammar rules. Both morphological and syntactic principles are learnt with semantic ones, which alone may guarantee their consistency.

We will take the stance that the existence of a backbone of rewriting rules with reference to recursion is inherently innate (see Hauser, Chomsky, 2002). However, together with Hinzen (2006;2007), we assume that syntactic structure should be underspecified with regard to the semantic (and pragmatic) task to be performed: "domain-general principles of organizing information economically lend themselves to semantic uses, they engender semantic consequences"(2007c). As will appear clear in the chapter on Text Generation, it is the Planning phase that organizes meaning structures which are then externalized by the Realization component where language-dependent syntactic constraints flesh out the appropriate surface forms.

At the same time, we claim that recursion is a mechanism driven by communicative needs, and in the last resort relates, to the second important goal of a psycholinguistic theory, that is the necessity the child has to communicate. Communicating with the external world will slowly make the child aware of the existence of a point of view which is external from his own.

Here by recursion we only refer to high sentence level recursion and not to the more technical concept of recursion in formal grammars, where it corresponds to the notion that recursion occurs every time a rewriting rule contains the same symbol in both right and left hand side. We are only concerned with recursive calls to Sentence level rules, which constitute a problem for parsers and an increase in complexity for sentence comprehension. From a linguistic point of view, recursion in utterances is represented basically by two types of structures: sentential complements which have a *reportive* semantic content, and relative clauses which have a *supportive* semantic content. Reportive contents are governed by *communication* predicates, which have the semantic content of introducing two propositions related to two separate situations in spatiotemporal terms. Supportive contents are determined by the need to bring in at the interpretation level a situation which helps better individuate the entity represented by the governing nominal predicate. Thus, we might assume that recursion is triggered by communicative processes and referential semantic properties of utterances and the underlying propositions.

The *Grammatical Theory* (hence GT) defines the way in which lexical entries need to be organized. However, the Lexicon is informed both by the Grammatical and the Semantic Theory which alone can provide the link to the Ontology or Knowledge of the World

Repository. As in LFG, we assume the existence of lexical forms where lexical knowledge is encoded, which is composed of grammatical information – categorial, morphological, syntactic, and selectional restrictions. These are then mapped onto semantic forms, where semantic roles are encoded and aspectual lexical classes are associated. In Analysis, c-structures are mapped onto f-structures and eventually turned into s-structures. Rules associating lexical representations with c-structures are part of GT. The mapping is effortless being just a bijective process, and is done by means of FSA – finite state automata. C-structure building is done in two phases. After grammatical categories are associated to inflected wordforms, a disambiguation phase takes place on the basis of local and available lexical information. The disambiguated tagged words are organized into local X-bar based head-dependent structures, which are then further developed into a complete clause-level hierarchically based structure, through a cascaded series of FSA which make use of recursion only when there are lexical constraints – both grammatical and semantic – requiring it. C-structure is mapped onto f-structure by interpretation processes based on rules defined in the grammar and translated into parsing procedures. It is a fact that Grammatical relations are only limited to what are usually referred to as Predicate-Argument relations, which may only encompass obligatory and optional arguments of a predicate. The Semantic Theory will add a number of important items of interpretation to the Grammatical representation, working at propositional level: negation, quantification, modality and pronominal binding. These items will appear in the semantic representation associated to each clause and are activated by means of parsing procedures specialized for those tasks. Semantic Theory also has the task of taking care of non-grammatical objects usually defined with the two terms, Modifiers and Adjuncts. In order to properly interpret meaning relations for these two optional component of utterance linguistic content, the Semantic theory may access Knowledge of the World as represented by a number of specialized lexical resources, like Ontology, for inferential relations; Associative Lexical Fields for Semantic Similarity relations; Collocates for most frequent modifier and adjunct relations; Idiomatic and Metonymic relations as well as Paraphrases for best stylistic purposes. In Generation, a plan is created and predicates are inserted in predicate-argument structures (hence PAS) with attributes – i.e. modifiers and adjuncts. Syntax plays only a secondary role in that they are hooked to stylistic, rhetorical rules which are genre and domain related. They are also highly idiosyncratic depending strongly on each individual social background. Surface forms will be produced according to rhetorical and discourse rules, by instantiating features activated by semantic information.

In particular, our theory of linguistic knowledge acquisition being strongly semantically founded, helps explain why lexical knowledge is coupled to the way in which words are used in sentences and how they are used to convey and comprehend knowledge of the world. In our perspective, lexical knowledge is gathered from and is constituted of the following semantic and pragmatic items:

- Events or Situations with Participants characterized by Semantic Roles, a Perspective or Point of View, a Temporal Extension of Event

As a consequence of that, we have a number of issues that are strictly related to lexical acquisition and need appropriate description in lexical entries – as they have in our lexicon:

a. Meaning of lexical entry is related to the actual world or not (factuality)
b. Events carry consequences on the state of affairs described (causality)
c. Relations of events to spatiotemporal locations of arguments may change or not (aspectuality)
d. Complexity of lexical meaning contained in the lexical entry (semantic decomposition)

The basic issue we will tackle in prospecting our theory is the way in which this knowledge is filtered from sentences as they are produced in the context of acquisition for the child. As we know from any semantic theory – but here we will be referring to Situation Semantics – sentences are to be interpreted as follows: sentential surface structures are propositions which contain among others, the following linguistic items for the semantic interpretation, organized into primary (i.) and secondary (ii.) items:

i. Predicates, Arguments, Adjuncts, Spatiotemporal Locations
ii. Modality, Negation, Conditionality, Quantification, Opacity.

From a computational point of view, we assume that to encode such knowledge, we need to posit the following 4 levels of lexical knowledge and consequent mapping operations which are organized by increasingly restrictive layers of representation, where syntax and morphology are used to provide starting elements, i.e. heads or lexemes for lexical encoding, which corresponds to 0 level:

I. Level 1. GRAMMATICAL FUNCTIONS – associated to each head/predicate from constituency labels by functional mapping and syntactic information (the subject being the NP that agrees with the verb in features) – SUBJect, OBJect, OBLique, ARG-MOD-agent, ADJunct, MODifier, PROPosition, etc.
II. Level 2. SEMANTIC MAPPING of each f-structure to a predicate-argument structure with modifiers and adjuncts – ARG0, ARG1, etc., and the other secondary components
III. Level 3. PRAGMATIC MAPPING from domain-bound definitions with semantically disambiguated meaning via an ontology-like knowledge base (WordNet) into a semantically structured representation.

As a consequence of that, there are two main tenets of the theory which are supporting the construction of the system: one is that it is possible to reduce access to domain world knowledge by means of contextual reasoning, i.e. reasoning triggered independently by contextual or linguistic features of the text or discourse under analysis. In other words, it adopts what could be termed the Shallow Processing Hypothesis: access to the Ontology is reduced and substituted whenever links are missing through inferences on the basis of hand-coded lexical and grammatical knowledge given to the system, which are worked out in a fully general manner.

In exploring this possibility we make one fundamental assumption and it is that the psychological processes needed for language analysis and understanding are controlled by a processing device which is completely separated from that of language generation with which it shares a common lexicon though.

In our approach there is no statistical processing, but only algorithms based on symbolic rules – even though we use FSA to help tag disambiguation and parsing. The reason for this is twofold: an objective one, statistical language models need linguistic resources which in turn are very time-consuming to produce and highly error-prone activities. On more general terms, one needs to consider that highly sophisticated linguistic resources are always language and genre dependent, besides the need to comply with requirements of statistical representativeness. No such limitations can be deemed for symbolic algorithms which on the contrary are more general and easily portable from one language to another. Differences in genre can also be easily accounted for by scaling rules adequately.

It is sensible to assume that when understanding a text a human reader or listener does make use of his encyclopaedia parsimoniously. Contextual reasoning is the only way in which a system for Natural Language Understanding should tap external knowledge of the domain. In other words, a system should be allowed to perform an inference on the basis of domain world knowledge when needed and only then. In this way, the system could simulate the actual human behaviour in that access to extralinguistic knowledge is triggered by contextual factors independently present in the text and detected by the system itself. This would be required only for implicit linguistic relations as can happen with bridging descriptions, to cope with anaphora resolution phenomena, for instance. In other words, we want to show that there are principled ways by which linguistic processes must interact with knowledgde representation or the ontology.

It is also our view that humans understand texts only whenever all the relevant information is supplied and available. Descriptive and narrative texts are usually self-explanatory - not so, literary texts - in order to allow even naive readers to grasp their meaning. Note that we are not here dealing with spoken dialogues, where a lot of what is meant can be left unsaid or must be implicitly understood.

In the best current systems for natural language, the linguistic components are kept separate from the knowledge representation, and work which could otherwise be done directly by the linguistic analysis is duplicated by the inferential mechanism. The linguistic representation is usually mapped onto a logical representation which is in turn fed onto the knowledge representation of the domain in order to understand and validate a given utterance or query. We shall comment and discuss some such systems in the book.

Thus the domain world model or ontology must be priorly built, usually in view of a given task the system is set out to perform. This modelling is domain and task limited and generality can only be achieved from coherent lexical representations, as will be discussed in the book. In some of these systems, the main issue is how to make the two realms interact as soon as possible in order to take advantage of the inferential mechanism to reduce ambiguities present in the text or to allow for reasoning on linguistic data, which otherwise couldn't be understandable.

We assume that an integration between linguistic information and knowledge of the world can/must be carried out at all levels of linguistic description and that contextual reasoning can be thus performed on the fly rather than sequentially. This does not imply that external knowledge of the world is useless and should not be provided at all: it simply means that access to this knowledge must be filtered out by the analysis of the linguistic content of surface linguistic forms and their abstract representations of the utterances making up the text.

As we said, the task we are faced with when trying to simulate human understanding of texts is to scientifically isolate the contexts in which external knowledge of the world should be made available to the system, as well as providing the tools to deal with this task adequately. There is a description of our task which deserves quoting, and is taken from P.Bosch contribution to a book by Herzog & Rollinger(eds), Text Understanding in LILOG, which we take to be the best example of the attempt to come to terms with the problem at stake. In his paper, the author makes the point of what he takes to be main problem to be tackled: i.e. identifying in a text "inferentially unstable" concepts which are to be kept distinct from "inferentially stable" ones. The latter should be analysed solely on the basis of linguistic description, while the former should tap external linguistic knowledge of the world. Before entering into a comment of this issue, we would like to quote from his Conclusions:

> "The central point of this paper is to try to give a direction to work on the interaction of linguistic analysis and knowledge representation in knowledge-based NL Systems. I have tried to argue and to demonstrate that without a full linguistic analysis there is little hope that we shall ever have reasonably general and portable language modules in NL systems. It has also become clear, I hope, that this is not a trivial task but requires a decent amount of empirical research for many years to come. But the linguistic research required is not isolated research in pure linguistics, but close cooperation with work on knowledge representation and - although this is a point I have not argued for - psychological work on conceptual systems, is imperative.
>
> The most difficult problem to overcome, I believe, is that the most generally held belief in the scientific community with respect to our problem is that the distinction between linguistic and conceptual facts is arbitrary and hence not a proper research question, but a matter of pragmatic decisions. It is this belief more than anything else that inhibits further progress of the kind Brachman found lacking."(p.257)

Our book can then be regarded as a contribution towards this final goal which we identify tout court with contextual reasoning, i.e. performing inferential processes on the basis of linguistic information while keeping under control the contribution of external knowledge in order to achieve understanding of a text.

2. THE SYSTEM GETARUN AND THE BOOKS

Getarun (General Text And Reference UNderstander) is a system for text understanding based manily on the resolution of referential processes, an extension of a previous system called ROSIE. It operates both with pronominal and nominal expressions, at sentence and text level. The aim of the system is to build a model world where relations and entities introduced and referred to in the text are asserted, searched for and ranked according to their relevance. In addition to that, the system is able to generate text, in the form of answers to queries, and in the form of short paraphrases or summaries of the input text(s). In some cases, it can also generate stories and Questions and Answers randomly from a plan and a Discourse Model.

The architecture of the system is strictly related to the structure of the books. To better describe it, we decided to dedicate one book to the lower level part of the system and another book to the higher level system components. In this way, each component or module is presented in at least one chapter of the book.

Thus, we can think of the book as being organized around two scientifically distinct but in fact strictly interrelated fields of research:

- sentence level linguistic phenomena
- text or discourse level linguistic phenomena

the former to be described by means of grammatical theories, the latter requiring the intervention of extralinguistic knowledge, i.e. knowledge of the world. This distinction is usually drawn for scientific purposes and is clearly artificial: the sentence being at the same time the smallest domain at which rigorous linguistic analysis can hopefully be applied; but also the basic complete semantic unit whereby meaning can be conveyed, depending on the text/discourse context. We are aware of the fact that this subdivision is mainly wrought out for scientific reasons and does not really imply that such a neat subdivision of tasks can be actually envisaged in real text processing. As shall be discussed in detail in the books, semantic issues need to be tackled already at the beginning. This notwithstanding, the separation has its own "raison d'etre" and we will try to validate it in the books.

The first part of Book I – Chapts. 1-4 - has been devoted to the discussion of sentence-level related linguistic issues, treating non directly explainable intruding discourse-level facts as exceptions or ambiguous cases, to be coped with by means of parsing strategies of one kind or another. There follows a central part of Book I – Chapts. 5-7 - which partakes of both issues and these are: quantification, semantic shallow interpretation, pronominally based discourse anaphora. Chapter 8 has been included to show that the system can be used fruitfully in a shallow version, by doing away with some of its components: indeed, in this version the quantity of semantic processing and the ensuing understanding achieved will be drastically reduced. In particular, Chapter I and Chapter II discuss the computational, the grammatical and semantic properties of the lexicon, the parser and their representation formalism. Chapter III discusses what is usually referred to as shallow parsing, which in our case coincides with a fully bottom-up version of a cascaded RTN parser also used in multilingual environments. Chapter IV describes the Anaphoric Binding module and its theoretical foundations. Chapter V, VI and Chapter VII discuss Anaphora Resolution at discourse and text level and outline a theory of discourse. Chapter V treats separately the question of quantifiers, which is however an all pervasive one. Chapter VIII introduces a full-fledged shallow version of the system, which however includes a discussion of a certain number of modules currently being deemed necessary to carry out Intelligent Sentence Extraction tasks as a first step towards Summarization.

Then Book II contains the following chapters which are strictly amenable to semantics, discourse-level issues, reasoning and generation. Chapter I and Chapter II introduce the Semantic Modules and the Interpreter. Chapter III discusses Spatio-Temporal Relations and their computation. Chapter IV discusses the module for the analysis of discourse and rhetorical relations. Chapter V deals with Text Generation, Chapter VI presents a shallow/hybrid version of the system which is used for Semantic Evaluation. Finally Chapter VII shows how the Discourse Model and Conceptual Representations can be used to produce reasoning and generate answers to queries, also on the basis of an ontology wrought in KL-ONE.

GETARUN is a general multilingual text and reference understander which represents a linguistically based approach to text understanding and embodies a number of general strategies on how to implement linguistic principles in a running system. As said before, the system addresses one main issue: the need to restrict access to extralinguistic knowledge of the world by contextual reasoning, i.e. reasoning from linguistically available cues.

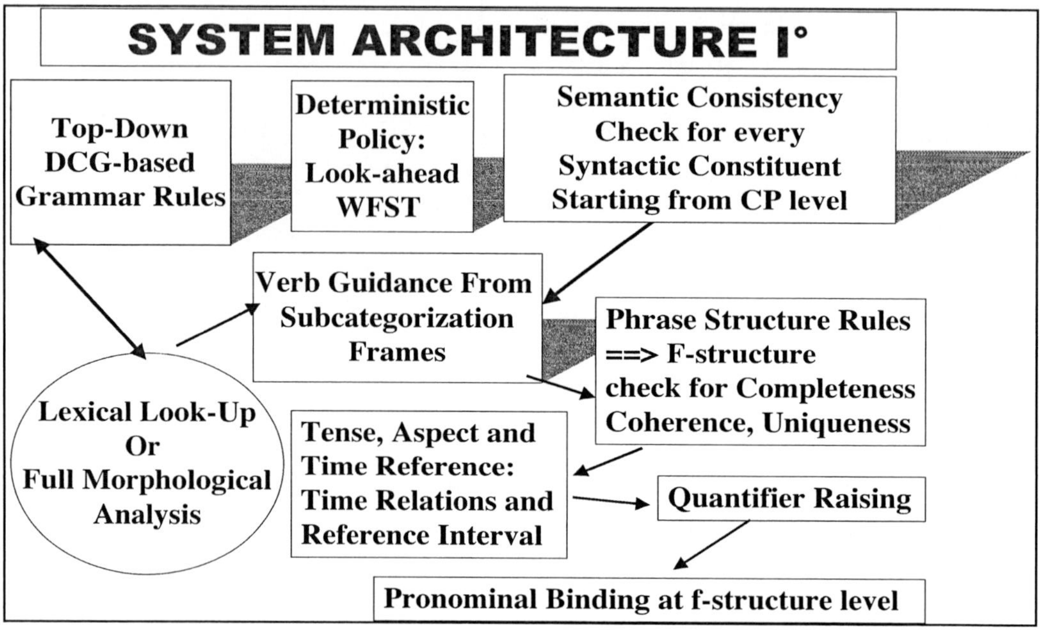

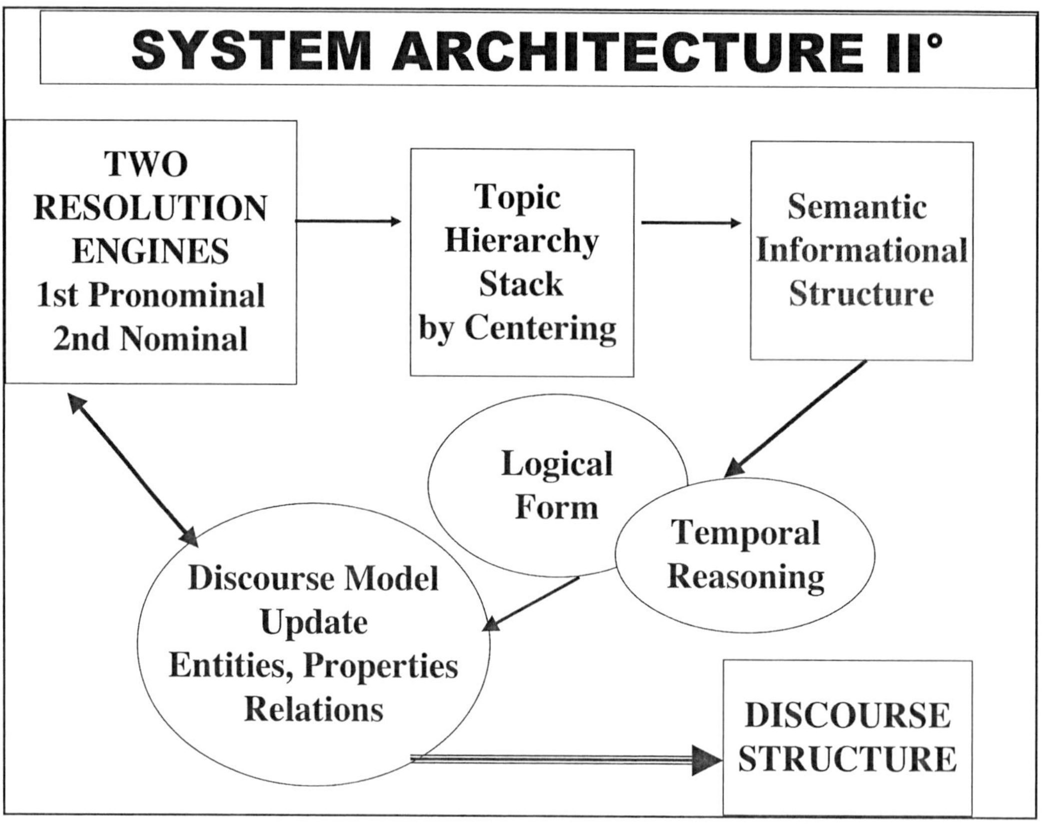

Figure 1 and Figure 2. Architecture of System I and II.

Another important issue addressed by the system is multilinguality. In GETARUN the user may switch from one language to another by simply unloading the current lexicon and loading the lexicon for the new language: at present only Italian, German and English are fully implemented. Work is under way for other Romance languages, such as French and Spanish. Multilinguality has been implemented to support the theoretical linguistic subdivision of Universal Grammar into a Core and a Pheripheral set of rules.

The system is organized around another fundamental assumption: the architecture of such a system must be modular thus requiring a pipeline of sequential feeding processes of information, each module providing one chunk of knowledge, backtracking being barred at intermodular level and allowed only within each single module. The architecture of the system is organized in such a way as to allow feedback into the parser from Anaphoric Binding: however, when pronominals have been finally bound or left free no more changes are allowed on the f-structure output of the parser.

Thus we can think of the system as being subdivided into two main meta-modules or levels: Low Level System, containing all modules that operate at Sentence Level; High Level System, containing all the modules that operate at Discourse and Text Level updating the Discourse Model. The Two subcomponents can be viewed in the preceding two figures, Figure 1 and Figure 2.

The book is organized as an experimental exercise: it contains both theoretical background and the output of the system, GETARUN that enacts and applies the theory. It is divided up into 8 chapters and each chapter addresses a single topic. However, it is sometimes hard to separate neatly strictly related semantic issues seen that they all contribute to produce the output of the system.

Five chapters are more theoretically bound – the first 4 chapters and chapter 6. The remaining 3 chapters are more application oriented. While dealing with foundational issues of semantics and reasoning, the theoretically bound chapters make use of the output of GETARUN in its complete and deep version, to illustrate and exemplify the theory. The application oriented chapters, on the contrary, are tied to GETARUNS – the "shallow" or partial version of the system, which is meant to cope with unlimited vocabulary or unrestricted text analysis, i.e. with no boundaries determined by domain or genre. This second version of the system will be introduced in chapter VII.

BOOK I: LOW LEVEL SYSTEM

2.1. Parser

The parser is based on LFG theoretical framework and has a highly interleaved modular structure. Basic grammatical representation modules are the Lexicon, and grammar rules to bind C-structure and F-structure which is internally represented as a graph. The Parser is a DCG which exploits the properties of Prolog as to its general parsing strategy - topdown, depth-first - and makes backtracking naturally available.

The internal architecture of the parser is organized on the basic idea of Universal Grammar, i.e. on the well-known fact that all languages share a common core grammar and may vary at the periphery: internal differences are predicted by principles. The DCG grammar allows the specification of linguistic rules in a highly declarative mode: it works topdown and by making a heavy use of linguistic knowledge may achieve an almost complete deterministic policy. Principles are scattered throughout the grammar so that they can be made operative as soon as a given rule is entered by the parser.

In particular, a rule may belong either to a set of languages, e.g. Romance or Germanic, or to a subset thereof, like English or Italian, thus becoming a peripheral rule. Rules are activated at startup and whenever a switch is being operated by the user, by means of logical flags appropriately inserted in the right hand side of the rule. No flags are required for rules belonging to the common core grammar.

Some such rules include the following ones: for languages like Italian and Spanish, a Subject NP may be an empty category, either a referential little pro or an expletive pronoun; Subject NPs may be freely inverted in postverbal position, i.e. preverbal NP is an empty category in these cases. For languages like Italian and French, PP or adverbial adjuncts may intervene between Verb and Object NP; adjectival modifiers may be taken to the right of their head Noun. For languages like English and German, tense and mood may be computed in CP internal position, when taking the auxiliary or the modal verb. English almost freely allows an empty Complementizer for finite complement and relative clauses, and negation requires do-support.

Syntactic and semantic information is accessed and used as soon as possible: in particular, both categorial and subcategorization information attached to predicates in the lexicon are extracted as soon as the main predicate is processed, be it adjective, noun or verb, and are used to subsequently restrict the number of possible structures to be built. Adjuncts are computed by semantic compatibility tests on the basis of selectional restrictions of main predicates and adjuncts' heads.

Syntactic rules are built according to some chomskyian paradigm with CP-IP functional maximal projections; however, the general underlying theoretical framework is cast into LFG theory. Thus, we build and process syntactic phenomena like wh- movement before building f-structure representations, where only anaphoric binding for pronominals takes place.

The parser makes use of Parsing Strategies and achieves a strong determinism thanks to a Lookahead mechanism, which has been finely tuned for each language. Lookahead may look the input stack for up to three symbols in sequence. The Hybrid architecture makes use of shallow c-structure information to predict when the verb is ready to be processed top-down.

2.2. Quantifier Raising

Since we know that quantifiers and quantified NPs usually take scope at propositional and NP level, we assume f-structure to be an adequate level of representation in which quantifer scope can be computed. In this we partially follow Halvorsen's proposal, which however requires a further mapping from f-structures to s-structures in order to do that. We proceed as follows: after assigning Q-Markers to quantifiers and quantified NPs and adding this information as attribute-value pair at f-structure, we perform Quantifier Raising by traversing f-structure until we reach a propositional or NP node. At that level we deposit a Quantifer-Operator(Q-Op), in an attribute that has a list as its value. Once Q-Ops have been produced, we are in a position to assign quantifier scope. In case more than one Q-Op is present in the list, the algorithm simply reorders the operators according to their quantifying force, and/or to grammatical function. Otherwise, a search downward is performed in the f-structure for other q-ops. When some q-marker is found another attribute-value pair is added at pred level indicating a quantified interpretation.

2.3. The Binding Module

The output of grammatical modules is fed then onto the Binding Module(BM) which activates an algorithm for anaphoric binding in LFG terms using f-structures as domains and grammatical functions as entry points into the structure. Pronominals are internally decomposed into a feature matrix which is made visible to the Binding Algorithm(BA) and allows for the activation of different search strategies into f-structure domains. Antecedents for pronouns are ranked according to grammatical function, semantic role, inherent features and their position at f-structure. Special devices are required for empty pronouns contained in a subordinate clause which have an ambiguous context, i.e. there are two or more possible antecedents available in the main clause. Also split antecedents trigger special search strategies in order to evaluate the possible set of antecedents in the appropriate f-structure domain. Special care is paid to pronominals bound by quantifiers or quantified NPs. The output of the BA is then passed on to an Interpretation Module which operates locally in order to spot the presence of conditions for Specific or Arbitrary Reading for pronominal expressions.

Finally, this information is added into the original f-structure graph and then passed on to the High Level System.

2.4. Anaphora Resolution

Anaphoric binding of free pronominals takes as input Discourse level information which is computed by a Module of Discourse Anaphora(MDA) and decides on the basis of semantic categories attached to predicates and arguments of predicates whether to bind a pronoun to the locally available antecedent or to the discourse level one.

Discourse Anaphora is computed by a system which is very close to the ones available in literature on the same topic, and presented by C.Sidner and B.Webber in their publications. Definite descriptions are computed by means of locally available information and, but only when required, by tapping external knowledge sources. However, a set of default rules are activated in lack of such knowledge which work simply on the basis of grammatical and semantic information.

This level of representation works on the basis of a list of candidates or possible arguments of discourse which includes all external pronouns and referential expressions. The algorithm creates a Weighted List of Candidate Arguments of Discourse(WLCAD).

The MDA detects Main, Secondary, Potential and Expected TOPIC in each utterance by weighting the list of external pronominals and of referential expressions made available by the grammatical representation. After the first utterance, the MDA tries to take advantage of discourse level internal cohesion and coherence mechanisms in order to check whether a given topic is reintroduced in the following text as a pronoun, a nominal substitute, a deictic and so on. The MDA is a finite state automaton that works strictly on the basis of two adjacent utterances; it has a set of six states available: Continue, Change, Resume, Shifting,

Retaining, Continue_Analyze. Special inferential mechanisms are activated at this local level by the presence of nonthematic functions, i.e. SUBJects or OBJects of copulative and other verbs which do not assign a semantic role to their arguments. The algorithm takes care of bridging descriptions using the Discourse Model and external world knowledge. The output of the MDA is a Rhetorical Structure with a list of all Topics in each utterance and a state.

2.5. Computing Information Structure

As a first step towards a semantic representation, the system builds Information Structure at clause level. Each utterance is decomposed into separate clauses to account for coordination and subordination. The output is a set of values associated to labels such as Clause Type, Point of View, Factivity, Change in State of the World, Relevance and Discourse Relations. Point of View may vary between Subjective, Subjective_Extensional, Subjective_Intensional, Objective; Change may be Null, Early, Culminated, Gradual and Setting; Relevance may be Foreground and Background. All these values are computed mainly on the basis of semantic, aspectual and temporal features associated with main verbal predicate at f-structure for each clause.

Information structure is passed, then, on to the Semantic Module and Discourse Relation Reasoning Module. In particular, the latter computes Discourse Relations on the basis of information structure, temporal interpretation and the model. The output of this module is a set of values, which include: Narration, Elaboration, Description, Parallel, Explanation, Cause, Result. The Discourse Model is consequently a database in which inheritance is easily computed at the end of the text. In addition, we created a mechanism of Relevance Score assignment which takes into account topicality and discourse relations in which a given entity was involved by computing a score with different weights. In this way, all entities appearing in the text are finally sorted in descending order according to their relevance, with the list of facts and situations each one shared.

2.6. Shallow and Partial Text Processing for Linguistic Information Extraction and Summarization

In this chapter we present a morphological analyser for Italian, a Tagger and the accompanying statistical and syntactically based Disambiguation algorithm; a Shallow Multilevel Syntactic Parser and an adaptation of the Higher Level Discourse and Semantic components of GETARUN to fit into a Partial Semantic Parser. This is both referred to grammar checking and the summarization problem. In the case of summarization, sentence extraction is viewed as a first step in the process of text summarization and as a means to achieve a reasonable reduction of information load when attempting text understanding tasks. Linguistic strategies can be fruitfully applied, as will be discussed, in order to postpone the use of a knowledge representation language for terminological reasoning, until the size of the text has been reduced to a percent of the original value - typically 25%.

BOOK II: HIGH LEVEL SYSTEM

2.7. Semantic Interpretation

Semantic interpretation is carried out in two phases: a static phase and a dynamic phase in the Semantic Interpreter.

The static phase starts by building wellformed-formula from a Logical Form where individuals and sets are taken care of to compute quantifier scope and build logical representations which are eventually linked together at propositional level, where temporal indeces are added to event/state quantified operators. At this level of computation we are still using syntactic indices; these are then turned into semantic indices by the second phase which takes as input the representation into wellformed-formulas realised by Logical Form, turns it into a situation semantics structure which contain relations, their arguments and their modifiers and adjuncts. At this level all syntactic indices are turned into semantic identifiers by accessing first the Discourse Model and taking into account the output of the anaphora resolution algorithm. Empty variables associated to syntactically controlled arguments are discarded and are substituted by their controller's semantic index. Arguments may also be added in case of passive agentless structures in order to preserve the integrity of predicate-argument structures as required by lexical and semantic forms. Other notable operations carried out at this level of computation regard idiomatic expressions and other locutions which discard pieces of logical representation related to semantically empty lexical elements and conflates them with their head – as for instance in "there_be" verbal predicate.

2.8. The World or Discourse Model

Reasoning is carried out in the Discourse Model into several separate modules: Discourse Relations, Temporal Reasoning and Situation Semantics Representations. Discourse Relations are built for each proposition by means of semantic information associated to main predicates and by the output of the Temporal Reasoner.

These information are eventually passed to the Semantic Module where a representation in terms of situation semantics is computed: each proposition has been translated by the Logical Form algorithm into a fact or a situation according to semantic conditions, and is now completed by a polarity, a spatio temporal location constituted by semantic indices inherited from the previous modules. The final ontology is made up by locations, individual entities which may also be treated as classes and set with a given cardinality, facts and situations about entities which may be attributes or roles according to their semantics. basically they are computed from grammatical functions and semantic roles associated to the argument or adjunct by the previous parse.

The Knowledge Base thus coincides with the dynamically built Discourse Model where extensionality and intensionality is computed according to the actual value of the main predicates in a given context. The External World Knowledge Base is tapped only when needed, and in particular whenever a singular definite NP is introduced with a special topicality in the discourse and no antecedent is available in the Model.

2.9. Spatio-Temporal Reasoning

Temporal aspectual interpretation is carried out intrasententially and intersententially on the output of f-structure representation and computes a complete interval logic coindexation of events and states at clause level on the basis of Reichenbach's tripartite model for temporal calculus. This is then passed on to the semantic module to serve for the understanding of Temporal Relations, which are cast on the basis of J.Allen's system for temporal logic notation, the Temporal Reasoner. The latter, is a module embodying J.Allen's ideas and Reichenbach's tripartite structure of temporal representation. According to the input received, the system may assign an interpretation in terms of discourse relations by means of a mechanism of Temporal Anaphora and Focus which takes into account information related to semantic roles associated with arguments of the predicates and matches them at first with the ones available in the previous proposition: a temporal anaphora or a new temporal focus is thus the outcome both of semantic and temporal reasoning.

2.10. Discourse Structure, Discourse Relations, and Point of View

Informational structure is used to build up discourse structures at clause level, by assigning each clause to an attachment point at the Same Level, or Down a previous clause. In case a new Topic is introduced or something happens in the world that interrupts the previous sequence or text stretch, an UP movement is used and a new discourse structure is begun. These structures may be used to bind deictic propositional pronouns like "this", "that", "it" in English. Discourse Relations are used to build discourse structure in an efficient way. Point of view is switched from the Narrator's to one or other character according to Domain information, which may be either Objective or Subjective, and to Topicality: Main Topic and Subjective Domain will trigger the assignment of Point-of-View to that character.

2.11. Causal Discourse Relations

This Chapter is devoted to Causal Discourse Relations, a special subtype of Discourse Relations discussed in the previous chapter. Causal Relations are usually signalled by the presence of specific discourse markers. However when these markers are missing or are highly ambiguous problems may arise as to the correct encoding of the Discourse relation. The chapter discusses in depth such cases and presents a working algorithm again based on a shallow version of GETARUN, and tested on available annotated corpora.

2.12. Text Generation

In this Chapter we review current unification-based generation systems and present our module for text generation which uses a Planner, Discourse Relations, Temporal Reasoning and Conceptual Representation to generate in Italian and English.

2.13. Linguistically-Based Semantic Evaluation for Text Entailment

Semantic processing is usually done in presence of meaning ambiguity, disambiguation processes being usually left for the final reasoning modules. What is being presented in this chapter is our approach to Text Entailment, a technique for deciding whether two text excerpts convey the same meaning or are semantically entailed in one another in an asymmetric way. To come up with such a decision, all lexical semantic inferences are fired in order to establish coherence and cohesion relations between main predicates and arguments of the two texts. The evaluation is carried out by associating penalties or rewards to synonymous and entailed linguistic material and by inducing failure whenever a contradiction ensues. In this chapter we present the shallow or robust complete parser which however will receive a much extended treatment in a dedicated chapter in Book I – to appear late in 2007.

2.14. Reasoning from a Text with Conceptual Representations and Discourse Model for Question/Answering and Text Paraphrasing

Eventually, the terminological reasoning system which takes as input the Discourse Model built by the Text Understanding System and uses lexical information encoded as Conceptual Representations to allow for queries about spatiotemporal locations of entities in the world of the text being analysed. This level of computation is made feasible by the presence of a fully consistent semantic representation. The important part of this Chapter is constituted by the generalized procedures that allow the system to instantiate all the objects needed by KL-ONE to build up its internal database for inferencing and consistency checking. These procedures testify to the solidity of the overall project, that of passing from linguistic representations onto knowledge representations automatically.

2.15. State of the Art and other Systems

There is a large number of well-documented systems in the literature which compare well with GETARUN, in particular TACITUS and KERNEL. However we will only comment on KERNEL as presented by Palmer et al.(1993). KERNEL's architecture is similar to ours in that syntactic, semantic and pragmatic tasks are segregated into separate processing modules but they are allowed to communicate: in particular many linguistic phenomena requiring interaction with knowledge representation and reasoning are channeled though lexical semantics.

KERNEL performs its analysis in two stages: first syntactic parsing "which has limited access to shallow semantic constraints for parse disambiguation"(ibid.,20) and second integrated semantic and pragmatic processing which has constrained access to external knowledge sources. However, syntactic processing is not itself performed by a context-sensitive semantically guided parser: it is basically a context-free grammar with restrictions, a grammar formalism called restriction grammar. In turn each clause is then translated or mapped into a functional-like representation with attribute-value pairs called ISR. Semantic interpretation is performed while building up ISR and requires among other things recovering unexpressed constituents like subjects or non obligatory prepositional phrases, as well implicit but essential and sometimes obligatory arguments of a given verb predicate when used in its nominalized form. Noun phrase analysis in addition has a separate mechanism from clause analysis in that the former but not the latter allows for reference resolution. This requires a search for a likely discourse referent. Here comes another important limitation in the system: since each constituent is interpreted in the order in which it is logically built, there are cases in which a pronoun in the matrix clause has its antecedent in the subordinate which however is not yet available for use in the interpretation process(ibid., 62). This rigidity of the system could be overcome in case the system could choose to delay reference resolution of all nouns as for instance in CANDIDE(see Pollack & Pereira). Actually the real problem with KERNEL is its inability to deal with adjunct semantic interpretation(ibid.,56) but only with the interpretation of arguments of a given predicate. In other words, there is no attempt at disambiguating prepositional phrase attachment for nominal structures, hence the requirement to apply directly pragmatic knowledge and reasoning or inferencing from discourse model and/or knowledge representation for the domain. Very much in the same way is resolved the problem of semantic interpretation: there is a first pass for semantic role assignment which is locally determined by some governing predicate. Then a second pass is performed that looks for inferred role fillers obtained as a by-product of reference resolution(ibid.,29). This way of interpreting noun phrases resembles very closely ours, in that we do a local interpretation first and then the current description may be found coreferring to some entity already in the domain model, thus automatically inheriting all previously asserted properties. KERNEL does not interpret spatial location but only temporal ones which are computed in a manner very similar to ours. Reference resolution is also handled in the same way except that we do not concentrate pronoun resolution in one single module as they do. They use a focus list which is a list of referents ordered by saliency: in addition, the entire previous utterance is regarded as the preferred potential focus. Reference resolution is also used to look for essential roles which have no syntactic realization in the utterance, which is recognized as a case of semantically implicit reference. In our case, the unexpressed agent role of a passive sentence is filled at f-structure level by an indefinite existential dummy quantifiers which is then used by the semantic interpreter to search the domain model for a suitable description. The conclusion the authors draw is that more inter-module communication is called for in order to cope with ambiguity at syntactic analysis level: but at present there are no choice point at which syntax is encouraged to query the discourse context about its structure. In this way, no contextual reasoning is performed.

3. The Stories

The theoretical basis of this book has been tested by means of GETARUN on a number of texts both in Italian and in English. We chose a selection of them that we report here below. More examples and texts are presented in the following chapters. Story 1 is the story of the three little pigs, an abridged version of the original much longer story, which we report partially in the first 24 utterances alone though - the most interesting part of the story - as Story 3. Then there is an abridged version of a newspaper article on a politician, Avveduti, which we report as Story 2. These are analyzed as Italian texts. We have also reported a number of English texts which are mainly taken from literary works. At the end we report an abridged version of an EC Council directive. We add a rough literal translation of each Italian text into English: translations have not been used to tune the system, however.

3.1. Italian Texts

La Storia dei Tre Porcellini / The Story of the Three Little Pigs

C'erano una volta tre fratelli porcellini che vivevano felici nella campagna. Nello stesso luogo però viveva anche un terribile lupo che si nutriva proprio di porcellini grassi e teneri. Questi allora, per proteggersi dal lupo, decisero di costruirsi ciascuno una casetta. Il maggiore, Jimmy che era saggio, lavorava di buona lena e costruì la sua casetta con solidi mattoni e cemento. Gli altri, Timmy e Tommy, pigri se la sbrigarono in fretta costruendo le loro casette con la paglia e con pezzetti di legno. I due porcellini pigri passavano le loro giornate suonando e cantando una canzone che diceva: chi ha paura del lupo cattivo. Ma ecco che improvvisamente il lupo apparve alle loro spalle. Aiuto, aiuto, gridarono i due porcellini e cominciarono a correre più veloci che potevano verso la loro casetta per sfuggire al terribile lupo. Questo intanto si leccava già i baffi pensando al suo prossimo pasto così invitante e saporito. Finalmente i porcellini riuscirono a raggiungere la loro casetta e vi si chiusero dentro sbarrando la porta. Dalla finestra cominciarono a deridere il lupo cantando la solita canzoncina: chi ha paura del lupo cattivo. Il lupo stava intanto pensando al modo di penetrare nella casa. Esso si mise ad osservare attentamente la casetta e notò che non era davvero molto solida. Soffiò con forza un paio di volte e la casetta si sfasciò completamente. Spaventatissimi i due porcellini corsero a perdifiato verso la casetta del fratello. "Presto, fratellino, aprici! Abbiamo il lupo alle calcagna". Fecero appena in tempo ad entrare e tirare il chiavistello. Il lupo stava già arrivando deciso a non rinunciare al suo pranzetto.Sicuro di abbattere anche la casetta di mattoni il lupo si riempì i polmoni di aria e cominciò a soffiare con forza alcune volte. Non c'era niente da fare. La casa non si mosse di un solo palmo. Alla fine esausto il lupo si accasciò a terra. I tre porcellini si sentivano al sicuro nella solida casetta di mattoni. Riconoscenti i due porcellini oziosi promisero al fratello che da quel giorno anche essi avrebbero lavorato sodo.

And this is a rough translation,

Once upon a time there were three little pigs who lived happily in the countryside. But in the same place lived a wicked wolf who fed precisely on plump and tender pigs. The little pigs therefore decided to build a small house each, to protect themselves from the wolf. The oldest one, Jimmy who was wise, worked hard and built his house with solid bricks and cement. The other two, Timmy and Tommy, who were lazy settled the matter hastily and built their houses with straw and pieces of wood. The lazy pigs spent their days playing and singing a song that said, "Who is afraid of the big bad wolf?" And one day, lo and behold, the wolf appeared suddenly behind their backs. "Help! Help!", shouted the pigs and started running as fast as they could to escape the terrible wolf. He was already licking his lips thinking of such an inviting and tasty meal. The little pigs eventually managed to reach their small house and shut themselves in, barring the door. They started mocking the wolf from the window singing the same song, "Who is afraid of the big bad wolf?" In the meantime the wolf was thinking a way of getting into the house. He began to observe the house very carefully and noticed it was not very solid. He huffed and puffed a couple of times and the house fell down completely. Frightened out of their wits,the two little pigs ran at breakneck speed towards their brother's house. "Fast, brother, open the door! The wolf is chasing us!" They got in just in time and pulled the bolt. Within seconds the wolf was arriving, determined not to give up his meal. Convinced that he could also blow the little brick house down, he filled his lungs with air and huffed and puffed a few times. There was nothing he could do. The house didn't move an inch. In the end he was so exhausted that he fell to the ground. The three little pigs felt safe inside the solid brick house. Grateful to their brother, the two lazy pigs promised him that from that day on they too would work hard.

La Storia di Avveduti /The Story of Avveduti

Fino a tre anni fa Franco Avveduti non si era mai immischiato col mondo della pubblica amministrazione. Come burocrate, era un immigrato che veniva dal di fuori. Figlio di buona famiglia, a venti anni decise di iscriversi alla accademia militare di cavalleria. Era un buon allievo con ottime qualifiche. Più tardi fu un ufficiale di successo. Poi nel 1945 Avveduti si dimise dallo esercito. I militari lo avevano deluso. Avveduti, deposta la divisa, si iscrisse alla università. Nel 1947 era laureato e nel 1948 era procuratore legale. Intanto a Verona aveva conosciuto Paola, figlia di Antonio Alberti, potente senatore democristiano, e la aveva sposata. Il senatore poteva considerarsi il più influente uomo politico veronese. Gli elettori lo mandavano al parlamento coprendolo di voti preferenziali. Al seguito di Alberti, che era diventato vicepresidente del senato, Franco Avveduti nello immediato dopoguerra si trasferì a Roma. Tuttavia, da principio si tenne lontano dalla sfera di interessi del suocero.

Gli piaceva parlare del suocero come di una facile occasione mancata che chiunque altro avrebbe sfruttato ma che lui, Avveduti, preferiva lasciare perdere. Solo verso il 1950 decise di accettare un posto nella organizzazione della fiera di Verona. Lo nominarono delegato cioè una specie di funzionario viaggiante con incarichi diplomatici di tenere i rapporti con le delegazioni commerciali, curare i produttori stranieri, le grandi ditte, la stampa. Questo era un compito che corrispondeva bene alla sua vocazione e nel quale Avveduti sapeva giostrare con notevole agilità. Quando il suocero morì, egli non perse il posto. A Verona il collegio di Alberti lo aveva ereditato Trabucchi e col collegio aveva ereditato la presidenza della fiera. Trabucchi continuò a valersi della collaborazione di Avveduti. L'ex-ufficiale del Novara-Cavalleria gli era simpatico. La sua distinzione lo impressionava. Lo confermò nell'incarico alla fiera. Avveduti funzionava benissimo come segretario particolare. Sapeva mobilitare prefetti e questori. Tutti gli invidiavano il suo segretario particolare.

And this is a rough literal translation,

Until three years ago, Franco Avveduti never got involved with the world of public administration. As a beaurocrat, he was an immigrant who came from outside. Son of a respected family, when he was 20, he decided to enroll at the Military Academy of Cavalry. He was a good cadet with excellent qualifications. Later on, he became a successful officer. Then in 1945, Avveduti resigned from the army. The military had disappointed him. Laid down his uniform, Avveduti enrolled in the University. In 1947 he graduated and in 1948 he became a solicitor. In the meantime, in Verona, he met Paola, the daughter of Antonio Alberti, powerful Christian Democrat senator, and he married her. The senator might be regarded the most powerful political man in Verona. The voters sent him to parliament covering him literally with preferential votes. At the suite of Alberti, who had become vicepresident of the Senate, Franco Avveduti in the immediate postwar moved to Rome. However at the beginning he kept himself aloof from the sphere of interest of his father-in-law. He liked to talk about his father-in-law as if he were an easy chance missed which anybody else would have exploited but which himself, Avveduti, preferred to let go. Only towards 1950 he grudgingly ended up by accepting a position in the committee of the Verona Fair. They appointed him delegate, i.e. a kind of travelling officer with diplomatic charges, to have relations with commercial committees, take care of foreign producers, the big corporations, the press. This was a task which fitted well with his inclination, and where Avveduti could joust with remarkable ease. In Verona, Alberti's college had been inherited by Trabucchi, and with the college he had inherited the chair of the Fair. Trabucchi continued availing himself of Avveduti's collaboration. To him, the Novara Cavalry officer was nice. His distinction impressed him. He confirmed him in the position at the Fair. Avveduti worked very well as special secretary. He knew how to mobilize prefects and questors. Everybody envied him his special secretary.

La Storia dei Tre Porcellini Rivisitata / The Story of the Little Pigs Revisited

Questa è la storia di tre porcellini che andarono per il mondo a cercare fortuna. I loro nomi erano Timmy, suonatore di flauto, Tommy, violinista e Jimmy, grande lavoratore. Giunti in un bel bosco, decisero di costruire ognuno una comoda casetta. A Timmy non piaceva per niente lavorare così pensò di costruirsi rapidamente una capanna di paglia. In breve la casetta fu pronta e Timmy decise allora di andare a vedere che cosa stavano facendo i suoi fratellini. Incontrò dapprima Tommy il violinista. Anche lui non aveva molta voglia di faticare così costruiva con dei pezzi di legno una semplice casetta. Ben presto anche la casa di legno fu pronta. Come quella di paglia, non era certo molto resistente. Ma i due porcellini scansafatiche se la erano sbrigata in poco tempo ed ora potevano tranquillamente divertirsi. Mentre Timmy suonava il flauto, Tommy lo accompagnava con il suo violino e insieme se la spassavano allegramente. Poi stanchi di fare baldoria, decisero di andare a vedere che cosa stava facendo il loro fratellino. Si misero in cammino e ben presto raggiunsero Jimmy. Il bravo porcellino stava costruendo anche lui la sua casetta. Ma poiché Jimmy era previdente e non aveva paura di lavorare sodo, la costruiva con mattoni e cemento. Jimmy voleva una casa robusta perché sapeva che il lupo cattivo viveva nel bosco vicino. Quando i due pigri porcellini videro Jimmy impegnato nel suo duro lavoro, si misero a ridere a crepapelle. Ma quei due sciocchi porcellini non pensavano al pericolo. Così continuarono a prendere in giro il saggio Jimmy, canticchiando e suonando con il flauto e il violino. I due porcellini, sempre suonando e ballando, tornarono ciascuno alla propria fragile casetta. Ma appena Timmy aprì la porta, sbucò fuori dal bosco il lupo cattivo. Il porcellino lo vide e tremante di paura si chiuse immediatamente in casa. Il lupo cattivo cominciò a chiamarlo. "Apri la porta e fammi entrare nella tua casetta di paglia."

And this is a rough literal translation,

This is the story of three little pigs who went around the world seeking their fortune. Their names were Timmy, flute player, Tommy, violinist, Jimmy, great worker. As they reached a nice wood, they decided to build each a comfortable little house. Timmy didn't like working at all, so he thought to build quickly a straw hut. Soon the little house was ready and Timmy decided then to go and see what his little brothers were doing. At first he met Tommy the violinist. Also he, himself, did not have much wish to toil, so he was building a simple little house with sticks of wood. Very soon, also the house of wood was ready. Like that of straw, it was not very resistant. But the two little pigs lazy had managed to finish their work in a short time and now they could enjoy themselves freely. While Timmy was playing the flute, Tommy accompanied him with his violin and together they were having a lot of fun. Then, tired to make merry, they decided to go and see what their little brother was doing. They started walking and soon they reached Jimmy. The clever little pig was building a little house. But since Jimmy was farsighted and did not fear working hard, he built it with bricks and cement. Jimmy wanted a sturdy house because he knew that the big bad wolf lived in the woods nearby. When the two lazy little pigs saw Jimmy busy in his hard word, they started laughing out of their wits. But those two silly little pigs didn't think about the danger. So they continued making a fool of the wise Jimmy, singing and playing the violin and the flute. Each of the two little pigs, always singing and playing, went back to its fragile little house. But as soon as Timmy opened the door, the big bad wolf got out of the woods. The little pig saw it and trembling with fear locked himself inside the house immediately. The big bad wolf started calling him. "Open the door and let me in your little house of straw."

3.2. English Texts

Virginia Woolf's Excerpts

Text 1.

John gave Mary a rose. She took it and put it in her hair. She knew that she had been given a present, something precious. When Steve faced them saying, "are you enjoying yourselves?". It was horrible! It was shocking! Not for herself. She felt only hostility and his determination to ruin that wonderful moment. John smiled and went away embarassed.

Text 2.

The three friends all went outdoors. As they were walking in the garden, John said to himself, "Sara will marry that man", without any resentment. Richard would marry Sara. He felt strongly about that. She was the right person for a man like Richard. For himself he was absurd. His demands upon Sara were absurd. She would have accepted him still if he had been less absurd. Richard began to sing.

Text 3.

Mary picked up the phone and called Jason. Her husband, she thought, would have considered such a move as untruthful and utterly base. Perhaps there was something bad in herself that she could not help but do the wrong thing at the wrong time. Jason answered immediately.

Psychological Statements: At the Restaurant

Text 1.

John went into a restaurant. There was a table in the corner. The waiter took the order. The air was nice and clean. He began to read his book.

A Legal Text

Council directive of July 1985 on the approximation of the laws, regulations and administrative provisions of the Member States concerning liability for defective products. The council of the european communities has adopted this directive. Having regard to the proposal from the commission. Whereas approximation of the laws of the Member States concerning the liability of the producer for damage caused by the defectiveness of his products is necessary because the existing divergences may entail a differing degree of protection of the consumer against damage caused by a defective product to his health or property. Whereas liability without fault should apply only to movables which have been industrially produced. Whereas protection of the consumer requires that all the producers involved in the production process should be made liable in so far as their finished product, component part or any raw material supplied by them was defective. Whereas, to the extent that liability for nuclear injury or damage is already covered in all member states by adequate special rules, it has been possible to exclude damage of this type from the scope of this directive. Whereas, in situations where several persons are liable for the same damage, the protection of the consumer requires that the injured person should be able to claim full compensation for the damage from any one of them. Producer means the manufacturer of a finished product, the producer of any raw material or the manufacturer of a component part and any person who, by putting his name, trade mark or other distinguishing feature on the product presents himself as its producer. The injured person shall be required to prove the damage, the defect and the causal relationship between defect and damage. This directive shall not apply to injury or damage arising from nuclear accidents and covered by international conventions ratified by the Member States. Where, as a result of the provisions of this directive, two or more persons are liable for the same damage. They shall be liable jointly and severally, without prejudice to the provisions of national law concerning the rights of contribution or recourse. A product is defective when it does not provide the safety which a person is entitled to expect, taking all circumstances into account. The liability of the producer arising from this directive may not, in relation to the injured person, be limited or excluded by a provision limiting his liability or exempting him from liability. Without prejudice to the liability of the producer any person who imports into the community a product for sale, hire or any form of distribution in the course of his business shall be deemed to be a producer within the meaning of this directive.

Whereas to protect the physical well-being and property of the consumer the defectiveness of the product should be determined by reference, not to its fitness for use, but to the lack of the safety which the public at large is entitled to expect. The liability of the producer may be reduced or disallowed when, having regard to all the circumstances, the damage is caused both by a defect in the product and by the fault of the injured person or any person for whom the injured person is responsible. However, if within three months of receiving the said information the commission does not advise the Member State concerned that it intends submitting such a proposal to the council, the Member State may take the proposed measure immediately. Any member state may provide that a producer's total liability for damage resulting from a death or personal injury and caused by identical items with the same defect shall be limited to an amount which may not be less than 70 million Ecu.

4. Acknowledgements

The book is largely taken from already published work, which has been fully revised and enlarged. In particular, Chapter I and Chapter II are taken from Delmonte R. 1999. Grammar and Structure; Delmonte R. Parsing with GETARUN; Delmonte R. 2000. Generating and

Parsing Clitics with GETARUN; a new enlarged version of Delmonte R. 1989. From Subcategorization Frames to Thematic Roles, in R.Delmonte(ed.), Lessico, Stutture e Interpretazione - Studi Linguistici Applicati I, Unipress, Padova, Chapt.IV,167-212, and also of Delmonte R. 1995. Lexical Representations: Syntax-Semantics interface and World Knowledge, in Notiziario AIIA (Associazione Italiana di Intelligenza Artificiale), Roma, pp.11-16; Chapter III is a revised and enlarged version of Delmonte R., D.Bianchi. 1991. Binding Pronominals with an LFG Parser, Proceeding of the Second International Workshop on Parsing Technologies, Cancun, 59-72; Chapter IV and Chapter V are a revised and enlarged version of Delmonte R., D. Bianchi. 1994. Computing Discourse Anaphora from Grammatical Representations, in Research in Humanities Computing, OUP; Chapter VI is a revised and enlarged version of Delmonte R., D. Bianchi (1992), Quantifiers in Discourse, in Proc. ALLC/ACH'92, Oxford(UK), OUP, 107-114; Chapter VII is partially taken from Delmonte R. 1991. Grammatica e quantificazione in LFG; Chapter VIII is a revised and enlarged version of ideas appearing in Delmonte R., Dibattista D. 1995. Switching from Narrative to Legal Genre, Working Papers in Linguistics, C.L.I., University of Venice, also published as Delmonte R., D.Bianchi. 1999. Determining Essential Properties of Linguistic Objects for Unrestricted Text Anaphora Resolution; Chapter IX is taken from Delmonte R. 1997. Lexical Representations, Event Structure and Quantification, Quaderni Patavini di Linguistica, 39-94; Chapter X owes something to Delmonte R. 1994. Inferences and Discourse Structure, in G.Ferrari(ed), Proc.IV Conference of the Italian Artificial Intelligence Association - AIIA, 11-14. Chapter XI, is taken from Delmonte R., E.Pianta. 1996. "IMMORTALE - Analizzatore Morfologico, Tagger e Lemmatizzatore per l'Italiano"; Delmonte R., E.Pianta. 1999. Tag Disambiguation in Italian. Eventually, Chapter XII owes something to Delmonte R., Pianta E.(1991), Generating Text with Relevance, ms. University of Venice, also published as Delmonte R., D.Bianchi. 1998. Dialogues From Texts: How to Generate Answers from a Discourse Model, and Delmonte R. 2000. Generating from a Discourse Model.

I must thank my colleague Dario Bianchi – who recently (September 2005) died - for providing a lot of ideas in the implementation of the system, and Emanuele Pianta who graduated and worked with me at the semantic interpretation. Ideas and implementation advances would have not been possible without the intervention of students at my Computational Linguistics courses which is the most valuable testbed for any theory.

Chapter 1

SEMANTIC INTERPRETATION AND LOGICAL FORM

1. INTRODUCTION

As said in the Introduction to the book, the task we are faced with when trying to simulate human understanding of texts consists in two steps: first to scientifically isolate the contexts in which external knowledge of the world should be made available to the system, in order to reduce access to WordNet and other similar resources; second, to provide tools to deal with this task adequately. In the following, we shall make our point in more detail, basically by discussing the work of other research groups. In particular we shall quote extensively from one publication, edited by Herzog & Rollinger, Text Understanding in LILOG, which we take to be the best example of the attempt to come to terms with the problem at hand.

We shall start by commenting on P. Bosch's contribution which we quoted in the Introduction. On a first reading, one could reach the conclusion that the author is unconditionally in favour of increasing the weight of linguistic research when creating NLU Systems, but this is not so: in fact, the Conclusions counterbalance the very start of the paper, where in the Abstract we can read more or less the opposite:

> "Linguistic parameters alone cannot determine the interpretation of natural language utterances. They can only constrain their interpretation and must leave the rest to other knowledge sources and other processes: language understanding is not just a matter of knowing the language, but also to a considerable degree a matter of logical inference and world knowledge. This is no news as far as the interpretation of referential expressions is concerned. Predicate expressions, however, tend to be treated as if they were functional or relational constrains that are directly interpreted with respect to a model. In this paper an attempt is made to treat them too as referential. The only real difference is that the referents of predicate expressions are of a different type: concepts rather than first-order objects.
> This generalized notion of reference gives us not only a natural way of understanding the interaction of knowledge representation and knowledge processing on the one hand and linguistic processing on the other, but also opens up a perspective for the modularization of NLU systems that provides for a very high degree of independence of the more strictly linguistic component from the specific tasks and domains of a particular application. The overall result should be a less language-dependent knowledge representation and less domain-dependent linguistic components, i.e. overall improved portability of the modules."(p.243)

We can subscribe here only to the second part of the abstract and the whole of the conclusions: the first part of the abstract, however, seems to imply that knowledge of the world is paramount and linguistic description can only achieve a subsidiary role in the overall task of text understanding.

This sounds a little bit contradictory if compared to the rest of the quoted text. Also, if one reads through the whole of Bosch's paper one has the feeling that the author is somewhat split between the two perspectives: giving higher prominence to the linguistic analysis, vs. the construction of a sound system for knowledge representation. The author reviews some of the most common examples appearing in the literature on linguistic semantics arguing that the mismatch between the output of the linguistic processor and the requirements of a semantic interpreter is so high that there is little hope to solve it in purely linguistic terms. At least this is what he admits after discussing a number of examples, ".. I want to make an attempt to weaken overdrawn expectations with respect to what linguistic meaning can do in processes of linguistic comprehension"(p.246).

In any text understanding task, there is a tension between what we might define following Bosch, "Inferentially unstable concepts" and "Contextual Concepts": it seems to me that this tension may be overcome only when we have in mind a particular application. In that case we should be able, by extensively studying the linguistic material concerning the domain to isolate the Inferentially unstable concepts and leave the Knowledge Representation Module and the Semantic Interpreter do the job of unravelling the appropriate interpretation in each case, given a sound linguistic analysis. The remaining cases are constituted by Contextual Concepts which should be fully under control of the system, in case a modularized system as the one we are proposing is available.

The importance of the Context must be stressed here: most ambiguities disappear when analysed in their context. Also we believe that ad hoc examples found in the literature do not help researchers in this field state the problem in the right way. Consider such cases as represented by the following examples taken from Bosch,

1. Five companies sold two hundred installations
2. Fred saw the woman with the binoculars
3. Visiting relatives can be boring
4. Pete went to the bank this morning
5. This paper is ten pages long
6. Faulkner is hard to understand

7a. The school made a major donation
  b. The school has a flat roof
  c. He enjoys school very much
  d. School is one of the pillars of our civilization

The problems to be tackled are not all the same, as can be easily noticed. In 1. we have a problem of quantifier scope, which we think is only solvable by allowing QR produce two different representations for the same f-structure and then letting the semantic component do the rest. However, QR would compute as a preferential reading the one in which the subject NP takes scope over the object NP when both are numerals. In case the ambiguity had to be solved in favour of the second reading a distributive floating quantifier (each) should be added. In 2 and 3 the parser would have come out with the most likely interpretation of the sentence and that might very well happen to be the wrong one: however the feeling one gets when discussing such sentences, is that they are very unlikely to be found in real texts - or at least this is what we assume. For sure, we would like our semantic component reject the parse and ask for another one: in our opinion, no backtracking should be allowed once f-structure has been completed. If we consider in more detail example 2, we can come out with a general default rule that prevents "binoculars" to be computed as an adequate adjunct of the head "woman", which is what at present our system does, and assigns it rather to the level of sentential adjuncts. There might however be special scenarios in which women walk around carrying binoculars around their neck: this does not happen in Venice, where everything can be comfortably looked at without binoculars, but could happen in the Grand Canyon where distances require it. In case our linguistic domain were a tourist guide for the Grand Canyon, the possibility of semantic compatibility between an internal adjunct whose head is "binocular" should turn out. Then the parser would simply choose this as the first parse, since the semantic matching would be successful in the most embedded structure, the NP. However, we should remark that the example does not certainly exhaust the possibilities of expressing the same concept, available at a linguistic level. In addition, linguistic variation due to typological differences should be taken into account. In Italian, the adjunct could well be inserted between the verb and the OBJect NP, as follows:

8. Franco vide con il binocolo la donna

which expresses more perspicuously the meaning we want. The same applies to German. As to English, consider a case of Heavy NP shift,

9.a. Fred saw with the binoculars the woman he met last night
b. ??Fred saw the woman he met last night with the binoculars

where we can see that the more appropriate linguistic form to assign to the utterance is now the disambiguating one. In other words, ad hoc examples may be very inadequate or rather biased to clarify a problem as the one we are now tackling.

As to 4. we are in presence of lexical ambiguity, which is however nonexistent in our system, since the semantic role would always be Locative, and the semantic features associated to the NP "bank" would have to accomodate for all lexical meanings: it is the task of the semantic component to look for the most adequate referent to the singular definite NP, in the model. Example 5. constitutes no problem at all, provided that a discourse module is available in the system, and we shall see examples in the following chapters.

Now consider 6. where we can either mean Faulkner as a person or rather his literary works: here again we take it to be the task of the semantic component to find out in the model whether we are dealing with the man talking, or simply with his works. This can be dealt nicely in our system where the predicate UNDERSTAND has the semantic role INFORMT, that is information, associated with the OBJect NP and that may select anyone source of information, be it spoken words or written text.

Coming now to the last set of examples, where the "school" is assigned a number of different meanings according to context. Again we may easily assume that the system of linguistic description – WordNet in this case - should cover the whole of them. In a. the school is the SUBJect of the predicate MAKE and this requires an Agent which may be a

Social_Institution, but not an object, i.e. a building, as is required by the meaning of the b. example. In this case, the meaning is not conveyed by the verb BE which has nonthematic arguments, but by contents of the predicate NP "the flat roof": this would be classified as [object, part_of], thus implying that the predication requires also an Object as its controller. In c. we have a psych verb "enjoy" which has an EXPERIENCER as SUBJect NP and a CAUSER_EMOT as OBJect NP. The school in this case will be assigned a semantic value by the semantic roles as happened with the a. example. The same applies to the c. example. In other words, it is the linguistic description which enables the semantic interpreter do its job properly by means of the conjoined information made available by semantic roles and semantic features.

Other examples we have not quoted here, regard the meaning of adjectives like "red", which we believe should be made available by WordNet: it is a matter of world knowledge that we understand "red wine" as being different from "red apple" or "red traffic lights": the inferences drawn by the system should be different and they should be triggered by the different conceptualization of the complex NP under analysis.

2. Defining the Contextual Domain or Discourse Model

In Webber(1983) and Sidner(1983) a theory for the treatment of anaphoric reference in natural language is put forward which tries to encompass cospecifiers which are both structurally identifiable and those identifiable by a discourse model. The underlying assumption made by the author is that in lack of structural cues, such as clefts or topicalizations, in order to find the antecedent or cospecifier of a pronoun, inferential processes can and must be activated every time the Focus Algorithm does not provide an adequate entity independently. Thus, Webber claims that definite pronouns and nominal expressions must be interpreted on the basis of a "discourse model". In her words:

> "...the assumption is that one objective of discourse is to talk about some situation or state of the real or some hypothetical world. To do this, a speaker must have a mental model of that situation of state. The ensuing discourse is thus, at one level, an attempt by the speaker to direct the listener in synthesizing a similar "discourse model" and by that, acquire information about the speaker's situation or state. (In this sense, I am equating "understanding" with "synthesizing an appropriate model")."

Informally, a DM may be described as the set of entities "naturally evoked" (or in Sidner's terms, "specified") by a discourse, linked together by the relations they participate in. They are called discourse entities, but may also be regarded as discourse referents or cognitive elements. We want to keep referring to what people do with language; evoking and accessing discourse entities are what texts/discourses do. A discourse entity inhabits a speaker's discourse model and represents something the speaker has referred to. A speaker refers to something by utterances that either evoke (if first reference) or access (if subsequent reference) its corresponding discourse entity. It is how the information is realized that determines what types of discourse entities are available when.

Now, a speaker is usually not able to communicate all at once the relevant properties and relations he may want to ascribe to the referent of a discourse entity. To do that he may have to direct the listener's attention to that referent (via its corresponding discourse entity) several times in succession. When the speaker wants to re-access an entity already in his DM (or another one directly inferable from it), he may do so with a definite anaphor (pronoun or NP). In doing so, the speaker assumes (1) that on the basis of the discourse thus far, a similar entity will be in (or directly inferable from) the listener's growing DM and (2) that the listener will be able to re-access (or infer) that entity on the basis of the speaker's cues. (For example, pronouns are less of a cue than anaphoric NPs). The problem then, at least for definite anaphora, is identifying what discourse entities a text naturally evokes.

What characterizes a discourse entity? Webber's view is that a discourse entity is a "conceptual coathook" (a term coined by William Woods) "... on which to hang descriptions of the entity's real world or hypothetical world correspondent. As soon as a DE is evoked, it gets a description. Over the course of the text, the descriptions it receives are derived from both the content of the speaker's utterances and their position within the discourse, as well as whatever general or specific information about the discourse entity the listener can bring to bear."(1983)

The initial description ID that tags a newly evoked DE might have a special status, because it is the only information about an entity that can, from the first and without question, be assumed to be shared (though not necessarily believed) by both speaker and listener alike. Even though certain types of DE must be derived from other ones inferentially, and that is the simplest way of account for anaphoric access to "generic set" DE.

The problem we set out to solve is transformed into (1) identifying the discourse entities a text evokes and (2) ascribing to them appropriate IDs.

Definite descriptions can be used like definite pronouns to access entities presumed to be in the listener's DM, or they can be used to evoke new entities into that model.

In McCawley(1981) we have an interesting definition of Partial Interpretation Model or Contextual Domain (hence CD). When discussing definite descriptions such as the ones contained in the following examples,

10a. The dog is hungry.
b. The dog likes all dogs.
c. The dog was barking at another dog.

he remarks that the restriction of attention cannot be a restriction of the universe of discourse, that is, of the set that is to provide the domains of ALL variables: if b. were used relative to a universe of discourse that contained only one dog, then it ought to convey the same meaning as "The dog likes itself", which it does not, and if c. were used relative to a universe of discourse containing only one dog, it ought to convey something that is guaranteed to be false, since there would be no other dog in that restricted universe for it to bark at. Clearly, all and another in b. and c. demand universes of discourse that can contain as many dogs as you want, and thus the dog cannot pick out its referent simply by virtue of a restriction on the universe of discourse. Further on (p. 266) he is more precise about what the contextual domain is. The CD at any point of a discourse will be the set of entities whose existence and identity the participants in the discourse take as established.

From examples like the following which we borrow again from McCawley,

11a. The dogs like all dogs.
b. The dogs were barking at another dog.

we can clearly see that a set may be a member of the contextual domain without all or even any of its members being a member of the contextual domain.

As to the interpretation of the definite NP “the dog”, it involves a search through the contextual domain for an entity that is a dog. In some cases, for an element to be picked out as referent of a definite description what is necessary is not that it be true but that it be included in the context.

In our system recency and topicality play an important role, which somehow answers some of the doubts McCawley expressed in his book(p.269), which we report here below:

> "Rather than being simply a set, the contextual domain must have different 'levels', with items on higher levels being, for the moment at least, more prominent than items on lower levels. As long as the temporary additions to the contextual domain are put on a higher level that its previous contents, the temporarily added discourse referents will be picked as the referents of the definite NPs... I have at the moment no general account of principles determining the relative prominence of the various discourse referents... it may change as the discourse proceeds and in some cases the speaker is free to decide which of two discourse referents is the more prominent. "

It is clearly not the whole story about coreferents, as McCawley himself notes. In the following example, for instance, we see that the reference of a plural definite NP is inferable from the presence of a collective NP in the previous portion of text:

12. Whenever I teach freshman linguistics, the girls do better than the boys.

The reference to freshman makes available a set as discourse referent which is coreferred by the two plural NP's the girls and the boys, as subsets of that set. Plural definite NPs may either be coreferred to an existing entity in the world or else, as this example shows, take the reference from a collective NP: this is due to the quantifier-like nature of plural NPs and collective NPs, the first one being computable as subset of adequate antecedents and the second ones as supersets. It is clear that knowledge of the world is needed to subsumes the "freshman" meaning and those of "boy" and "girl". However in our system, we allow for the generation of default properties from selectional restrictions associated to arguments of a predicate: in the above example, this could be done simply on the basis of the fact that “fresman”'s inherent semantic features are [+human, +young].

Semantic peculiarities concern genre specialization that affect the way in which the interpretation process is tied up with linguistic forms. It is a fact that linguistic structure and form is the first means by which meaning is conveyed to language users, and it is often contingent upon genre.

Generally speaking, building a Discourse Model is a precondition for any reader or generic addressee of the contents of a legal text to enable reference to entities and events contained in the text. A DM is clearly only a part of the overall process of understanding which makes heavy use of background mutual knowledge on the side of the adressee in order to carry out the complex inferences required by this genre.

In line with current assumptions about the ontological status of entities and events referred to in any legal texts, we also assume that they are spatiotemporally disanchored and they have no counterpart in the real present world: in other word, their referential status is abstracted from spatiotemporal restrictions. Nonetheless, the DM will be represented as a list of facts and sits very much in the same way in which it would happen in narrative texts. The reason for this is very simple, the DM constitutes the semantic informational representation of the linguistic structure of any text or discourse. It aims at simulating the processes underlying anaphora and reference resolution within the text, thus registering and storing information in a given formal format which is the actual interpretation related to entities and events contained in the text.

For instance, a norm, directive or other legal text might contain Obligations which are expressed by a specialized use of the modal "shall" and as is the case with Permissions which are highlighted by the presence of the modal "may", are treated as facts in the DM; in turn, Hypotheses do not count as extensional objects and are carefully set apart from Conditions which assume a similar syntactic pattern but have a different semantic marker.

If we take reference to classes as the norm in legal language we still must allow for individuals - the current directive is one such case - or sets, the commission or the European community, or still the Member states.

Strzalkowski and Cercone(1989)(hence S&C) in their work introduce the problem of reference from a semantic computationally feasible point of view. This is how they define their proposal:

> "... we introduce a layered model of reality (the universe) as perceived by a discourse participant, and define relative singularity of objects in this universe as an abstraction class of the layer-membership relation. Subsequently, linguistic descriptions and names are classified as *singular*, *measurably singular*, or *non-singular* depending upon what they are assumed to denote in the universe. The relationship between objects referred to in discourse and classified into different layers (levels) of the universe model has a particular significance for resolution of certain types of cohesive links in text. We call these links *remote reference* because they cross level boundaries."(p.172)

The tripartipe classification of entities in the model reflects our proposal where we have generic entities, classes and individuals. As in S & C they are partially ordered by the relation "more informative than": intuitively, they introduce a relation of relative singularity among objects that allows us to break down the universe of objects into classes or levels, where a lower level L0 consist of manifestations, extensions, instances of objects at level L1. In fact S & C always speak of the existence of three main levels, one for each type of denotation: if L0 contains objects with a measurable singular interpretation, L-1 may contain the same object with a specific or singular interpretation - if possible at all, and L+1 will contain referring expressions - nouns, definite descriptions, pronouns but also other nominals denoting objects which are non-singular. If level L+1 contains generalizations of objects from L0, then level L-1 will contain their specializations of extensions (ibid., 177). Any non singular object can potentially be decomposed into instances in many ways, depending upon the relation that bind the two objects, or coordinate - part_of, instance_of, genus, specimen etc.; also, and more generally, whenever a higher-level object is decomposed with two different coordinates, the resulting sets of instances need not belong to the same level(ibid., 178).

However, we will assume that natural language users, when introducing referring expressions in a text or discourse will abide the wellknown maxim that requires them not to be ambiguous. In particular, in our model the spatiotemporal location indices assigned according to semantic and linguistic criteria are the only possible coordinates but cannot be used to partition our discourse model into layers or levels, with respect to some current level, corresponding to the level of reference at a present point of discourse. We do not find any convenience in introducing such layers into the overall computation of entities and their reference. In turn S & C do not describe in detail how one could compute remote reference in discourse, apart from establishing an obvious definition that relates two objects by means of remote reference in case they have different kinds of singularity. Naming an object previously existing in the discourse model may end up simply with a coreferring operation, or with the need to create a supercontext in case it is less informative than the existing entity, or a subcontext in case it is an instance of the previously existing entity (ibid., 182).

3. The Model and the Interpreter

In order to build an adequate Discourse Model we rely on a version of Situation Semantics which takes perspectives as the higher node in a hierarchical scheme in which there is a bifurcation between factual and non-factual situations. Partially following Burke(1991) we assume that the notion of perspectives is significant in situation theory insofar as the very same situations can be viewed by an agent (or by different agents) from different perspectives, hence situations may support different and perhaps conflicting kinds of information(ibid.,134). We want to accomodate the fact that the theory is concerned with finite agents with limited information-handling capabilities: different agents carve the world up differently into objects, properties and relations according to their respective experience. To this end, we introduce the notion of Subject-of-Consciousness (as will be discussed at length in Chapter V of Book 1 to appear) which has two main functions: on the one hand it tells us that the point of view from which situations are viewed may be associated to some speaker which is not the narrator's, and it gives us the identity of the new speaker; on the other hand it tells us that situations are not factual in an objective sense, but are only such from the new speaker's perspective. This mechanism allows us to change Point-of-View accordingly, so that we can differentiate what the narrator's believes or makes the reader believe about a certain situation and the participants thereof, from what each character believes.

Situations are characterized in terms of "infons", or better the infons that they support. In turn we distinguish between *facts* and *concepts* where the former have to do with concrete ostensive entities which yield information that are referential, in that they explicitly involve objects in the world relative to a given perspective. On the contrary *concepts* constitute a piece of general information about the world relative to a given perspective, which does not directly refer to any particular entity or object, nor is it specific to particular ostensive entities.

A basic *infon* consists of an *issue* together with a polarity; an issue in turn consists of a relation and an assignment of appropriate arguments to the argument roles of that relation. The dual of a basic infon is that infon consisting of the same issue resolved with the opposite polarity. An infon is an object which is appropriate to stand in the support relation with a situation: that is, an infon is something which may or may not hold in a situation.

We also assume with Cooper R.P.(1991) that infons have the property of persistence, which is meant to capture the notion that if a piece of information is supported by some situation, then it is supported by all larger situations - no amount of further information can deny the original information. To produce this result we assume that the domain of situations comes with a partial ordering $\leq$, corresponding to the part-of type that holds between situations to be defined in pure extensional terms. Infon persistence is just a special case of this property. Natural language statements involving quantification over events, states or processes should correspond to non-persistent infons: as Cooper puts it, "if every kitten is meowing in one situation then there is no guarantee that every kitten must be meowing in every larger situation". In particular, universally quantified infons need not be persistent and similarly for the duals of existentially quantified infons: persistence should only apply to basic infons or *facts*.

In our system, *facts* may describe information relative to a *subjective* or an *objective* discourse domain: subjective facts are thus computable as situations viewed from the perspective of a given agent, in our case corresponding to the Main Topic of discourse. On the contrary, objective facts are reported from the perspective of the text's author. However, to highlight the difference existing between subjective and objective information in the model, we decided to call *facts* only objective infons; subjective infons are called **sit**; finally, generic assertions are called *conc*.

These main constituents of situations are further described by taking individuals, relations and locations as primitives and by using set theory as logical notation. Thus, individuals and inferences on individuals are wrought out in set theory notation, which is very straightforward when using Prolog as programming language: we use *ind* for a unique individual, *set* for a collection of individuals which can be individuated by means of membership, *card* for every set with a numerical or indefinite quantified value, in order to indicate membership, *class* for generic sets which can be made up by an indefinite quantity however big enough to encompass sets, subsets, classes or individuals, and *ensemble* to indicate mass nouns whose internal structure is made up only of subsets. Each entity is assigned a constant value or *id* and an *infon* which are uniquely individuated by a number. As said above, infons are made up of an issue, which in turn contain a main relation: relations may be properties, social or relational roles, events or states, locational modifiers or specifiers, etc.. Simplex properties predicate some property of a given identifier; complex properties take individuals and propositions as their arguments and in this case individuals may be assigned a semantic role. Semantic roles are inherited from the lexical form associated to a given predicate in the lexicon and transferred into the f-structure of the utterance under analysis. Semantic roles are paramount in the choice and construction of conceptual representations.

Infons are built according to situation theory: they have a location which is made up of a couple of indices anchoring the event/state/processes to a given spatiotemporal location and a polarity.

Inferences are produced every time a given property is reintroduced in the story in order to ascertain whether the same property was already present in the model world and should not be reasserted, or whether it should be added to it. In particular, in the Story of the 3 Little Pigs, we know at the beginning of the story that a little pig possesses a certain house, a certain name and is evaluated by a given attribute: these properties are used in the following text to individuate one little pig from the other, or even one house from the other. Inferences are then fired every time an individual reappears in order to check the persistence of the information it carries in the story. Properties may be anchored to a given location or be universally anchored: a name, is a rigid designator in that it is computed as a property associated to a given individual and has a universal locational anchoring, meaning that the same individual will always be individuated by that name in the story. The same would apply to permanent properties like the substance or matter constituting an object, like a house, or other such properties.

Persistence may then be computed both for entities, properties, relations and locations and from a separate module that computes information structure for each simplex utterance we get a *Relevance Score.* In this way complex situation and courses of events or eventualities may be constructed and checked.

The Semantic Module is responsible for the interpretation of the text in that it extracts from f-structure representation all the information relevant for the construction of the model. In particular, as will be shown below, we use all the information contained in the SPECifier: definiteness, cardinality, partitivity, the quantifier if present, the focalizer if present; Number; the Pred or the lexeme; the grammatical Function label and the semantic Role label; the semantic categories or inherent features associated to each Pred; the Referential Table where the feature ±ref is contained. In the Semantic Module there are a number of procedures to map the relevant information extracted from f-structure representation onto the model. These procedures are absolutely general and may be applied to any text whatsoever: in other words the semantic interpretation is not contextualized, in that it abstracts from the actual meaning in the world of the lexemes used in the text. Contextual reasoning is however required sometimes in order to produce inferences which call for encyclopaedic knowledge or knowledge of the world. For instance, when the bad wolf is struggling to get hold of one of the little pigs, the text refers to it as "pasto"/meal which fires an inference on the little pigs being the wolf's food, which in turn may constitute its meal. However, we want to keep contextual reasoning as an exceptional procedure called for every time is needed and only then: in this sense, the presence of a definite NP with a possessor triggers the inferential machine, after the default inferences on facts and sits present in the model have failed.

The actual model is built in two steps: at first, logical form is called in order to construct wellformed formulas and terms out of f-structure representation discussed below in details. The result of this computation is the list of facts and sits which constitute the propositional level representation of the utterance under analysis. At this level we also compute the sentence level modifiers of the situation of the event/state. At the same time, the internal structure of each proposition is passed onto the Interpreter which divides up arguments of each predicate, filtering out modifiers and adjuncts, and builds up an array made up of the semantic attributes listed above. The list attached to each argument of a predicate is the input to the Interpreter which works its way through the algorithm in order to assign an interpretation.

The interpretation is the conjoined effort of the actual information attached to the argument semantic attribute list, the discourse module anaphora resolution results, and the state of the model. The discourse module has the information that a given argument is a coreferential NP, because the result of the resolution has been previously asserted and is now available. Since a noun or a pronoun may have been used to corefer, we simply take advantage of that information by preventing the Interpreter from asserting the existence of a new entity in the world. In this case, we simply assert in the rhetorical structure that an individual already present in the model is now being reintroduced in the discourse as a topic. The rhetorical structure associated to that utterance will then show a topic with the model identifier and a label for it, taken from the discourse module which includes the following: EXPECTED, MAIN, SECONDARY, POTENTIAL. Each of these labels causes the Relevance Score to produce a different computation in the total figures associated to that identifier.

In case nothing has been asserted relatively to the argument under analysis, the Interpreter activates different procedures according to the definiteness feature present in the semantic array. At least the following four main categories of NPs are possible:

1. indefinite NPs;
2. definite NPs - singular and plural are treated separately, and proper names;
3. common nouns with empty specifier or naked NPs;
4. quantified NPs, quantifiers, mass nouns.

Category one usually leads to the creation of a new individual in the model; category two and category three may lead to the creation of a new entity in case the common noun is a newly introduced property for a given individual. This may be detected in a number of different ways, listed below,

Case 1. directly from the model - the property is new;

Case 2. from the model and the semantic categories associated to the argument - the NP denotes a relational property and is not asserted in the model;

Case 3. from the grammatical function and the semantic role - the NP is an open function, XCOMP and must be computed as a property associated to the controller, a nonargument or nonthematic function;

Case 4. the NP is in a possession relation with an individual already asserted in the model and the relation is a new property - or not, according to the model. Note that possession is not intrinsically specified as to cardinality, and in case the possessed object has more than one possessor, this may cause the Interpreter to produce more than one entity possessed;

Case 5. from the grammatical function and the semantic role - the NP is an open adjunct, XADJ, and must be computed as a property associated to the controller, a closed function;

Case 6. from the grammatical function and the semantic role - the NP is a closed adjunct and may introduce a relation of comparison between two entities, one of which is coreferred in the previous text. The identifier of one of the members of the comparison has to be recovered from the property associated to the pronoun.

As to category four, in case the quantifier is a nominal substitute like "maggiore"/the elder, or "altri"/the others inferential processes are required in order to compute the membership and the subset relations intervening between the entities already present in the model and the newly asserted ones. As to quantifiers, they only introduce entities which are classes or ensembles: these in turn may be used to establish inclusion relation with other classes or ensembles, even though we have not coped with any of these cases in our texts.

4. Definite NPs

In the analysis we are about to propose, the interpretation of definite descriptions involves a search not through the universe of discourse but through the contextual domain. Singular definite NPs are cases which require a search throughout the current knowledge base, and in case of failure, constitute the trigger for a search outside the model, into the external or encyclopaedic knowledge available to the system. In this, we follow McCawley(1981) suggestions, discussed at length below. Inferences can be very complex to work out, particularly in case a metaphor is used: for instance, in our texts, there is a case in which the little pigs are coreferred by the singular definite NP "il pasto"/the meal. Before accessing external knowledge, the interpreter tries to match semantic features associated to the definite NP to those of other NPs used with a semantic role which requires those semantic features, in a relation in which the participants were the same individuals. Failure of both a search into the model and of any other inferential mechanisms available will cause tapping the external world knowledge.

This is in line with McCawley's ideas about dividing up the model into different layers thus reflecting the level of recency or prominence of the individuals present in the Contextual Domain, where we take the bottom level to correspond to the external knowledge, which we report here below:

"If a search for a referent for a definite description fails to yield one on any of the levels of the Contextual Domain that have some prominence, it will continue on the bottom level, and if there is exactly one element on that level having the given property, that element will be picked out as the referent of the definite description." (p. 270)

There is an extensive literature dealing with how definiteness contributes to the understanding and generation of texts. We shall review briefly only two contributions, i.e. Clark & Marshall(1981) and Appelt(1985). In the former paper there is a classification of definite nongeneric expressions which in turn is taken from Hawkins(1978) which in a sense is on the same line with Appelt's classification, and we believe can help in understanding how we treat definiteness in our system. The authors characterize definite NP usage in the following list of the eight major uses:

4. *The anaphoric use:*
   - I bought a lathe, but the machine didn't work right.

where the NP a lathe sets up the background against which the reference to the machine is understood.

5. *The visible situation:*
   - Pass me the bucket.

where the referent is visible to both speaker and listener.

This modality will be commented below in the discussion of text genres. However, it is not present in narrative and descriptive texts.

6. *The immediate situation use:*
    - Don't feed the pony.

where the pony is not visible, but its existence can be inferred from the situation. Again a discourse situation. However, such a situation can be found in our texts: in particular in Story 1, where a set of houses is introduced as an intensional object and in the subsequent text reference to "the little house" can be inferred to belong to this shared set of objects.

7. *The larger situation use based on specific knowledge:*
    - I'm going to the store.

where it is understood a particular store shared by both speaker and listener.

8. *The larger situation use based on general knowledge:*
    - I wonder where the city hall is.

where reference to the city hall can be recovered because it is known as a general fact about towns of a certain size that they have a city hall. This is present in our texts, but is not built as a fact rather as a sit(uation) or as an intensional object because of its linguistic usage. Definite expression not introduced as Topics do not contribute to the active construction of the facts relevant to the world model, even though they might in other texts. This is also commented in Appelt's paper, with the following example (his (5)),

- Turn left at the third block past the stoplight

which is a case where the speaker gives instructions to the hearer, even though "they have no mutual belief at the time of the utterance about the location to which the speaker intends to refer". However, as Appelt notes, the speaker knows that the hearer can formulate a plan that will guarantee that he will have identified the referent when needed. This modality is always connected to discourse situations. As Appelt comments, definite NPs can be viewed as concept activation actions, which in this case imply that, even though the hearer does not share the denotation of the description contained in the utterance, the speaker intends the hearer to be able to realize the perlocutionary effects of the utterance, and be able to identify the speaker's intended referent. Another related case is when the speaker knows of a plan the hearer can execute that will lead to the identification of the referent at the appropriate time, as in the following example (his (7)),

- Get me the largest tomato from the garden

As Appelt suggests, this definite NP constitutes an attributive description rather than a referential one, in the sense that the speaker is not referring to a particular tomato, but to whatever tomato fits the description.

9. *The associative anaphoric use*:
   - A car just went by and the exhaust fumes made me sick.

where the car can be considered the trigger to the associate exhaust fumes, again a means to constitute a shared set of objects. This is also present in our texts and is treated as a case of tapping external knowledge of the world.

10. *The unavailable use*:
    - Bill is amazed by the fact that there is so much life on earth.

in which the fact that... introduces new information unknown to the listener or reader. This is commented by the authors as being a similar case to the use of restrictive relatives as in,

- The woman whom Max went out with last night was nasty to him.

which is present in our texts and constitutes a relation which is presupposed as a fact and added to the world model. Note that in order for a restrictive relative to be treated as a specifying relation, it must be "factive": which in this case amounts to evaluating the import of tense, aspect and temporal adjuncts. However, there might be cases in which the modality introduced by the restrictive relative is nonfactive, thus contributing to merely establishing the existence of an individual whose identity is not yet available, or not known to the world model. This is what happens in an example proposed by Appelt, example (1), which we report here below,

- The runner who wins tomorrow's race will qualify for the semifinals

which is dubbed as a case where the existence of an individual is simply presupposed, due to the use of future tense and the presence of a deictic temporal modifier in the restrictive relative, like "tomorrow" which is unable to specify the identity of "the runner". Thus, even though the description "the runner who wins tomorrow's race" is not referential it can still be used to support an ID in the model world, provided it is not treated as extensional but rather as an intensional entity.

11. *The unexplanatory modifier use*:
    - The first person to sail to America was an islander

where the definite expression picks out a unique person, whoever he may be, from the set of people who sailed to America - which in this particular case might be wrong, in view of the fact that Cristoforo Colombo was not an islander!! However, in this case, the predicate nominal may be used as a property to either identify the name of this person, or else to set up the Initial Description for that person, which might be identified by the usual means assigning it a name,

- He was Colombo

4.1. Definiteness and Text Genre: Technical Manuals

Generally speaking, definite NPs should always be conceived of on a par with other discourse level anaphors, in that they cannot possibly be considered the appropriate syntactic means for introducing new individuals in a text. However, this only applies as long as the text typology is one in which the identity of the extension of the Noun being denoted is strictly derivable from the text itself. In every other case, referential conditions may even be reversed.

Descriptive and narrative texts are standard and normal cases in question: here, new entities must be introduced in the world according to some default procedure which treats indefinite NPs as their typical syntactic realization. On the contrary, in such texts as instruction manuals for the maintenance or use of any kind of appliance be it electronic or mechanical equipment, things must be computed differently. The text is only understandable by the user in case he is in presence of the object the description will deal with. This could be regarded as an ostensive description, in the sense that referents of NPs are not to be found within the description itself but in the external object, which is in front of the user. It is a norm that locations for some referents are to be understood in terms of the object rather than in their intrinsic linguistic value, which if abstracted from the ostensive process are meaningless. In such texts, definite NPs are used to introduce new entities in the description, and indefinite NPs are usually non referential generic entities introduced only for comparison.

The same happens with spoken dialogues, where the participants in the communicative exchange may refer to new entities with definite NPs in case these are part of their mutual knowledge of the world. This might fail, and some recovering action should be undertaken by the speaker.

We shall now present a small excerpt from Macintosh 12" RGB Display, Owner's Guide, section "Connecting the display", pp.6-7,

Segment A.

"Your display connects to a built-in video port or a video card connector on the back panel of the computer and to a power source. Here's how to connect the display:

1. Position the display and computer so that you can easily get at the back panel of each.
2. Connect the end of the display's video cable to the appropriate video socket on the computer (as shown in Figure 2).
    - If your computer has a built-in video port, plug the cable into the video port - it's the horizontal socket on the computer's back panel that's marked with the video icon.
    - If you have installed a video card, plug the cable into the vertical connector on the video card.
3. Tighten the thumbscrews.

    Tightening the two thumbscrews keeps the connection from coming loose and helps prevent radio and television interference.
4. Plug the power cord into the monitor's power socket then plug the display's power cord into a power source.

    The socket is on the left side of the back panel. It's marked with the power icon.

- If your Macintosh has an auxiliary power outlet (located next to its power receptacle), plug the other end of the power cable into this outlet.
- If your Macintosh does not have an auxiliary power outlet, you should have received an extra power cord with your computer which plugs into a (three-hole) grounded AC outlet. If you did not receive a second power cord, contact your Apple dealer."

In the first paragraph we can see at work the principles we proposed: the possessive is used to introduce the entity being focussed upon, the display, and the indefinite NPs are used to introduce indefinite entities which not necessarily exist in the world of the user being referred to: in particular "a power source" is understood as "any" existing power source, in case it exists. There is also a reference to "the computer" which should be existent in force of the fact that a video display is only a display for a computer: the reference to "the back panel" is only understandable under these conditions. In the following instructions, reference to new entities is always carried out by definite NPs: this happens with "the display's video cable", "the appropriate video socket". Notice that the indefinite NPs we found at the outset of this section, are used in a conditional "if" clause, thus indicating that they need not be existent in the model world - even though one or the other should be present. However, indefiniteness cannot be computed as a syntactic clue for the introduction of a new entity in the world! Notice now the reference to "the video port", which is extensively commented in order to allow the user understand it, by checking directly on the object for the relevant locational parameters, i.e. "it's the horizontal socket on the computer's back panel that's marked with the video icon"; the same applies below to the reference to "the monitor's power socket" which is extensively commented by "The socket is on the left side of the back panel. It's marked with the power icon." Subsection 3. introduces a new entity "the thumbscrews" again by a definite NP. And again, in the final paragraph reference to entities which could possibly exist in the world, but not necessarily do so, is carried out by indefinite NPs in conditional clauses: "an auxiliary power outlet", "an extra power cord", "a (three-hole) grounded AC outlet". In case all these indefinite NPs are computed as intensional entities of the world, they could however contribute to referential mechanisms - even though with some special means - if we consider that in the last sentence, reference to "an extra power cord" is achieved within an if-clause by the indefinite NP "a second power cord".

Here then we see that semantic interpretation should be tailored to text genre. Even though some mechanism could remain invariant across textual varieties, as for instance is the case with the use of possessive pronouns, which establish the existence of the object in the world model it is clear that the use of referential indices like definiteness must be parameterized.

4.2. Predications and Properties

Generally speaking(see Talmy, 1973), a predicate may never be more referential than its subject. The referential is less general than the attributive, while the definite is less general than the indefinite. A predicate may never be less general than its subject. In particular, then, referential subjects may take either referential or attributive nominal predicates, but nonreferential subjects may take only nonreferential (attributive) predication.

13a. Women are angels/ tutte le donne sono angeli
b. *Women are the angels we saw/*Tutte le donne sono gli angeli che abbiamo visto

This implies that nominal expressions do not have inherent referential power, but inherit it from the clause in which they are embedded or the predicate in relation to which they are interpreted, compositionally within a certain f-structure, or proposition.

However, we must distinguish what applies to OBJect nominals from what applies to SUBJect nominals: the latter seem to possess referentiality unless some opacity operator prevents it from being operative, e.g. in a copulative context (be, become, elect, etc.) in case the SUBJect is not a proper noun, i.e. a uniquely referring individual in the world - or a referential subject, i.e. a SUBJect that is presupposed to have a unique referent. OBJect nominals on the contrary are dependent on the verb. Thus we might say that a nominal is always interpreted referentially, if it is a SUBJect, unless it falls under the scope - directly or indirectly - of opacity produced by a modality operator. Given no opacity operator, one would expect that if a non-definitional proposition is presupposed to be true, the nominals involved in it are therefore presupposed to have referentiality. Referentiality and opacity are discussed below in more detail.

Yes-no questions: is one of the most obvious opaque environments, allowing the use of any in English to mark the nonreferential noun. No factive presuppositions are attached to sentences embedded in this construction, since presumably the speaker has deferred his judgement assuming that the proposition in question may be either true or false. Thus a nominal within a proposition that is not held to be true could not be obligatorily interpreted referentially, and this applies to both SUBJect and OBJect nominals. In turn, in copulative constructions, the referential NP is less general than the attributive, while the definite is less general than the indefinite, less general corresponding to more specific. We might use Talmy's(1973,45) principle regarding referential expression which is the following,

14. A predicate may never be less general than its subject.

In other words, a SUBJect of a copular construction must always be more specific than its predicate, in case it is an Ncomp. One of the most obvious context in which one may find the referential/nonreferential contrast is in nominal predicates. This is so because nominal predicates may be used to perform two functions: they either are attributive and thus describe the properties of the subject or else they are referential and identify the subject.

15a. John is a student(attributive)
b. John is the student(referential)
c. John is the student who passed your exams.

The referential expression above clearly presupposes that a certain student exist and is well-known to the speaker (and hearer). The expression is thus used to identify one referential noun (John) with another (the student). In the attributive expression, on the other hand, no such presupposition exists. We treat such constructions as assigning a role to the referential expression which is the subject, while at the same time establishing the existence of a new individual in the world: the reason is quite obvious, the attribute "student" is also a property of John, and may be assigned certain other properties or attributes which are independent of the individual John, as the following text shows:

16a. John was a student.
b. He used to attend my lessons with little interest.

Sentence a. and b. above describes what used to be John's inherent attributes at some period in the past. Thus there can be an indication in the world or discourse model that that property held for a certain period of time. The past tense in a. may indicate remoteness of reference and the fact that the property no longer holds for the individual John.

In our system we compute *default properties* automatically from selectional restrictions: these properties are generalizations or general properties which the current individual is an instance of. Thus, nouns which are computed as [umano/human] will be classified as *inst_of* [class:man] in case their gender is masculine, or *inst_of* [class:woman] for feminine. Objects, animals [ferocious and edible], and many other default properties can be easily worked out from the lexicon and added to model to be used for generic statements.

5. Inherent Semantic Features and WordNet

First of all it is important to say that nouns, adjective, verbs, adverbials are all treated as predicates in our system as they are in WordNet. In other words, they may all be associated with some semantic classification which can be used subsequently by the system to restrict their occurrence in some specific context. Apart from adverbials, the remaining predicates may also and must, in the case of verbs, be associated with a list of arguments which carry syntactic and semantic information, as well as selectional restrictions. This topic is discussed at length in chapter I of Book I to appear. Here below we show in detail the classification we use for nouns. Adjectives and verbs have no inherent features associated with their lexical form: they only have syntactic and semantic classifications.

The classification that we use is partly been used as an experimental prototypical representation. In the experiment, we wanted to verify how efficient a feature based classification could be for the analysis and understanding of extended texts. The same classification was used for text generation in the restricted domain of traffic messaging. Most of our features are the usual features one finds in linguistically based systems. In particular we followed Dahlgren's suggestions in that we attempted to introduce a cross-classification, which is listed below, where more specific features are presented and discussed. Most features are self-explanatory: however notice the use of body-part which can trigger a part_of relation inference in the DM. Features like "edible, ferocious" might be used in the planning to understand more closely the implication of one or the other action. A feature like "relational" is used to trigger special routines in the semantics: however, it is clearly still to be regarded as a generalization: "fratello"/brother must be treated differently from "padre, madre"/father, mother since the type of relational role is completely different. Some features are used in couple, for instance, as happens with "time,duration", to be kept distinct from "time,unreal" or "time,iterative" Here below is the first list:

1. hum	human	21. state	state
2. anim	animate	22. time	time
3. obj	object	23. durat	duration
4. abstr	abstract	24. repet	iterative
5. social	social	25. unreal	unreal
6. eval	evaluative	26. neg	negative
7. emot	emotional	27. neg_prop	negative property
8. edible	edible		
9. body-part	body_part	28. deict	deictic
10. subst	substance	29. surname	surname
11. feroc	ferocious	30. means_trans	means of transport
12. instr	instrument		
13. meas	measure	31. nquant	quantity noun
14. matter	matter		
15. relat	relational	32. danger	danger
16. event	event	33. exort	exortation
17. place	place	34. exclam	exclamation
18. activ	activity	35. greet	greeting
19. instit	institution	36. atm_dang	atmospheric danger
20. milit	military		

The second set of inherent features is built according to a fixed scheme of cross-classification in which each position has always a certain attribute with a fixed number of values. We also assume that the ontology we are creating has certain internal properties: in particular, each attribute is in a subsumption relation with the attribute/s on its left, which in other words is a generalization of the attribute on its right. This classification is due to work carried out in connection with Dahlgren's. Slot 4 is an open-ended list which might be changed according to domain requirements.

SLOT 1:	ind	=	individual	temp	=	temporal
	coll	=	collective	state	=	state
	hum	=	human	instit	=	institution
SLOT 2:	real	=	real	event	=	event
	abst	=	abstract	activ	=	activity
SLOT 3:	nat	=	natural	hum_set	=	human set
	art	=	artifact			
	min	=	mineral	anim	=	animal
	soc	=	social	veget	=	vegetable
	mil	=	military	part	=	part
	quant	=	quantity	sol	=	solid
SLOT 4:	hum	=	human	liq	=	liquid
	role	=	role	body_p	=	body_part
	relat	=	relational	stuff	=	stuff

subst	=	substance	meas	=	measure
vehi	=	vehicle	mann	=	manner
prod	=	product	locat	=	location
tool	=	tool	gen_loc	=	generic location
edib	=	edible			

We include here below some examples of classification derived from our lexicon and related to Avveduti's story.

- [ind, real, nat, hum], uomo/man, paola
- [ind, real, soc, role], laureato/graduated, procuratore/barrister
- [ind, real, nat, relat], figlia/daughter
- [ind, real, mil, role], militare/military, ufficiale/officer
- [ind, abst, quant, temp], 1945
- [ind, abst, soc, state], successo/success, qualifica/qualification
- [ind,abst,soc,event], carriera/carreer
- [ind, real, soc, instit], università/university
- [ind,real,soc,nonliv], voto/vote
- [ind,real,quant,gen_locat], italia/italy, veneto/veneto
- [ind,real,phys,nonliv], nota/note, divisa/uniform
- [coll,abst,soc,event], amministrazione/administration
- [coll, real, soc, event], fiera/fair
- [coll,real,soc,set], mondo/world
- [coll, real, soc, instit], senato/senate, parlamento/parliament
- [coll, real, soc, hum_set], seguito/followers, famiglia/family
- [coll, real, mil, hum_set], esercito/army
- [coll,real,quant,gen_locat], estero/foreign
- [hum, abstr, soc, role], elettore/voter

Lately – from 2000 onward - we worked on WordNet 1.6 at different levels. The idea was to create a more "friendly" and updatable version of the synsets and their inferential links. We produced a manual labeling of WordNet 120,000 entries by adopting a set of 72 semantic labels partially derived from CORELEX, the freely downloadable lexicon of English made available at the University of Pennsylvania. We report here below the main lexical fields we individuated:

*act, activity
100020977-100860774
*mathematic & education
100558391-->100562186 counting,assessing / aatt
100567704-->100577380 education / aatt
100577495-->100583338 representation, model
*places
100821498-->100860774 battle place names /bloc
*animal, fauna

100861689-->102155158 / anim
*artifact
102155313-->103642095 / str
*attribute
103642179-->104055000 / attr
*body
104055158==>104345779 / bod
*cognition, knowledge
104345975-->104728238 / kabs
*communication
104728391-->105158630 / inf
*event, happening
105363971-->105560569 / hev
*feeling, emotion
105560772-->105617136 / emot
*food
105617228-->105955129 / edib
*group, grouping
106023733==>106262375 / coll
*location
106262545-->106659365 locations, places / locs
106700800-->106848534 mountains,lakes,rivers / nloc
*natural object
106666185-->106700800 / nmat
*motivation, motive
106659588-->106665994 / amot
*natural phenomenon / events
107764306-->107851373 / nev
*person, human being / hum
106938180-->107764175
*relation, social roles / rel
107356184-->107693242
*famous names
107693483-->107764175 / fhum
*plant flora
107851510-->109525373 / fmat
*possession
109525525-->109669733
*process
109669871-->109756140
*quantity amount
104597590-->104622100 maths
105097156-->105129593 marks, numbers formulas
109756361-->109986859
*abstract
105020842-->105032036 titles / thum

105158776-->105251837 nationalities, languages / nhum
105251961-->105363868 art, literature, linguistics / latt
106848705-->106938058 imaginary beings,characters / uhum
*shape
109986997-->110034997
*state
110035141-->110446732
*substance
110446867-->110843517
*time
110843624-->110989410

The main body of WordNet included only certain semantic fields so we had to supplement those areas which where present in the top hierarchy but were then poorly represented. We report here below the set of features we used in our mapping of the main body of WordNet:

ach – change, beginning, destroying, removing, concluding, abandoning, avoiding, discarding
acl legal activities
act general activities, deverbal
anm animate beings, animals
atm modifying activity, change of dimension-joining, separating, accumulating, thinning
bod body parts
btl battles, events, locations
chd change of direction, change of state-turning, shaking, rearranging, shifting, sliding, rising
chp change of position, walking, transforming, packing, journeying, restoring, cleaning
col collective entities, groups, groupings
edb edibles and drikables
emt emotional
evl abstract evaluations, evaluative states
evn events natural
fac physical activities, related to body
lat learning activities, games
lcg general locations
lng locations natural
loc locations
mab mathematical and other abstracts
mac mental activities - sciences
mat trees, natural objects
mnt mental activities
mst mental states
mtf mathematical formula

mus	music
nat	negative actions
nev	natural events
nfa	activities related to information processing
nfl	linguistic information, software, publishing
nft	information transmission
nhm	wellknown people
nlg	languages and geografical names
pos	possessions, money, gifts
pro	processes
qua	quantities
rel	social roles, human relations
sac	social activities
sha	shapes
sta	states
str	objects, instruments, artifacts
sub	substances
tit	titles and jobs
tme	times, dates
unr	unreal entities
sur	surnames
nmm	masculine names
nmf	female names

To these 48 more specific features we added the following general features which are mainly related to the top level entities of WordNet hierarchy: they can also be called Basic Concepts. We use these Basic Concepts as features in some application, by activating a small inferential procedure that we report below:

abs	00012670	abstraction 0
amb	00008030	animal 0 animate_being 0 beast 0 brute 0 creature 0 fauna 0
art	00011607	artifact 0 artefact 0
atr	00017586	attribute 0
ecn	00126393	economy
evt	00016459	event 0
eng	00607693	engineering
fod	00011263	food 0 nutrient 0
frm	00014558	shape 0 form 0
hum	00004865	person 0 individual 0 someone 0 mortal 0 human 0 soul 0
hvt	00020977	human activity
inf	04734700	information
leg	00765298	legal
lfr	00002728	life_form 0 organism 0 being 0 living_thing 0
mtt	04026286	matter
plt	00008894	plant 0 flora 0 plant_life 0
pho	00009469	object 0 inanimate_object 0 physical_object 0

psy	00012517	psychological_feature 0
qun	00020056	quantity
sts	00016185	state
tec	00064182	technology
unb	00017487	unbound action

This was supplemented by another 150,000 entries related to the lexical fields of Economics, Mathematics, Computer Science, Technology which we took from freely downloadable dictionaries on the web. Finally the last features associated to the additional semantic fields:

cmp	computer, logic and technology
adv	language of advertising

For compatibility criteria we then mapped the semantic features into our internal features, which are a subset of the ones reported above. We also produced an inheritance scheme, this to be used solely for inference purposes in lack of other inferential cues.

```
translwncats(ach, event, [n]).
translwncats(acl, activity, [n]).
translwncats(acl, legal, [n]).
translwncats(act, activity, [n]).
translwncats(anm, animated, [n]).
translwncats(atm, event, [n]).
translwncats(atm, change, [n]).
translwncats(bod, body_part, [n]).
translwncats(bod, object, [n]).
translwncats(btl, place, [np]).
translwncats(btl, event, [n]).
translwncats(chd, event, [n]).
translwncats(chp, event, [n]).
translwncats(chd, change, [n]).
translwncats(chp, change, [n]).
translwncats(col, human, [nh]).
translwncats(col, institution, [nh]).
translwncats(com, abstract, [n]).
translwncats(sac, social, [nh]).
translwncats(com, activity, [n]).
translwncats(ecn, legal, [n]).
translwncats(edb, edible, [n]).
translwncats(emt, emotive, [n]).
translwncats(evl, abstract, [n]).
translwncats(evn, event, [n]).
translwncats(fac, activity, [n]).
translwncats(lat, activity, [n]).
translwncats(lat, informtn, [n]).
translwncats(lcg, place, [np]).
translwncats(lng, place, [np]).
translwncats(loc, place, [np]).
translwncats(mab, abstract, [n]).
translwncats(mab, informatn, [n]).
translwncats(mac, activity, [n]).
translwncats(mac, informatn, [n]).
translwncats(mat, plant, [n]).
translwncats(mnt, activity, [n]).
translwncats(mnt, informatn, [n]).
translwncats(mst, state, [n]).
translwncats(mst, abstract, [n]).
translwncats(mtf, abstract, [n]).
translwncats(mtf, measure, [n]).
translwncats(mus, abstract, [n]).
translwncats(mus, activity, [n]).
translwncats(nat, danger, [n]).
translwncats(nat, activity, [n]).
translwncats(nev, event, [n]).
translwncats(nfa, informatn, [n]).
translwncats(nfa, activity, [n]).
translwncats(nfl, informatn, [n]).
translwncats(nfl, activity, [n]).
translwncats(nft, activity, [n]).
translwncats(nft, informatn, [n]).
translwncats(nhm, human, [nh]).
translwncats(nlg, place, [np]).
translwncats(nlg, human, [nh]).
```

translwncats(pos, object, [n]).
translwncats(pro, activity, [n]).
translwncats(qua, nquant, [n]).
translwncats(rel, relat, [nh]).
translwncats(rel, human, [nh]).
translwncats(rel, social, [nh]).
translwncats(sac, social, [nh]).
translwncats(sac, human, [nh]).
translwncats(sha, abstract, [n]).
translwncats(sta, state, [n]).
translwncats(str, object, [n]).
translwncats(str, instrument, [n]).
translwncats(sub, substance, [n]).
translwncats(tit, social, [nh]).
translwncats(tit, human, [nh]).
translwncats(tme, temporal, [nt]).
translwncats(unr, human, [nh]).
translwncats(unr, abstract, [n]).
translwncats(cmp, informatn, [n]).
translwncats(cmp, techno, [n]).
translwncats(adv, informatn, [n]).
translwncats(adv, public, [n]).
translwncats(lfr, animated, [n]).
translwncats(hum, human, [nh]).
translwncats(amb, animated, [n]).
translwncats(plt, plant, [n]).
translwncats(pho, object, [n]).
translwncats(mtt, substance, [n]).
translwncats(fod, edible, [n]).
translwncats(art, object, [n]).
translwncats(art, instrument, [n]).
translwncats(abs, abstract, [n]).
translwncats(psy, abstract, [n]).
translwncats(psy, informatn, [n]).
translwncats(llc, place, [np]).
translwncats(frm, abstract, [n]).
translwncats(evt, event, [n]).
translwncats(hvt, change, [n]).
translwncats(unb, activity, [n]).
translwncats(atr, abstract, [n]).
translwncats(sur, human, [nh]).
translwncats(nmm, human, [nh]).
translwncats(nmf, human, [nh]).

The system contains the following 24 basic concepts for general inference:

- abstract;
- human;
- relat;
- informatn;
- state;
- temporal;
- social;
- change;
- legal;
- instrument;
- substance;
- body_part;
- activity;
- nquant;
- institution
- plant;
- measure;
- edible;
- event;
- object;
- place;
- animate;
- public;
- emotive

We also elaborated an inferential hierarchy for WordNet 72 conceptual labels which we attach below, where the features at the left hand side of the arrow include or are supersets – mostly taken from the top hierarchy above - of the labels at the right hand side of the arrow:

abs --> emt, evl, mab, mst, mtf, mus, psy, sha, sts
art --> pos, str
evt --> ach, atm, btl, chd, chp, evn, hvt, nev
fod --> edb
hum --> bod, col, emt, nhm, nlg, nmf, nmm, rel, sac, sur, tit, unr
inf --> adv, lat, mab, mac, mnt, nfa, nft
leg --> acl
lfr --> amb, anm, hum, mat, plt
llc --> btl, lcg, lng, loc, nlg, tme
mtt --> fod, sub

pho --> bod, mat
qun --> mtf, qua
sts --> mst, sta
tec --> cmp
unb --> act, fac, lat, mac, mnt, mus, nat, nfa, nfl, pro, sts

6. Logical Form Representation

In order to produce a semantic interpretation from the output of the grammar or parser we must adopt a uniform meaning representation which is usually called Logical Form. In other terms we have to map our f-structures into a linear propositional formalism that can capture the basic meaning relations of the structural units of grammatical representation and turn it into a LF. This must necessarily be a predicate logic of first order with restricted quantification and no additional variables apart from those introduced by the syntax and the QR algorithm. Those variables have already been bound by syntactic control, by anaphoric control or by discourse anaphora resolution strategies and there will be no unbound variables. The remaining elements of this FOPL are "constants" or atoms representing word senses describing objects of the world including abstract objects such as events and situations which are built as "terms"; constants that describe relations and properties are called "predicates" (see also Allen, 234). Well formed formulas or propositions in this language, corresponding to an utterance, are formed from a predicate followed by an appropriate number of terms as their arguments. We also use a number of constants called "logical operators", such as the negation operator NOT or the conjunction operator AND.

Overall we will follow a Davidsonian approach, with Event variables in order to treat Tense appropriately, i.e. as an operator that quantifies over Events. In this case we intend to take advantage of Higginbotham's(1983) suggestions that finite tense introduces quantification over the event.

Quantifiers will all be represented as terms, which in our language are a three part generalized quantifier notation, or a complex term,

Quantifier, Variable, Restriction

where the Restriction is again a formula. Our LF is taken from Hobbs & Shieber(1987)(hence H&S) algorithm and is in line with Alshawi(1990) ideas on QLF resolution. A complex term is an ordered triple where the restriction represents the predication that is grammatically subordinated to the variable(H&S, 49). We do not use four part quantified expressions like the one used in H&S simply because our expressions are already scoped. In particular we only consider fully scoped quantifiers and resolved referring expressions, seen that in our modularised system QR takes place before anaphoric binding. We also assume that parsing has made explicit the predicate-argument relations and the relation of grammatical subordination and adjunction in f-structure representation.

Here below we include the main call of the LF transducer: the starting node is the propositional node, where mood and tense are both available. All arguments are searched first, by looking for grammatical functions: notice that f-structures containing semantic role

Form are excluded from LF. These f-structures correspond to idiomatic expressions, as well as to pleonastic elements like "it", "there" in there-sentences and “si-clitic” in predicates with ethic dative expressed.

```
xlate(Node,LF) :-
    (node(Node)::mood::Mood,
    node(Node)::sogg/prop::_ ),
    node(Node)::pred::Pred,
    node(Node)::index::Ind,
    node(Node)::cat::CatV,
    node(Node)::mood::Mood,
    node(Node)::tense::Tense,
    findall(N, (member( F,
            [sogg,sogg_top,sogg_foc,topic,focus
            ogg,ogg2,obl2,obl1,obl,ogg_avv,adv,
            pcomp,acomp,ncomp,vpred,vcomp,fcomp]),
    node(Node)::F/Role::node(N),Role\=form ),
    La1),
    maplist(xlate,La1,La2),
    sentential_adjuncts(Node,Ind, Adjs),
```

After argument f-structures are mapped in appropriate logical terms, i.e. by computing internal adjuncts and/or arguments, the algorithm looks for sentence level adjuncts, which in LFG terms, might be computed as both open and closed adjuncts. These two syntactic constructions receive a different treatment in the semantics, seen that closed adjuncts have only a modifying import on the Event variable associate to the main predicate. On the contrary, open adjuncts have both an Event variable and an argument variable which they modify: this information is represented in f-structure by the presence of an (usual) internal Subject variable, functionally controlled by the governing head NP. An example will be reported below and discussed in details. Subsequently, the algorithm calls for the event restriction building subroutine, which is reported here below.

```
build_event_restrictions(Tense, Ind, Adjs, EvState, TQuant, EventRes),
    (on(CatV, [result_state,achiev_irr,achiev,achiev_tr,accomp])
    ->
    EvStato=ev,
    TQuant=definite,
    append(La3,[term(event,Ind,EventRes)],Args)
    ;
    CatV=activity,
    EvStato=pr,
    TQuant=indefinite,
    append(La3,[term(process,Ind,EventRes)],Args)
    ;
    EvStato=st,
    TQuant=indefinite,
```

```
append(La3,[term(state,Ind,EventRes)],Args) ),
(find_forms(Node,Pred,Pre),
LF1 = wff(Pre,Args)
;
LF1 = wff(Pred,Args) ),
(node(Node)::adjs::neg::Neg,
LF2 = wff(not,[LF1]), !
;
LF2 = LF1 ),
(Mood=inf,
LF=LF2, !
;
node(Node)::focus::tipo_focus::interrogative,
LF=LF2, !
;
LF= wff(situation,[LF2]) ).

build_event_restrictions(Tense, Ind, Adjs, EvStato, TQuant, EventRes) :-
    EventRes = wff(and, [wff(isa,[Ind, EvStato]), EventRes1]),
    TimeRes = wff(and, [wff(isa,[TInd, tloc]), wff(Tense, [TInd])]),
    Time = wff(time,[Ind, term(TQuant,TInd, TimeRes) ]),
    gen_sym(t, TInd),
    (Adjs = []
    ->
    EventRes1 = Time
    ;
    EventRes1 = wff(and,[Time, Adjs]).
```

6.1. Some Examples

LF representations are used to produce a semantic analysis for an utterance and represents its interpretation in context and also its truth conditions. Once it is produced, the system generates a situation semantics mapping which is used to update the Discourse Model of currently salient discourse entities, or new properties of already existing entities.

In order to produce a semantic interpretation of each utterance we proceed as follows:

A. we start from DAGs available for each utterance which we used to produce f-structure and perform pronominal binding and anaphora resolution at discourse level;
B. each CLAUSE in a DAG is turned into a well-formed-formula with restricted quantification, positive literals, no variables except for those introduced at a syntactic level.
C. each wff is an expression of logical form which is made up of a predicate and a number of arguments, "p(arg_1, ..., arg_n), where 'p' is a constant and 'arg' may a complex term. A term is made up of a quantifier, a variable and a restriction, "term(quant,var,restr)" where the quantifier may be a real natural language quantifier

existing in a NP or a time operator like "time"; the variable is a syntactic index assigned to the phrase in the f-structure representation by the parser; the restriction is the structure on which the quantifier/operator takes scope which might coincide with the phrase or clause of f-structure representation or be a logical expression built for that aim at logical form level, as happens for time formulas.

D. in order to reach an adequate representation for our discourse model we generate a generic "situation" predicate for each tensed clause we compute and we build a complex term for time representation.

Let's look at an example: we shall show the complete computation at LF and at semantic representation of the first of the Texts we dubbed as “Psychological Statements” in the Introduction, which was taken from a paper by Garrod and Sanford(1988) - now "At the Restaurant", which we report again here below:

"John went into a restaurant. There was a table in the corner. The waiter took the order. The atmosphere was warm and friendly. He begun to read his book."

The following is the LF for the first utterance: John went into a restaurant.

```
wff(situation, [
    wff(go, [term(definite, sn2, wff(isa, [sn2, john])),
             term(definite, sn5, wff(isa, [sn5, restaurant])),
             term(event, f5, wff(and, [wff(isa, [f5, ev]),
                    wff(time, [f5, term(definite, t1,
                            wff(and, [wff(isa, [t1, tloc]),
                            wff(past, [t1])]))])]))  'term-event'
                                   ]) 'wff-go'
                                   ])'wff-situation'
```

Generic 'isa' relations are introduced into wffs for NP's and the quantifier is represented by the translation of the content of the NP's specifier. In addition, indefinite NP are turned into 'definite' operators in case no scope ambiguity in the clause may arise due to the absence of ambiguity inducing quantifiers. Tense specifications are transformed into a complex term which has a semantic operator that translates the contents of semantic aspect after undergoing the computations that have transformed the lexical static value of aspect into its corresponding dynamic propositional import. We use three different operators: event, process, state. These operators then have a complex restriction, represented by a conjoined number of wffs, where we indicate both the location in time - tloc - and its specificity.

This LF representation is then converted into a situational semantic representation where syntactic identifiers are turned into semantic identifiers and all logical predicates are omitted except for the conjunction 'and'. Semantic identifiers might be derived from the discourse model in case the linguistic form represents an entity already existing or known to the world of the DM. Situation semantics builds infons for each unit of information constituting the situation denoted by the proposition being represented in the formula. In addition, for each individual or set entity we record the semantic role already assigned at f-structure level by the grammar. A generic 'arg' is associated to arguments of time predicate. Notice then that a polarity argument has been added at the end of each expression.

```
sit(event, id4, go,
    [ind(definite, id3, and([infon(att, infon8, isa, [id3, john], [], 1)]), agent),
    ind(indefinite, id2, and([infon(att, infon9, isa, [id2, restaurant], [], 1)]), locat)],
          and([infon(att, infon10, isa, [id4, ev], [], 1),
                infon(att, infon13, time, [id4,
                ind(definite, id5, and([infon(att, infon11, isa, [id5, tloc], [], 1),
                infon(att, infon12, past, [id5], [], 1)]), arg)], [], 1)]), 1),
                      fact, 1, id1, id2, prop, rels
```

Finally the content of this representation is asserted in the DM as a set of 'facts' or 'sits' in case they are not already present. Factuality for situational types - events, processes and states - is computed from propositional level informational and semantic characteristics. Semantic roles inherited from f-structure representation make explicit, in a declarative way, semantic relations which are not computed in the LF.

The final translation in the DM introduces the objects of our ontology which, as said above are made up of the following literals: fact, sit, loc, ind, set, card, in, class. The structure of each situation semantic expression is different according to their semantic role: loc, locations has no polarity and no spatiotemporal location indices; ind, in, card, set, class are type denotators and have no internal structure. Fact and sit have an internal structure which is made up of the following arguments:

- an infon ranked number; a relational type specifier; a list of arguments expressed as a role:identifier pair; a polarity, spatiotemporal indices

Facts and sits corresponding to main propositional relations have no infon: in its place they have a semantic unique identifier.

```
loc(infon3, id1, [arg:main_tloc, arg:tr(f5_r01)])
loc(infon4, id2, [arg:main_sloc, arg:restaurant])
ind(infon5, id3)
fact(infon6, inst_of, [ind:id3, class:man], 1, univ, univ)
fact(infon7, name, [john, id3], 1, univ, univ)
ind(infon8, id2)
fact(infon9, isa, [arg:id2, arg:restaurant], 1, id1, id2)
fact(id4, go, [agent:id3, locat:id2], 1, tes(f5_r01), id2)
fact(infon10, isa, [arg:id4, arg:ev], 1, tes(f5_r01), id2)
fact(infon11, isa, [arg:id5, arg:tloc], 1, tes(f5_r01), id2)
fact(infon12, past, [arg:id5], 1, tes(f5_r01), id2)
fact(infon13, time, [arg:id4, arg:id5], 1, tes(f5_r01), id2)
```

This is an example of a binary predicate "take" which however becomes ternary due to the presence of the usual 'event' argument which in our case is a process.

```
[The waiter took the order]
wff(situation,
          [wff(take, [term(definito, sn1, wff(isa, [sn1, waiter])),
```

```
                        term(definito, sn4, wff(isa, [sn4, order])),
                        term(process, f5, wff(and, [wff(isa, [f5, pr]),
                                    wff(time, [f5, term(indefinito, t3,
                                           wff(and, [wff(isa, [t3, tloc]),
                                           wff(past, [t3])]))])]))])])
sit(process, id13, take,
     [ind(definito, id11, and([infon(att, infon46, isa, [id11, waiter], [], 1)]), agent),
    ind(definito, id12, and([infon(att, infon47, isa, [id12, order], [], 1)]), theme_aff)],
          and([infon(att, infon48, isa, [id13, pr], [], 1),
            infon(att, infon51, time, [id13, ind(indefinite, id14,
             and([infon(att, infon49, isa, [id14, tloc], [], 1),
               infon(att, infon50, past, [id14], [], 1)]), arg)], [], 1)]), 1),
                fact, 3, id1, id2, prop, rels
ind(infon42, id11)
fact(infon43, inst_of, [ind:id11, class:[social_role]], 1, univ, univ)
fact(infon44, isa, [ind:id11, class:waiter], 1, id1, id2)
fact(infon45, role, [waiter, id2, id11], 1, id1, id2)
fact(infon47, isa, [arg:id12, arg:order], 1, id1, id2)
fact(id13, take, [agent:id11, theme_aff:id12], 1, tes(f5_r03), id2)
```

Consider now a copulative construction, where we find a SUBJect of a predication and the predication itself, which in our case is constituted by a pair of conjoined adjectives. The predicate is not built as a term, rather it is a wff with a predicate and a number of arguments, in our case one argument.

```
[the atmosphere was warm and friendly]
wff(situation,
     [wff(be, [term(definito, sn1, wff(isa, [sn1, atmosphere])), wff([warm, friendly],
      [sn1]),
        term(state, f5, wff(and, [wff(isa, [f5, st]),
             wff(time, [f5, term(indefinito, t4,
                     wff(and, [wff(isa, [t4, tloc]),
                      wff(past, [t4])]))])]))])])
sit(state, id17, be,
   [ind(definito, id16, and([infon(att, infon60, isa, [id16, atmosphere], [], 1)]),
    theme_bound),
        infon(att, infon61, [warm, friendly], [id16], [], 1)],
        and([infon(att, infon62, isa, [id17, st], [], 1),
           infon(att, infon65, time, [id17, ind(indefinite, id18,
           and([infon(att, infon63, isa, [id18, tloc], [], 1),
              infon(att, infon64, past, [id18], [], 1)]), arg)], [], 1)]), 1),
              fact, 4, id15, id2, prop, rels
loc(infon59, id15, [arg:main_tloc, arg:tes(f5_r03)])
fact(infon60, isa, [arg:id16, arg: atmosphere], 1, id15, id2)
fact(infon61, [warm,friendly], [arg:id16], 1, id15, id2)
fact(id17, be, [prop:infon61], 1, tes(f5_r04), id2)
```

Now a more complex example: an open complement which is an infinitive, i.e. a VCOMP in LFG terms. In addition, there are two pronouns one of which has no local antecedents, and is encoded as antecedent-external - whereas the other has the index of its antecedent included in a two argument structure. Thus antecedenthood is encoded in LF as a wff again, i.e. as a structure which has a predicate and two arguments, in particular, a first argument which is the index of the pronoun and a second argument which is the index of the antecedent. Now look at the infinitival which has a big Pro as a subject and a controller which is the functional control structure added at f-structure by the grammar. As for antecedent structure, control structure are built as wff with two indices as arguments, the controllee and the controller's. The second pronoun is a possessive, which in LF counts as an adjunct: adjoined structure are built as additional restrictions of the term constituting the logical structure of the governing head. In our case 'his book' has 'book' as governing head and 'his' as adjoined structure: both are terms with a 'definite' operator, however the possessing relation is the one governing the adjunction of the pronoun. Adjunctions at LF are all realized by means of the logical operator 'and'. Now, if syntactically we might regard the infinitival as a separate structural phrase and functionally also a separate f-structure, i.e. VCOMP, from the logical perspective we end up with only one term, the subject of the main clause and a relation expressed by the VCOMP as a wff.

```
[he began to read his book]
wff(situation,
     [wff(begin, [term(definite, sn2, wff(and, [wff(isa, [sn2, he]),
                    wff(antecedent, [sn2, external])])),
                    wff(read, [term(definite, sn22, wff(and, [wff(isa, [sn22, pPro]),
                              wff(controller, [sn22, sn2])])),
                              term(definite, sn13, wff(and, [wff(isa, [sn13, book]),
                                wff(poss, [sn13, term(definite, sn19,
                                   wff(and, [wff(isa, [sn19, his]),
                                     wff(antecedent, [sn19, sn2])]))])])),
                             term(process, finf1, wff(and, [wff(isa, [finf1, pr]),
                                  wff(time, [finf1, term(indefinite, t5,
                                    wff(and, [wff(isa, [t5, tloc]),
                                       wff(pres, [t5])]))])]))]),
              term(event, f3, wff(and, [wff(isa, [f3, ev]),
                              wff(time, [f3, term(definite, t6,
                              wff(and, [wff(isa, [t6, tloc]),
                              wff(past, [t6])]))])]))])])
sit(event, id6, begin,
     [ind(arbitrary, id2, and([infon(att, infon6, isa, [id2, he], [], 1)]), agent),
          infon(process, id4, read,
               [ind(definito, id2, and([]), agente), ind(definito, id3,
                  and([infon(att, infon7, isa, [id3, book], [], 1),
                       infon(att, infon8, poss, [id3,
                            ind(arbitrary, id2, and([]), poss)], [], 1)]), theme_aff)],
                  and([infon(att, infon9, isa, [id4, pr], [], 1),
                       infon(att, infon12, time, [id4, ind(indefinite, id5,
```

```
and([infon(att, infon10, isa, [id5, tloc], [], 1),
 infon(att, infon11, pres, [id5], [], 1)]), arg)], [], 1)]), 1)],
and([infon(att, infon13, isa, [id6, ev], [], 1),
 infon(att, infon16, time, [id6, ind(definite, id7,
 and([infon(att, infon14, isa, [id7, tloc], [], 1),
 infon(att, infon15, past, [id7], [], 1)]), arg)], [], 1)]), 1),
 fact, 1, id1, univ, prop, rels
fact(infon76, isa, [arg:id19, arg:book], 1, id15, id2)
fact(infon77, poss, [arg:id19, poss:id3], 1, id15, id2)
fact(id20, read, [agent:id3, theme_aff:id19], 1, tes(finf1_free_a1), id2)
fact(id22, begin, [agent:id3, prop:id20], 1, tes(f3_free_a1), id2)
```

In the following example we see both how a relative clause and an open adjunct is treated in LF: in particular the sentence analysed is the first one of Story 1 of the Three Little Pigs that says approximately "Once upon a time there were three little pigs who lived happily in the countryside" where "happily", an adverbial, is the English for "felici", ad adjectival which in f-structure is computed as an open adjunct. Both the "living" and the subject "little pigs" are understood to be happy in the countryside. This is realized by having a double controller

```
wff(situation, [wff(esserci,
 [term(plural, sn9, wff(and, [wff(isa, [sn9, porcellino]),
 wff(and, [wff(isa, [sn9, fratello]),
 wff(imply, [wff(situation, [wff(vivere, [term(plural, sn15,
 wff(and, [wff(isa, [sn15, pro]),
 wff(and, [wff(felice, [term(definite, sn21,
 wff(and, [wff(isa, [sn21, vbl]),
 wff(controller, [sn21, sn15])]))]),
 wff(controller, [sn15, sn9])])])),
 term(definite, sn16, wff(isa, [sn16, campagna])),
 term(state, f4, wff(and, [wff(isa, [f4, st]),
 wff(and, [wff(time, [f4,
 term(indefinite, t17,
 wff(and, [wff(isa, [t17, tloc]),
 wff(imp, [t17])]))]),
 wff(felice, [f4])])]))])])])])])),
 term(state, f5, wff(and, [wff(isa, [f5, st]),
 wff(and, [wff(time, [f5,
 term(indefinite, t18, wff(and, [wff(isa, [t18, tloc]),
 wff(imp, [t18])]))]), wff(nil, [f5,
 term(indefinite, sn5, wff(isa, [sn5, volta]))])])]))])])
```

The result is a semantic representation where the state of being happy is both associated to the subject id3, and to the event/state id4.

```
sit(state, id6, esserci,
 [ind(plural, id3, and([infon(att, infon10, isa, [id3, porcellino], [], 1),
```

```
                    infon(att, infon11, isa, [id3, fratello], [], 1),
    sit(state, id4, vivere, [ind(plural, id3,
      and([infon(att, infon12, felice, [ind(definite, id3, and([]), nil)], [], 1)]), actor),
      ind(definito, id2, and([infon(att, infon13, isa, [id2, campagna], [], 1)]), locat)],
          and([infon(att, infon14, isa, [id4, st], [], 1),
            infon(att, infon17, time, [id4, ind(indefinite, id5,
            and([infon(att, infon15, isa, [id5, tloc], [], 1),
              infon(att, infon16, imp, [id5], [], 1)]), arg)], [], 1),
              infon(att, infon18, felice, [id4], [], 1)]), 1)]), theme_nonaff)],
      and([infon(att, infon19, isa, [id6, st], [], 1),
        infon(att, infon22, time, [id6, ind(indefinite, id7,
        and([infon(att, infon20, isa, [id7, tloc], [], 1),
          infon(att, infon21, imp, [id7], [], 1)]), arg)], [], 1),
          infon(att, infon24, nil, [id6, ind(indefinite, id1,
          and([infon(att, infon23, isa, [id1, volta], [], 1)]), non_punct)], [], 1)]), 1),
           fact, 1, id1, id2, prop, rels)
```

This LF is then translated into a series of facts which we report here below integrally:

```
loc(infon3, id1, [arg:main_tloc, arg:volta])
loc(infon4, id2, [arg:main_sloc, arg:campagna])
set(infon5, id3)
card(infon6, id3, 3)
fact(infon7, fratello, [ind:id3], 1, id1, id2)
fact(infon8, felice, [nil:id3], 1, id1, id2)
fact(infon9, inst_of, [ind:id3, class:animale_cibo], 1, univ, univ)
fact(infon10, isa, [ind:id3, class:porcellino], 1, id1, id2)
fact(infon14, isa, [arg:id2, arg:campagna], 1, id1, id2)
fact(id4, vivere, [actor:id3, locat:id2], 1, tes(f4_po01), id2)
fact(infon15, isa, [arg:id4, arg:st], 1, tes(f4_po01), id2)
fact(infon16, isa, [arg:id5, arg:tloc], 1, tes(f4_po01), id2)
fact(infon17, imp, [arg:id5], 1, tes(f4_po01), id2)
fact(infon19, felice, [arg:id4], 1, tes(f4_po01), id2)
fact(id6, esserci, [theme_nonaff:id3], 1, tes(f5_po01), id2)
fact(infon20, isa, [arg:id6, arg:st], 1, tes(f5_po01), id2)
fact(infon21, isa, [arg:id7, arg:tloc], 1, tes(f5_po01), id2)
fact(infon22, imp, [arg:id7], 1, tes(f5_po01), id2)
fact(infon24, isa, [arg:id1, arg:volta], 1, tes(f5_po01), id2)
fact(infon25, isa, [arg:id6, non_punct:id1], 1, tes(f5_po01), id2)
included(tr(f5_po01), id1)
during(tes(f4_po01), tes(f5_po01))
```

Chapter 2

DISCOURSE MODEL AND INFERENTIAL PROCESSES

1. INTRODUCTION

As shall be made clear by the chapters on the same topic contained in Book I to appear, the problem of assigning a suitable antecedent to pronominals can be solved by a number of interleaved procedures which first search in the same utterance, then in the previous utterance's topic hierarchy (or local history list) - and this first process has been dubbed grammatical binding. In case this search fails the full history list will be searched, to look for another explicitly mentioned occurence of the nominal head to corefer with, or the pronominal head to agree with and in case this fails some inferential mechanism must be activated - and we may dub this semantic binding or Bridging.

To do Semantic Binding, there are a number of possible processes that we have been using in our system successfully and we will deal with here, and they are:

- Indirect Reference
- Implication
- Equality Match
- Membership Match
- Meaning Postulate Inferences
- Set Reference
- Domain Point-of-View Reference
- World Knowledge Inferential Reference

We shall discuss all these phenomena in this chapter in the following sections. However, before going into the description of what the system does, it is important that we point out what mechanisms are usually adopted in a knowledge representation and artificial intelligence environment, and have not been introduced in our system.

In particular, we are neither using frames nor plans to reason about the world, all our knowledge is encoded in WordNet and in lexical forms. As to the latter, we use inherent semantic features associated to noun predicates, and selectional restrictions to verb and adjective argument slots if present. The semantic module takes advantage of semantic roles and sometimes of grammatical functions to carry out its tasks; inherent features are used for instance to deal with relational nouns or with collective nouns. So we do not rely on scripts or on expectations generated by the previous context. In fact, we are not interested in building a dialogue system, nor do we actually want to ascertain whether the text conforms to a specific plan structure. As said above, we are only interested in narratives, stories, newspaper articles, etc. which should all make their internal plot, and text structure clear to the reader.

When needed, the knowledge base access has been heuristically built around a number of phenomena that make use of inferential processes that call for domain dependent external knowledge of the world, sometimes but not always made available by WordNet. Conditions on this access are very strict:

(A) no match has been found by grammatical and semantic binding procedures;
(B) the nominal expression must be a definite singular NP.

In particular it is used for the following specific tasks:

- to infer the meaning a nominal head, not mentioned in the previous discourse, as for instance is required by a relational complex noun like "father-in-law";
- to infer the referential import of attributes associated with a nominal head, and not mentioned in the previous discourse;
- to associate an adequate coreferential entity for metaphorical nominal heads;
- to reason about actions and causality in order to establish the appropriate discourse relation in a given clause.

We could summarize our introduction in the following two schemata:

How Inferential Processes are Activated

1. Grammatical properties of linguistic objects
    - Functional Features of NPs
    - Selectional Restrictions of NPs
    - Grammatical Functions of NPs
    - Semantic Roles of all Phrases
    - Semantic classes of propositions
    - Aspectual and Temporal Representations of propositions
    - Quantifier scope operator-variable pairs
2. Topic Hierarchies for referential expressions
3. Domains of Point_of_View and Subject_of_Consciousness
4. Discourse Model of facts locs and sits
5. Spatiotemporal locations for scenario effects
6. External World Knowledge Base

Goals and Aims of Inferential Processes

1. Execute Anaphora Resolution
2. Ascribe properties and roles to entities in the model
3. Determine non-extensional entities from a computation of opaque and intensional propositional domains
4. Determine superset, subset and inclusion relations
5. Determine spatiotemporal locations of entities and relations
6. Build up discourse structure, assign discourse relations and build reference intervals for temporal relations

2. SEMANTIC BINDING

The perspective we are working for however requires us to cope with these problems from the context. Anaphora is a general term for a range of expressions that are context-dependent in that they either specify entities in an evolving model of the discourse that the listener is constructing, or they depend on other entities in the discourse model. They are called Discourse Anaphors(DA) in Webber's paper on Tense (1988).

The dependency of a DA on a discourse entity may result from the ontological status of the specified entity, as well as from discourse structure and its focusing effect.

It has been argued extensively in the literature that definite NPs are exclusively used to corefer or cospecify entities already in the DM, whereas indefinite NPs can be used to introduce new entities in the world. However, we shall stress the need to ensure that both definite and indefinite NPs can be used to corefer or cospecify entities and relations in the DM. Besides, we should also note that both kinds of NPs can be used to introduce new entities in the world.

We now comment Webber's example 5. where a definite NP is introduced as a new entity associated to an existing discourse entity:

1a. A bus came round the corner.
 b. I signalled to the driver to stop.

The definite NP "the driver" is here understood as an entity associated with the "bus" mentioned in the previous sentence. In our system this is achieved by an inference on the main location of the text. The driver is related to the bus, since there is the setting of a scenario by mentioning the location in which the driver could be inferred as being a part of, or better a role linked to that frame. Better examples of this problem are constituted by the text we dubbed "At the Restaurant" – we partially commented in the previous chapter, where the scenario effect is more marked:

2a. John went into a restaurant.
 b. There was a table in the corner.
 c. The waiter took the order.
 d. The atmosphere was warm and friendly.

The scenario is set at the beginning of the text, either by a title “At the restaurant”, or by explicitly mentioning the restaurant as an Oblique argument of a “GO” relation where the main Topic is also introduced. Sentence b. is not just meant to indicate the presence of a table in a corner of a restaurant which is a fairly redundant and irrelevant fact in the text, but it has another important goal: it tells the reader that the main Topic, John, is now sitting at a table and ready to order. This implied additional information can be triggered by assuming that the presence of TABLE as new Topic of discourse, introduced in the PRESENTATIVE structure by the verb THERE_BE is not a suitable topic – being classified as THING in inherent features - and is less important than John. In turn the TABLE induces the SIT relation for the now Main Topic John to be asserted as an implicit relation which can only apply however, in case the Main Location is RESTAURANT. To ascertain that the main location is not changed, another important inference has to be triggered, and is the one generated by CORNER, which is in a meronymic relation with RESTAURANT.

When we get to the definite NP “the waiter”, an inclusion relation inference has already being fired by the location “the corner” which is understood as being a part of the main location, the RESTAURANT – a meronymic relation, which remains the main location of the story. Thus, “the waiter” can now be computed as being in an inclusion relation with “the restaurant”, being a role pertaining to that scenario or frame. Another important side effect of the analysis is that the Main Topic, John, is not discarded in favour of the new entity “the waiter”, but persists in the Topic Hierarchy – see Book I, Chapts. 4/5. Thus, in case the text continues with what the authors call “psychological atmosphere statements”, we may impute the subjective judgment on the Main Topic, John, rather than on a possible Expected Topic, the waiter.

More complex examples can be derived from our texts, in which more than one character is present. In particular, the “Story of the Three Little Pigs” has the most intricate plot we found, since we are given at the same time six possible entities to be used for further processing. This is the beginning of an abridged version:

Segment B.

Once upon a time there were three little pigs who lived happily in the countryside. But in the same place lived a wicked wolf who fed precisely on plump and tender pigs. The little pigs therefore decided to build a small house each, to protect themselves from the wolf. The oldest one, Jimmy who was wise, worked hard and built his house with solid bricks and cement. The other two, Timmy and Tommy, who were lazy settled the matter hastily and built their houses with straw and pieces of wood. The lazy pigs spent their days playing and singing a song that said, "Who is afraid of the big bad wolf?"

And these are the entities already present at this point of the computation:

i. a set of three little pigs
ii. a set of three little houses
iii. an individual, member of the set of little pigs, whose name is Jimmy
iv. a subset made of two little pigs, always members of the set of three little pigs, whose names are Timmy and Tommy
v. a single little house, member of the set of three little houses, made of bricks and cement, owned by Jimmy

vi. a subset of two little houses, included in the set of little houses, made of straw and little pieces of wood, owned by the subset of two little pigs, named Timmy and Tommy

As the text proceeds, coreference is activated by evoking one of the entities either by a property, the fact of being brothers or being pigs, or by explicitly indicating cardinality.

Segment C.

And one day, lo and behold, the wolf appeared suddenly behind their backs. "Help! Help!", shouted the pigs and started running as fast as they could to escape the terrible wolf. He was already licking his lips thinking of such an inviting and tasty meal. The little pigs eventually managed to reach their small house and shut themselves in, barring the door.

Consider the deictic singular NP "such an inviting and tasty meal", which requires knowledge of the world to compute the metaphor. We should also note that the sentence is a case of idiomatic expression computed by the parser at grammatical level. Reference to houses in the following text, is expressed in the form of a singular little house associated to the two lazy pigs, rather than a plural noun. We should still be talking about a set of two houses, and this is suggested by the possessor's cardinality. However the following text, reverts this decision, in that it makes us understand that the two little pigs are now both in the same house.

Segment D.

In the meantime the wolf was thinking a way of getting into the house. He began to observe the house very carefully and noticed it was not very solid. He huffed and puffed a couple of times and the house fell down completely. Frightened out of their wits, the two little pigs ran at breakneck speed towards their brother's house.

Problems at this point arise in the reasoning mechanism since the only singular little house available is the one built by the wise brother, Jimmy, which could be picked up for coreference. This is clearly wrong, because this is not the house that gets destroyed since it is still there in the last sentence of Segment D. In order to prevent a failure in the reasoning process, we simply allow reference to a little house to be inferable as belonging to the set of two little pigs under discussion, on the assumption that it is the closest one and is available for coreference in the previous portion of text. The inferential mechanism is always driven by a recency checker which estimates which is the closest topic being asserted: on that basis an inference is fired, and in case it is successful that topic is taken as being coreferent – see Book I, Chapts. 4/5.

Another interesting case is exemplified by the second version of the story of the three little pigs, where we see that a definite NP is used to introduce one the main characters in the story. Differently from what happens in the first story, where the big bad wolf is presented in the world at the very start together with the little pigs, in the second story the wolf only appears after the little pigs have built their houses. The story refers to the wolf as an intensional entity whose presence in the woods nearby is taken for granted:

3a. Jimmy wanted a robust house because he knew that the bad wolf lived in the woods nearby

This reference to the wolf is understood by the system as an *infon* related to an individual, and an appropriate identifier is assigned to it. In the following text, when the wolf reappears on the scene, it is a definite NP again and a fact is asserted. Coreference is enabled thus by virtue of the fact that an intensional entity was available in the model:

b. But as soon as Timmy opened the door, the bad wolf appeared out of the woods.

Another interesting case is suggested by Webber(1988, her example 4.) where a plural pronoun is made to corefer to a class related to a singular NP in the previous discourse by inferential processes,

4a. The dachshund down the block bit me yesterday.
b. They are really vicious beasts.

The pronoun is computed as the controller of the property "beasts" which is in the open complement of the verb "be"; this in turn should be taken as a generic property associated to the definite NP "the dachshund" which the sentence evokes. Clearly this case requires the presence of an ISA Relation in the ontology of the entities, constituting the extra-linguistic knowledge of WordNet required to understand the relations intervening in the text at hand.

2.1. Indefinite NPs

Consider now indefinite NPs: they may cospecify some previously asserted relation or they may introduce some generic property which is already inferable from the model:

5a. John gave Mary a rose.
b. She took it and put it in her hair.
c. She knew that she had been given a present, something precious.

While in a. the indefinite NP is actually a new entity in the DM, in c. "a present" cospecifies the previous NP "a rose" and must be computed as a class entity in which "a rose" is included.

6a. Mary picked up the phone and called Jason.
b. Her husband would have considered such a move as base.

The NP "a move" is an event noun coreferring to a discourse segment as Webber(1990) suggests discussing the role of deictics in discourse; in our system this is achieved at discourse structure where discourse segments are produced and can be recovered from the model.

7a. They appointed John managing director.
b. This was a position he had been longing for ages.

The NP "a position" is an activity noun cospecifying the role property "managing director" asserted in the previous discourse segment and associated to John.

8a. Richard would marry Sara.
 b. He felt strongly about all this.
 c. She was the right person for a man like Richard.

The NP "a man" is a generic noun which corefers with Richard, while the deictic is again coreferring with the previously built discourse segment.

9a. Once upon a time there were three little pigs.
 b. They decided to build a little house each.

The NP "a little house" is asserted as a sit and not a fact – the building is just decided and not terminated - and a cardinality is assigned to this set due to its being in the scope of the distributive quantifier "each". In turn, the floating quantifier is computed as an open adjunct controlled by the subject "They" which corefers with the antecedent NP "three little pigs" in the previous segment of discourse. In another version of the same story, the little house becomes a straw hut and then a little house again, as shown in the following excerpt:

10a. As they reached a nice wood, they decided to build each a comfortable little house.
 b. Timmy didn't like working at all, so he thought to build quickly a straw hut.
 c. Soon the little house was ready.

The NP "a straw hut" is understood to be one of the little houses already introduced in the previous discourse segments. However, knowledge of the world is called for in order to make the appropriate inference. Also notice that the following sentence uses a definite NP to corefer with the previous indefinite NP, and here again the same problem arises: the hut becomes a little house. For sure, we want the DM to be consistent and to understand that there is only one little house under discussion, which however is a_kind_of house, a hut.

Finally the most interesting case: an indefinite NP which is understood as a generic property of an entity introduced in the model by the same relation.

11a. John gave Mary a rose.
 b. She took it and put it in her hair.
 c. She knew she had been given a present, something precious.

The NP "a present" cospecify the NP "a rose" which has been previously introduced in the model by a "GIVE" relation. The dependency is contextually determined by the presence of an entity Mary which is assigned the same semantic role in both sentences: she is always the Patient argument of the predicate GIVE. The system can also recover the Agent argument which has been omitted and is represented in f-structure as a lexically-bound existential quantifier "exist". At the end of the computations, we know that "a rose" is also "a present" which has been given to Mary by John. In order for the inferential mechanism to draw the relevant inference, tense is used: the past perfect can be regarded as a presuppositional tense, i.e. a tense that indicates that some fact or event took place in the previous portion of text.

This can be assumed also by the presence of a presuppositional verb "know" that governs the sentential complement clause in which the giving relation is used.

The second story refers to Jimmy's house as an intensional entity which is however not yet fully in existence:

12. Jimmy wanted a sturdy house because he knew that the bad wolf lived in the woods nearby

The system introduces in this case a set of infons which are computed as sits and are then ascribed to the perspective set up by Jimmy.

2.2. Possession Relations

The presence of a possessor is a property which adds some specificity to the head noun. In particular, it could enable the system to identify a certain object in the world, by the fact of its belonging to a certain possessor. In the text we analysed, the possessor is used frequently to tell different objects included in a set apart, on the basis of the identity of the possessor. In particular, if we consider Segment D. again, where the text introduces a plural reference to house with the possessive pronoun "their", there are two possible inferences:

a. either the text refers collectively to a set of houses with two members;
b. or they are referred to disjointly and there is no set, contrary to the linguistic form used in the text, "their houses".

In fact, if we keep ourselves to the distributive reading induced by the presence of "each" in the previous portion of text, we are led to the conclusion that there should be three separate entities of the class "house" in the world.

However this is not actually what the text does, since we take the subsequent reference to a single house for Jimmy and a plural set for Timmy and Tommy to imply that we should consider the initial set as made up of two subsets. Since the two lazy pigs are always treated as a plural entity which is a set, also their possessions - their little houses - are so treated in the text. Thus, we know that each little pig has built its own little house and that there are three individual entities in the world, but for coherence and cohesion principles, coreference is activated only in relation to a subset of two such entities. This is the reason of the transformation of a set with two members into a single entity, which can be used to corefer to the plural NP "their houses" in Segment B. with the NP "their small house" in Segment C. without any further specification. In turn, this latter NP is coreferred in Segment D. simply as "the house" being the more prominent house locally available or last mentioned due to recency effects.

In the same segment we note then that in order to distinguish the reference to this now singular "house" from the other little house present in the model, the latter is evoked with a possessor's specification, "their brother's house".

To recover the identifier of that entity we let the system infer a property belonging to the class "brother" and search for a fully specified individual - someone who has been given a name - and possesses a house which has been introduced as a single entity. In case every little house were introduced both as set and as single individual there would be no straightforward way to draw the necessary inference. Or at least the inferential process required to recover that individual little house would have been by far more complicated.

In particular, one would have been obliged to compute first the individual entities who possess the property of being "brother"; then, by subtraction, calculate from the possessors' identity - or their names - the single brother the genitive is now indicating. At this point the identity of the little house could be established.

We might regard the procedure by which we reached the conclusion to generalise the description of a set to the description of a single entity as a linguistically driven sloppy reading. There are empirical reasons that drove our decision: if we look at the longest version of the story of the three little pigs, we discover that it justifies our stance. This is the relevant portion of text:

Segment E.

This is the story of three little pigs who went around the world seeking their fortune. Their names were Timmy, flute player, Tommy, violinist, Jimmy, great worker. As they reached a nice wood, they decided to build each a comfortable little house. Timmy didn't like working at all, so he thought to build quickly a straw hut. Soon the little house was ready and Timmy decided then to go and see what his little brothers were doing. At first he met Tommy the violinist. Also he, himself, did not have much wish to toil, so he was building a simple little house with sticks of wood.

Segment F.

Very soon, also the house of wood was ready. Like that of straw, it was not very resistant. But the two little pigs lazy had managed to finish their work in a short time and now they could enjoy themselves freely. While Timmy was playing the flute, Tommy accompanied him with his violin and together they were having a lot of fun.

Segment G.

Then, tired to make merry, they decided to go and see what their little brother was doing. They started walking and soon they reached Jimmy. The clever little pig was building a little house. But since Jimmy was farsighted and did not fear working hard, he built it with bricks and cement.

The story starts by introducing the set of little pigs; then it assigns them names, and establishes thus their individuality. Also the little houses are introduced as sets, again by the use of a distributive quantifier. As the story continues, we see that each little pig builds its own little house separately. The identity of each little house is now preserved only by its specific properties: in particular in Segment F. we see that in order to cospecify each of the two little houses previously introduced in text as single entities, the linguistic form used is "the house of wood", even though this was the house now under discussion. The following sentence, uses a pronoun "it" to corefer to the most recently mentioned little house and a deictic with a property, "that of straw" to corefer to the other singular little house already existing in the model. The specification of some distinctive property is now required simply because in the model there are two entities of the same class "house", both singular in number, i.e. existing as individuals, which are being further specified as "not very resistant". This property, in force of the linguistic form used in the text, is thus distributed over the two single entities.

As the story proceeds, in Segment G. we see that coreference with the little brother (Jimmy) is achieved as in the previous version of the story, by the use of a possessive pronoun. In this case, we might deem that the identity of the individual brother is recovered by subtraction: first, the identity of the possessor is recovered, i.e. an inference is required from the property "brother" to that of their names; then, a singular brother is searched for, whose name does not match with the ones already assigned to the possessor. However, we might also consider the possibility that the use of "brother" here is simply due to the need to assert this property and to extend it to the set of little pigs. In fact, the following sentence makes it clear to the reader that the topic is now set to Jimmy.

An important thing to notice, at this point, is the fact that the introduction of another single entity belonging to the class "house" requires the use of an indefinite NP: another possibility could have been the use of a possessive, "his little house". In both cases, the system understands that it should add a new individual of the class "house" to the model, since Jimmy does not yet own a little house - the first mention to a set of three houses is computed as an intension, or a sit, and not as a fact. However, we take the use of an indefinite NP a much simpler way to achieve the same goal. In this case, the factivity of the proposition in which the NP is used, requires the indefinite NP to be regarded as a new entity, which however is included in the set of the three little houses mentioned at the beginning of the story.

2.3. Proper Names

Differently from what happens with definite or indefinite NPs, notably the fact that both types can be used either extensionally or intensionally to denote some entity, in the case of proper names we know that we are always dealing with rigid designator of the same individual in all possible worlds, as Kripke defined them. A proper name fixes the reference to an individual in that it designates unambiguously that individual for any further reference in the text.

However, the mechanism by which a proper name is used in a text is something that deserves further scrutiny. In our texts, there are at least two ways to associate proper names with individual entities. The first and more canonical method is the one that is represented by a copulative construction, as in,

Segment H.

This is the story of three little pigs who went around the world seeking their fortune. Their names were Timmy, flute player, Tommy, violinist, Jimmy, great worker.

Another method, is the one represented by a predicative adjunct, a vocative, as in,

Segment I.

The oldest one, Jimmy, who was wise, worked hard and built his house with solid bricks and cement. The other two, Timmy and Tommy, who were lazy, settled the matter hastily and built their houses with straw and pieces of wood.

These might be considered as more or less direct methods for name association with a property already existing in the world. A more subtle and indirect way of obtaining the same result is shown in the following example,

Segment J.

The three friends went all outside. As they were walking in the garden, John said to himself "Sara will marry that man", without any resentment. Richard would marry her.

In this latter example, the association is implicitly achieved by the semantic import of the structural organisation of the utterance. A pronoun is used in the subordinate clause to corefer to the property "friends" in the previous text; then, the subordinator indicates coincidence of temporal relation between the main and the subordinate clause. The main clause, in turn makes the pronoun explicit and introduces proper names as prominent characters. The inference we are naturally drawing at this point is that the Subject pronoun "they" and the Subject of the main clause point at the same individual. However since the pronoun corefers with a set of cardinality 3, we are allowed to make further inferences: we assume that also "Sara" is the name of one of the entity denoted by the set of friends. The same applies to the appearance of "Richard" in the following sentence.

How are these assumption and inferences caused: I take the association rule for proper names to be formulated as follows:

Rule for Proper Names Association

Whenever a Proper Name appears in the world, check in the model if there is already some entity associated with that name;

In case the search fails, check whether there is an explicit (direct/indirect) association link with some entity in the current clause;

Else, check whether there is an implicit indirect association link with some entity in the local context.

In other words, we always require Proper Names to be associated with some previously asserted property in the local context. However, narratives show that a proper name could be simply introduced as such, and be a new individual in the world, as for instance in,

13. Mary picked up the phone and called Jason.

or as in,

14. John went into a restaurant.

In these last two example, proper names are used to introduce some new entity in the world and the property assumed is simply a generic class specification derived by default properties rules from selectional restrictions associated to that NP as argument of a given predicate.

Names are used freely in the following text to recover coreference to a given individual. In particular, they may be used in place of a pronoun, when the text would make its use ambiguous. In the first version of the story of the little pigs, names are introduced in the story, however no other mention is needed in the following text to recover the corresponding individuals. This is simply due to the fact that they are well distinguished as being either a set of three little pigs, a set of two little pigs, and a single individual: thus, the use of names becomes redundant.

However, the second version of the same story introduces the three little pigs at first as a set of cardinality three; but as the story progresses, each of the three little pigs is introduced separately by its name. This is possible because previously there has been an explicit association of names to each member of the set of three. At a certain point of the story, it would seem that talking of a single little pig induces ambiguity, however this is not so, as shown by Segment K, which we report here below,

Segment K.

Then, tired to make merry, they decided to go and see what their little brother was doing. They started walking and soon they reached Jimmy. The clever little pig was building a little house. But since Jimmy was farsighted and did not fear working hard, he built it with bricks and cement.

Rather than using the name for the first occurrence of a reference to Jimmy, we see that the text uses "their little brother", which is clearly less individuating as the three little pigs are all brothers: but the use of the possessive makes coreference clear. In the following sentence, we see however that a name is used: is this required or is it redundant? We take the use of the proper name to be not cognitively but textually required, since the use of a common name like "the little pig" would sound unnatural. Also, note that the use of a pronoun is impossible, since "their little brother" has not been established as a current Topic.

3. Inferences and Triggers

In a more schematic way we list here below the most interesting cases of inferential processes performed by the system:

Case 1 - Individual to Set Inference

The three friends went all outdoors.

As they were walking in the garden, John said to himself, "Sara will marry that man", without any resentment.

TRIGGER: Free pronoun "they" coreferent with "friend" a set with cardinality 3 in a fronted subordinate clause temporally coincident with the main.

INFERENCES TO BE DRAWN: Proper nouns introduced in the main clause should cospecify the members of the set of friends

Case 2 - Domain of Point-of-View

Richard would marry Sara.

He felt strongly about that.

TRIGGER: Free pronoun “he” to be coreferred to the subject_of_consciousness rather than to the locally available masculine proper noun “Richard”. The deictic pronoun “that” with clausal reference.

INFERENCE TO BE DRAWN: The first utterance is to be computed as belonging to John’s domain of point_of_view: this would allow the system to continue the same Main Topic which will be made available to the following utterance, thus correctly coreferring “he” to John rather than to Richard.

Discourse deixis is triggered by the presence of an external pronoun with indefinite antecedent: discourse structure will be invoked and a discourse segment will be taken as coreference to “that”.

Case 3 - Domain of Point-of-View

She was the right person for a man like Richard.

For himself he was absurd.

TRIGGER: external pronouns ‘“she”, “he”.

INFERENCES TO BE DRAWN: both pronouns require a search in the Discourse Model from where to recover the antecedent of “she”; as to “he”, the domain of point_of_view is used and the subject_of_consciousness taken as the antecedent to which the pronoun corefers.

Case 4 - Predicate-argument equality match

John gave Mary a rose.

She took it and put it in her hair.

She knew that she had been given a present, something precious.

TRIGGER: external pronoun “she” and the dummy logical predicate “exist” added by the grammar to account for the missing agent of the passive sentence. The search in the Discourse Model is also activated by the indefinite NP "a present" in presence of a governing presuppositional predicate “know”, in addition to tense Pluperfect in which the passive is expressed.

INFERENCES TO BE DRAWN: to recover the complete propositional content of the passive sentence a search in the Discourse Model is performed to look for a similar relation, “give” in a previous portion of text in which the same participant, “Mary” was involved with the same semantic role that of “Patient”. In addition the indefinite NP "a present" is computed as a property cospecifying "a rose" and not as a new property in the DM.

Case 5 - Set to Individuals Inference

When Steve faced them saying: are you enjoying yourselves?.

TRIGGER: the external pronoun “them”.

INFERENCES TO BE DRAWN: in the Discourse Model there must be two fully identified individuals - i.e. which have been assigned proper names - apart from the one currently being nominated which is however obviative with the reference of the pronoun.

They shall have to be built into a set to be used as antecedent of the pronoun “them”. It uses the History List made up of most recent topics.

Case 6 - Domain of Point-of-View

It was horrible! It was shocking!

Not for herself.

TRIGGER: an external pronoun “it” with indefinite reference subject of copulative constructions with evaluative predicates; a logophoric anaphora “herself” which has no local antecedent in the adjacent portion of text.

INFERENCES TO BE DRAWN: the indefinite pronoun “it” should be treated as a case of discourse deixis to be bound to an appropriate discourse segment independently organized by discourse structure. As to the anaphoric “herself” the subject_of_consciousness will be as usual assumed to be the antecedent coreferent with it, in this case, Mary.

Case 7 - Recency Constraint

She felt only hostility and his determination to ruin that wonderful moment.

TRIGGER: the external free pronoun “his”.

INFERENCES TO BE DRAWN: no indication whatsover in the previous portion of text tells us who should be the antecedent for the pronoun, apart from the meaning of the text which however requires in itself quite a lot of understanding. The antecedent is picked out on a recency criterion: the most recent possible antecedent is Steve and there is no other intervening Topics which interfere with this decision. We use the History List again and look for an individual entity which has been fully specified.

Case 8 - Selectional Restrictions Membership Match

Mary picked up the phone and called Jason.

Her husband, she thought, would have considered such a move as untruthful and utterly base.

TRIGGER: the deictic NP “such a move” realized linguistically as an Object semantically dependent on the predication.

INFERENCES TO BE DRAWN: the grammatical nature of the NP is such that it does not allow it to be computed as an independently referring entity, so the previous discourse is searched for. Actually, the semantic class to which the predicate “move” belongs is an Event, this will cause the semantic interpretation to search for an event in the previous DM, and the relation “call” will be taken to be the cospecifying one.

Case 9 - Selectional Restrictions Membership Match and Meaning Postulate

Più tardi fu un ufficiale di successo.
Poi nel 1945 Avveduti si dimise dall'esercito.
I militari lo avevano deluso.
Avveduti, deposta la divisa, si iscrisse all'università.

TRIGGER: singular definite NP "l'esercito" and plural definite NP "i militari".

INFERENCES TO BE DRAWN: the reference to "esercito"/army is recovered in the global context by looking up into the DM for an instance of a domain dependent individual/set/role of the kind "military": in this case "ufficiale" is the role which has been asserted as being an instance of an individual belonging to a "military" class. Selectional restrictions associated to "esercito" include "coll, hum_set" which allow the system to assert the fact of the superset nature of "esercito" if related to "ufficiale". At the same time, the plural definite NP "militari" in the third utterance is also understood as coreferring with "esercito" even though with a different grammatical number. The same applies to "divisa"/uniform in the fourth utterance which is also understood as a metonimic expression, thus included semantically in the meaning of "esercito"/army.

In addition, an important inference is drawn in the second utterance due to the present tense of the achievement verb "dimettere"/resign. In force of the meaning of the main predicate - a meaning postulate - the role "ufficiale" is a property no longer applicable to the individual it was associated with. Thus, there will be a new fact in the DM with polarity set to "0" asserting that the property of possessing the role of "ufficiale" is no longer applicable to the same individual from a given spatiotemporal location.

We give here below the complete semantic representation of the DM:

```
[più tardi fu un ufficiale di successo]
loc(infon113, id23, [arg:main_tloc, arg:più_tardi])
ind(infon114, id24)
ind(infon115, id25)
fact(infon116, inst_of, [ind:id25, class:[ind, abst, soc, state]], 1, univ, univ)
fact(infon117, isa, [ind:id25, class:successo], 1, id23, id14)
fact(infon118, di, [arg:id24, specif:id25], 1, id23, id14)
fact(infon119, role, [ufficiale, id24, id2], 1, id23, id14)
fact(infon120, inst_of, [ind:id24, class:militare], 1, univ, univ)
fact(infon121, isa, [ind:id24, class:ufficiale], 1, id23, id14)
fact(infon122, ufficiale, [nil:id2], 1, id23, id14)
fact(id26, essere, [prop:infon122], 1, tes(f3_avv05), id14)
fact(infon125, isa, [arg:id26, arg:st], 1, tes(f3_avv05), id14)
fact(infon126, isa, [arg:id27, arg:tloc], 1, tes(f3_avv05), id14)
fact(infon127, pass_rem, [arg:id27], 1, tes(f3_avv05), id14)
included(tr(f3_avv05), id23)
contains(tes(f3_avv05), tes(f3_avv03))

[poi nel 1945 avveduti si dimise dallo esercito]
loc(infon136, id28, [arg:main_tloc, arg:id28])
loc(infon137, id29, [arg:main_sloc, arg:esercito])
```

```
set(infon138, id30)
card(infon139, id30, >100)
fact(infon140, inst_of, [ind:id30, class:militare], 1, univ, univ)
fact(infon141, isa, [ind:id30, class:esercito], 1, id28, id29)
in(infon142, id24, id30)
fact(infon143, role, [ufficiale, id24, id2], 0, id28, id29)
fact(id31, dimettere, [actor:id2, actee:id2, locat:id30], 1, tes(f4_avv06), id29)
fact(infon146, isa, [arg:id31, arg:ev], 1, tes(f4_avv06), id29)
fact(infon147, isa, [arg:id32, arg:tloc], 1, tes(f4_avv06), id29)
fact(infon148, pass_rem, [arg:id32], 1, tes(f4_avv06), id29)
fact(infon150, isa, [arg:id33, arg:1945], 1, tes(f4_avv06), id29)
fact(infon151, in, [arg:id31, nil:id33], 1, tes(f4_avv06), id29)
fact(infon152, adj, [temp_seq:id31], 1, id28, id29)
fact(infon153, poi, [prop:infon152], 1, id28, id29)
included(tr(f2_avv06), id28)
after(tes(f4_avv06), tes(f3_avv05))

[i militari lo avevano deluso]
loc(infon163, id34, [arg:main_tloc, arg:tes(f4_avv06)])
fact(id35, deludere, [causer_emot:id30, experiencer:id2], 1, tes(f3_avv07), id29)
fact(infon166, isa, [arg:id35, arg:ev], 1, tes(f3_avv07), id29)
fact(infon167, isa, [arg:id36, arg:tloc], 1, tes(f3_avv07), id29)
fact(infon168, trap_pross, [arg:id36], 1, tes(f3_avv07), id29)
included(tr(f3_avv07), id34)
before(tes(f3_avv07), tes(f4_avv06))

[avveduti, deposta la divisa, si iscrisse alla università]
class(infon173, id37)
fact(infon174, inst_of, [ind:id37, class:cosa], 1, univ, univ)
fact(infon175, isa, [ind:id37, class:divisa], 1, id34, id29)
fact(infon176, part_of, [divisa, id37, id30], 1, id34, id29)
fact(infon178, isa, [arg:id38, arg:università], 1, id34, id29)
fact(id39, iscrivere, [actor:id2, theme_unaff:id2, goal:id38], 1, tes(f3_avv08), id29)
fact(infon179, isa, [arg:id39, arg:ev], 1, tes(f3_avv08), id29)
fact(infon180, isa, [arg:id40, arg:tloc], 1, tes(f3_avv08), id29)
fact(infon181, pass_rem, [arg:id40], 1, tes(f3_avv08), id29)
included(tr(f3_avv08), id34)
after(tes(f3_avv08), tes(f4_avv06))
```

Case 10 - Meaning Postulate

Intanto a Verona aveva conosciuto Paola, figlia di Antonio Alberti, potente senatore democristiano, e la aveva sposata.

......

Gli piaceva parlare del suocero come di una facile occasione mancata che chiunque avrebbe sfruttato ma che lui, Avveduti, preferiva lasciare perdere.

TRIGGER: the singular definite NP "suocero"/father-in-law.

INFERENCES TO BE DRAWN: the head noun is taken together with the pronominal "gli" and two suitable antecedents are searched in the local context, but an inference is required in order to determine the reference of the definite NP. A meaning postulate is used, which is made up of a number of interleaved "facts" to be checked against the DM.

Here below we give the details of the implementation of this particular case of anaphora resolution: it is performed in the Discourse Anaphora module which checks both disjointness and activates an inferential process to look for the entity that satisfies the meaning constraints specified in the call. It is important to notice that in this call the head of the Referential Expression to be matched must correspond to a given linguistic element "father-in-law":

```
resolve_two(StN,RefList,Est1,Ext2,ListOut) :-
    back_state(StN,PrecStN,[continue, cont_analyze, retaining]),
    on(ref_ex(Ext1,father-in-law,_,_,_,_,_,_)/_,RefList),
    find_antecedents(StN, PrecSN,Est1,Ext2, father-in-law, RefList, [main-sec, sec-
      main], ListOut),!.
find_antecedents(StN, PrecStN, SnX, SnY, father-in-law, ListArgs, Types, L4) :-
    on(ref_ex(SnX,T,Ta,P,G,N,C,F/R)/Px, ListaArgs),
    on(ref_ex(SnY,T1,Ta1,P1,G1,N1,C1,F1/R1)/Py, ListArgs),
    check_disjoint(PrecStN, father-in-law, G1, Types, Head1, Head2),
    append([est(SnX,Head1),est(SnY,Head2)],ListArgs,L3),
    modify_head(L3,L4).
check_disjoint(PrecStN, father-in-law, Gen, [main-sec, sec-main], Head1, Head2):-
    fact(_,relat,[daughter,Id,Id1],1,Temp1,Loc1),
    (fact(_,isa, [ind:Id1, class:Head1], 1, Temp, Loc)
    ;
    fact(_,name,[Head1, Id1], 1, _ ,_)),
    fact(_, marry, [agent:Id2, theme_aff:Id],1,_,Loc1),
    (fact(_,isa, [ind:Id2, class:Head2], 1, Temp2, Loc2);
    fact(_,name,[Head2, Id2], 1, _ ,_)),
    (
    main(ref_ex(_,Head1,_,_,_,_,_,_)),
    topic(PrecStN,,secondary,Id2),
    secondary(ref_ex(_,Head2,_,_,Gen,_,_,_))
     ;
    secondary(ref_ex(_,Head1,_,_,_,_,_,_)),
    topic(PrecStN,,main,Id2),
    main(ref_ex(_,Head2,_,_,Gen,_,_,_))
    ),
    check_gender(Gen, Id2),
    Head2 \= Head1, !.
```

In particular, the meaning of the expression father-in-law is made to correspond to a name or property who has a daughter which has associated the constant semantic identifier Id, who is married to an individual entity Id2, who also has a name or property associated in the DM, and either he was a Secondary Topic and the father-in-law's name was asserted as Main Topic in the previous utterance, or the opposite applies. Then gender is checked against the DM, to ensure we are not taking the wrong partner of the marriage, and finally disjointness is checked.

Case 11 - Selectional restrictions membership match

Solo verso il 1950 decise di accettare un posto nella organizzazione della Fiera di Verona.

Lo nominarono delegato cioè una specie di funzionario viaggiante...

Questo era un compito che...

TRIGGER: the empty subject pronoun with plural number. Then the predicative nominal "delegato" and the predicative indefinite nominal "compito".

INFERENCES TO BE DRAWN: there is a collective noun which can be the antecedent even though its grammatical number is singular: this is taken care by the agreement procedure of the anaphora resolution module at discourse level, which sets the number of nouns classified as "institutions" at a selectional restrictions level as plural if needed.

In the same vein is captured the cospecifying relation of the social role "delegato" to the previous "posto" a generic name for an occupation. The same process is at stake with the predicative indefinite NP "un compito", computed as an "activity" at selectional resctrictions lexical level.

Case 12 - Selectional restrictions membership match

Lo confermò nell'incarico alla Fiera.

TRIGGER: the definite NP "incarico".

INFERENCES TO BE DRAWN: this NP is physically removed from the source reference by quite a number of utterances; the DM is searched for and the matching element is again the selectional restriction, "activity" assigned to both "incarico" e "posto" or "delegato" the antecedent to be picked up. In this way an inferential chain is created between "posto" and "delegato", "compito", "collaborazione", "incarico", which are all related to Avveduti's social role.

Case 13 - Implication

L'ex ufficiale del Novara Cavalleria gli era simpatico.

TRIGGER: The presence of a singular definite NP with a prefix modifier "ex", and of a free external pronoun "gli".

INFERENCES TO BE DRAWN: In the case of the pronoun "gli" this is correctly assigned as coreferent to the Main Topic, being the best candidate and the state of the automaton "Continue". However, the definite NP requires a complex chain of inferences: in fact Avveduti was mentioned at the beginning of the story as being an officer, but then as resigning from this activity to become a lawyer. The prefix “ex” is understood by the system as requiring a given property to be no longer applicable to a certain individual: in other word, the property of being an officer should exist in the Model but there should also be an explicit indication that it no longer applies. This is derived by the presence of a second fact about the same role “ufficiale” which is temporally subsequent to the first fact and asserts that the property has polarity “0”, see above for the relevant portion of the DM.

Case 14 - Recency Constraint

Lo confermò nello incarico alla fiera.
Avveduti funzionava benissimo come segretario particolare.
Sapeva mobilitare prefetti e questori.
Tutti gli invidiavano il suo segretario particolare.

TRIGGER: The presence of a free external pronoun “gli” and a definite NP “segretario particolare” which is obviative in reference with the pronominal “gli”.

INFERENCES TO BE DRAWN: There is a singular definite NP “il segretario particolare” which is coreferent with Avveduti, being a property already assigned to him in the previous portion of text and derivable from the DM; thus the pronoun “gli” cannot possibly be referred to the same antecedent. A search is made in the stack of Main Topics to find the most recent one, which is different from the current one, and “Trabucchi” is found, a character already asserted in the DM as being an instance of a “man”: in this way the masculine reference of “gli” is correctly recovered.

4. Reference and General Nouns in Legal Texts

In this section we will refer to General Nouns as they are being used in legal texts, such as the one that can be found in the Appendix of the Introduction. As required in that text, we will focus on human entities, which are addressed both in their social roles and in their general properties. In particular, we want to differentiate generic from defining descriptions or properties; in turn these descriptions, which might be exemplified by “consumer” or “producer” in our case, are roles attached to default properties or general nouns like “person” or “man” which are computed as generic entities. A side effect of the special use of referential expressions in legal texts is their lack of referential content: in other words, legal texts do not refer extensionally to entities in the world but deal with generic entities or with classes of individuals; proper nouns may only refer to institutions and as such they can be treated as collective entities or sets; common nouns may deal with abstract concepts belonging to the vocabulary of law or to concrete individuals or objects which could be found in the world but needn’t do so. Usually, when common nouns are introduced in a directive or bill they are individuated by a specific definition: this is particularly so, when those nouns are the addressee or the main topic to which the norm applies.

The general noun “person” should be referentially empty in legal contexts: consider its lack of gender specification and its inherent generic nature if compared to common nouns related to social roles. It is heavily used to refer either to actual or to potential addressees: in particular, we might be talking about "producers" and "consumer", and then go on talking about "the injured person" or "two or more persons" which can cause damage. In fact, "person" can be used both with modifiers and without them, as a definite NP or as an indefinite one. When it is used as a definite NP, it requires some modifier to be properly coreferred; no bare NPs can be created in association with such a generic head.

While common nouns may refer either to individuals or to classes, singular definite NPs with a generic head cannot be computed as individuals but only as classes and this must be inferred from the modifier or adjunct that specifies it adequately.

Plural definite NPs with generic heads are computed as classes, and can be used to corefer to other singular generic nouns or to specific nouns which they share default properties with.

Differently from what happens in narrative texts, legal texts introduce indefinite NPs not to assert the existence of some individual or set but to refer to classes or to generic entities.

Now consider the problem of general nouns: person, man, individual etc. They constitute the most common and most frequent noun in our texts and this is due to their referential properties: they can pick the maximum set of human entities available when used with no attribute or modifier; they can also be used to corefer to single classes of individuals by adequate modification. In other words, the concept "person" will be present at different levels of generality in the DM and it will be instantiated with a different semantic identifier according to its "dattrs" (see Woods and Brachman). Reference to one or the other of the instantiations of "person" will depend upon the way in which the discourse entity is described, in other terms on its "dattrs", i.e. attributes, properties, parts, constituents, features, relations and so on. Notice that in our DM every entity has a description in terms of situation semantics, with a polarity and a spatiotemporal anchorage in terms of indices for main spatial and main temporal location.

Let's now go back to general nouns: in any text, "person" should be introduced effectively only whenever a number of possible specific entities which might be subsumed by "person" already exist in the DM. In the texts we analyzed, this is what happens: in particular, the Council Directive we used and implemented which is discussed in more detail at the end of this paper, has the following textual structure:

1. introduce main topics and addressee of its contents, which are "producers" and "consumers" living in the "Member States"; the directive concerns the protection of consumes and the producers' liability in relation to injury or damage which might result from defective products. Importers of products who present themselves as producers are also regarded as such.
2. subsequently, both main topics are coreferred by means of the general noun "person".

On first appearance of common nouns which might be subsumed by "person", the system checks whether there is any such entity in the DM: in the affirmative case it simply inherits its identifier and in the negative case, a generic entity is asserted in the DM. This entity is not an individual nor a set but has the following properties:

- it may subsume other generic entities of the same kind;

- it may be used to infer the nature of references to individuals by means of "person" and some specific attribute or property.

In particular, in the following text we find "several persons liable" and "injured person". The first referring expression is computed as "producer" and the second one as "consumer". In order to get this interpretation, which is the one intended in the Directive, an inferential process must be carried out on the basis of external knowledge of the world. However, the trigger to start this process is constituted by the attribute "injured" which is computed in the property checker algorithm as a possible new property to be associated to some entity already existing in the DM. The search starts from a referring expression that has some attribute or modifier which is a property not yet asserted for the corresponding entity. Consider the case of "injured person": by looking into the DM the algorithm recovers the identifier associated to "consumer" on the basis of the inference that he is a "person" which is expressed in the following list of facts:

```
class(_, Id)
class(_, Ind)
fact(_, isa, [_:Ind, class:person], 1, _, _)
fact(_, ist_of, [_:Ind, class:man], 1, _, _)
fact(_, role, [consumer, Id, Ind], 1, _, _)
fact(_, isa, [_:Id, class:consumer], 1, _, _)
in(_, Id, Ind)
```

When the Id of "consumer" is recovered from the DM by the property checker that looks for correspondences between literal predicates and their relations in the DM, the "injured" attribute and the Id is passed on to the following inference engine that collects knowledge of the world associated to the trigger and checks to see whether it applies to the current identifier and its properties in the DM.

```
infer_process(Trigger, Id):-
  infer_trig(Trigger, Props),
  infer_rels(Id, Props).
```

This is done by means of an inferential process that takes as input external knowledge of the world – WordNet, but also manually added synsets -, where we deposit information related to implicit knowledge, mutual knowledge and specialized information which could be part of a T-box component in a knowledge base understanding system. In those inheritance networks (see Woods, 1978), each concept that the system understands is represented in a network of concepts, which have to cope with the problem of internal recursion - i.e. of a concept defined in terms of another concept. Our taxonomy for this domain is constituted by a small list of facts which might be regarded on a par with an axiom made up of a certain number of logical implications and the portion that interests us now is represented as follows:

```
infer_trig(injured, [cause(damage, 0) & has(protection, 1) & liable(Id, 0)]).
infer_trig(liable, [cause(damage, 1) & has(liability, 1)]).
```

Each term is made up of a trigger, "injured", "liable" which are the properties by means of which the general noun "person" is modified; in turn each trigger is associated with a set of relations and properties which have as argument either a class predicate and a polarity, or a variable and a polarity.

In the text, we learn that "injured person" is only used to corefer to "consumer"; we also know that in order to be interpreted as "injured" a person has not to have caused the damage, nor to be "liable" for it, and finally be the one that is given "protection". By definition, then, a person is liable in case "he caused damage" and in case " he has liability".

```
infer_rels(Id, [Prop(Id, 1)|Props]):-
    fact(_,Prop, [_:Id], 1, _, _),
    infer_rels(Id, Props)
;
infer_rels(Id, [Prop(Id, 0)|Props]):-
    (not fact(_,liable, [_:Id], 1, _, _))
    ;
fact(_,liable, [_:Id], 0, _, _)))
    infer_rels(Id, Props)
    ;
infer_rels(Id, [Rel(Prop, 1)|Props]):-
    fact(_, Rel, [_:Idx, _:Id], 1, _, _),
    fact(_, isa, [_:Id, class:Prop], 1, _, _)
    infer_rels(Id, Props)
    ;
infer_rels(Id, [Rel(Prop, 0)|Props]):-
    fact(_, Rel, [_:Idx, _:Id], 0, _, _),
    fact(_, isa, [_:Id, class:Prop], 1, _, _) ).
```

5. The Basic Algorithm

In our system, the problem of assigning properties to entities in narrative genre is carried out in two main phases: first only referring expressions (ref_exs) asserted as best candidates for topichood and ranked as Main, Secondary, Expected or Potential Topics by the Topic Hierarchy Mechanism are considered. This might or might not apply to legal genre, on the basis of the assumption that there is no plot nor main character to focus on. However, legal texts contain pronominals which refer in the previous discourse segment and cannot be done away with. In case no such coreferent is found, the remaining DM is searched for. Generally speaking, there are four possible ways in which the problem might be solved:

Case A-there is already at least one such entity in the Discourse Model (DM) with the same class restrictions which could be used to corefer or cospecify the current ref_ex disregarding its possible contextually determined properties and considering only the Initial Description (ID);

Case B-the entity to be picked up as possible coreferent or cospecifier must be semantically equal: i.e. we consider number of the current ref_ex and if plural, check whether the entity has the same cardinality or is asserted as a class; and if singular look only for individuals;

Case C-the entity and the ref_ex must have the same attributes, roles or other properties assigned to it in the DM and present in the current ref-_ex;

Case D-works as case C and in addition it looks only for properties associated to entities asserted as Topics of discourse in the previous text; in case no such property is present, a new entity is entered in the DM;

It is easy to notice that, case D is the most restrictive but also the most genre bound procedure: in fact, it is only useful in case the text is a narrative one.

The first question is discovering whether the current ref_ex is already present in the DM, i.e. if it has already been explicitely mentioned. If the problem at hand were that of matching the current linguistic form of the predicate or concept with those present in the DM this would be easily solved. However this procedure is clearly insufficient and leads to mistaken matches in case cardinality, definiteness, or simply the modifiers of the current linguistic use of a certain entity present in the DM does not coincide semantically with it.

The overall framework is further complicated by the presence of generic entities and by the fact that what we are dealing with are usually entities which might be easily subsumed by them or constitute a specific subclass. A "consumer" or a "producer" is clearly such a subclass in case the general noun "person" has already been introduced in the DM. However, problems will arise when the contrary applies, i.e. whenever a general noun is introduced with specific properties added by adjunction or modification: in this case it would both represent a subclass of a generic entity and a coreferent of a some class of individual or role.

The general problem to be solved might be coped with by the following algorithm:

1. find all semantic identifiers associated in the DM with the predicate of the current referring expression starting from the most recent ones in the stack of ids' associated with some previous topic;
   1.i. search all ids' starting from the most recent one and make a list;
   1.ii. then for each id, look whether the current predicate head is associated to some property in the DM;
      a.1. no identifier associated with the head, goto 2.
      a.2. there is at least one identifier associated with the head;
   b. verify whether the set of adjuncts, modifiers and other property functional assigners, MODS associated to the current head is empty or not
      b.1. if it is empty, goto f.;
      b.2. if it is nonempty, find all predicate heads associated to MODS;
   c. search the DM for properties associated to the predicate head other than the head itself and the default properties;
      c.1. if no property is found in the DM goto f.;
      c.2. if the list of properties in the DM is nonempty:
   d. make the intersection between the two sets of properties: set1 from MODS, set2 from DM;
      d.1. if the intersection is empty goto e.;

d.2. f the intersection is nonempty and the property/ies found is/are equal to the one/s contained in set1 then fail;

d.3. else continue.

e. check in the external knowledge of the world whether the two sets contain properties which are synonymous or which are inferentially derivable from other properties;

e.1. if there are some such properties, remove them from the list;

e.2. if not continue;

f. check whether the two sets of properties are nonempty; then, check number, and if plural check cardinality and then

f.1. if it is the same, assert the set of properties in MODS;

i. a singular is compatible with inds;

ii. a plural is compatible with sets and classes

•in legal genre, a singular is compatible both with singular and with classes!!

f.2. if it is different fail;

g. search for other ids associated to the current head;

g.1. if no other id is present goto end;

g.2. if some other id is present goto b.

2. find all semantic identifiers associated in the discourse model (DM) with the predicate of the current referring expression which are not included in the list of the topic identifiers;

2.i. if it is empty, goto 3.

2.ii. if it is nonempty goto b.

3. find all semantic identifiers associated in the External Knowledge Base with the predicate of the current referring expression;

3.i. if it is empty, goto end.

3.ii. if it is nonempty goto b.

end.

6. DM and Inferences: Some Examples

We will show here below the DM relatively only to three entities: consumer, producer and their general noun "person" subsuming both. In utterance 4 with first appearance of "consumer and producer" the system generates a generic entity "person" which subsumes both: the inclusion relation is registered by the fact in(_, A, B) where A is the semantic identifier or initial description of the superset or superobject, and B is the subsumed entity:

[Whereas approximation of the laws of the 'Member' 'States' concerning the liability of the producer for damage caused by the defectiveness of his products is necessary, because the existing divergences may entail a differing degree of protection of the consumer, against damage caused by a defective product to his health or property.]

ent(infon102, id22)

fact(infon103, isa, [arg:id22, class:person], 1, univ, univ)

class(infon104, id23)

```
class(infon105, id24)
fact(infon106, cause, [causer:id5, arg:id24], 1, univ, univ)
fact(infon107, inst_of, [ind:id24, class:abstract_state], 1, univ, univ)
fact(infon108, isa, [ind:id24, class:damage], 1, univ, univ)
fact(infon109, against, [arg:id23, malefactive:id24], 1, univ, univ)
fact(infon110, inst_of, [ind:id23, class:man], 1, univ, univ)
fact(infon111, isa, [ind:id23, class:consumer], 1, univ, univ)
in(infon112, id23, id22)
fact(infon113, role, [consumer, id23, id22], 1, univ, univ)
fact(infon114, cause, [arg:id4, damage:id24], 1, univ, univ)
class(infon115, id25)
fact(infon116, inst_of, [ind:id25, class:man], 1, univ, univ)
fact(infon117, isa, [ind:id25, class:producer], 1, univ, univ)
in(infon118, id25, id22)
fact(infon119, role, [producer, id25, id22], 1, univ, univ)
class(infon133, id29)
fact(infon134, differing, [ind:id29], 1, univ, univ)
class(infon135, id30)
fact(infon136, has, [experiencer:id23, arg:id30], 1, univ, univ)
fact(infon137, inst_of, [ind:id30, class:abstract_state], 1, univ, univ)
fact(infon138, isa, [ind:id30, class:protection], 1, univ, univ)
fact(infon139, of, [arg:id29, specif:id30], 1, univ, univ)
fact(infon140, inst_of, [ind:id29, class:[measure]], 1, univ, univ)
fact(infon141, isa, [ind:id29, class:degree], 1, univ, univ)
```

In utterance 6 we learn that the producer should be made liable at certain conditions, and this is registered as an additional fact about producers:

[Whereas protection of the consumer requires that all the producers involved in the production process should be made liable in so far as their finished product, component part or any raw material supplied by them was defective.]

```
fact(infon248, liable, [nil:id25], 1, univ, univ)
```

In utterance 8 the text introduces an undefined set of "several persons" which are liable for a certain damage and are related to protection of the consumer in the same context. The system assigns to "injured person" the same identifier as the consumer, creates a new class of entities "person" which are liable and cause "damage", included in the same superset of producers:

[Whereas, in situations where several persons are liable for the same damage the protection of the consumer requires that the injured person should be able to claim full compensation from any one of them.]

```
fact(infon323, injured, [ind:id23], 1, univ, univ)
class(infon324, id73)
fact(infon325, full, [ind:id73], 1, univ, univ)
fact(infon326, inst_of, [ind:id73, class:legal], 1, univ, univ)
```

fact(infon327, isa, [ind:id73, class:compensation], 1, univ, univ)
fact(infon328, cause, [arg:id25, damage:id24], 1, univ, univ)
class(infon329, id74)
fact(infon330, liable, [nil:id74], 1, univ, univ)
fact(infon331, cause, [arg:id74, damage:id24], 1, univ, univ)
in(infon332, id25, id74)
fact(infon333, inst_of, [ind:id74, class:man], 1, univ, univ)
fact(infon334, isa, [ind:id74, class:person], 1, univ, univ)
class(infon335, id75)
fact(infon336, inst_of, [ind:id75, class:abstract_state], 1, univ, univ)
fact(infon337, isa, [ind:id75, class:situation], 1, univ, univ)
fact(id76, claim, [experiencer:id74, theme_aff:id73, source:id74], 1, tes(finf1_aq4), univ)

In utterance 10 liability for damage is charged on the producer: the system looks for a similar predication in the knowledge base and finds the one related to infon248, which was asserted in utterance 6 above:

[The producer shall be liable for damage caused by a defect in his product.]
fact(infon382, cause, [arg:id25, damage:id24], 1, univ, univ)
class(infon383, id84)
fact(infon384, in, [arg:id84, locative:id5], 1, univ, univ)
fact(infon385, inst_of, [ind:id84, class:legal], 1, univ, univ)
fact(infon386, isa, [ind:id84, class:defect], 1, univ, univ)
fact(infon387, cause, [causer:id84, arg:id24], 1, univ, univ)
fact(id85, be, [prop:infon248], 1, tes(f3_dd07), univ)

In utterance 11 we find "the injured person" again, and the system picks up id23 associated to consumer. Notice the computation of the meaning for "relationship" which has "causal" as modifier: the system understands it as a relation and finds infon387 which is associated to a fact in the knowledge base asserted in the previous utterance and saying that there is a "cause" relation between "defect" and "damage". This was expressed in terms of semantic roles, i.e. the defect is interpreted as a "causer" and its argument is id24, the "damage". In the new utterance, this is linguistically formulated in terms of "relationship", where there is a semantic marker "between" which expresses a relation, and the relation has two arguments:

[The injured person shall be required to prove the damage, the defect and the causal relationship between defect and damage.]
ind(infon423, id95)
class(infon424, id96)
fact(infon425, inst_of, [ind:id96, class:abstract_state], 1, univ, univ)
fact(infon426, isa, [ind:id96, class:defect_damage], 1, univ, univ)
fact(infon427, between, [arg:id95, relation:id96], 1, univ, univ)
fact(infon428, cause, [arg:id95, relation:infon387], 1, univ, univ)
fact(infon429, inst_of, [ind:id95, class:abstract_state], 1, univ, univ)
fact(infon430, isa, [ind:id95, class:relationship], 1, univ, univ)

fact(infon433, [defect, damage, relationship], [arg:id97], 1, univ, univ)
fact(id98, prove, [actor:id23, prop:infon433], 1, tes(finf1_dd07), univ)
fact(id100, require, [actor:id23, prop:id98], 1, tes(f4_dd07), univ)

In utterance 12 the same predication is present, "be liable" and the same infon248 is picked up:

[Where, as a result of the provisions of this directive, two or more persons are liable for the same damage.]
fact(id104, be, [prop:infon248], 1, tes(f49_dd08), univ)

In utterance 13 a pronoun is introduced intersententially to corefer to the same persons, associated to the class of producers:

[They shall be liable jointly and severally, without prejudice to the provisions of national law concerning the rights of contribution or recourse.]
fact(id109, be, [prop:infon248], 1, tes(f3_dd10), univ)

In utterance 14, we find a reference to the superset of persons, the one introduced as generic entity, since the system does not find any hint in the utterance by means of which "a person" could be interpreted as belonging either to the class of consumers or to the class of producers:

[A product is defective when it does not provide the safety which a person is entitled to expect, taking all circumstances into account.]
fact(id116, expect, [experiencer:id22, theme_unaff:id111], 1, tes(finf1_dd10), univ)
fact(id118, entitle, [theme:id22, prop:id116], 1, tes(f6_dd10), univ)

Finally, in utterance 17, a new set of "person" is introduced which "imports a product" and according to the interpretation assigned by the utterance to this set it is included in the superset of the class of producers:

[Without prejudice to the liability of the producer any person who imports into the community a product for sale, hire or any form of distribution in the course of his business, shall be deemed to be a producer within the meaning of this directive.]
class(infon631, id132)
in(infon633, id25, id132)
fact(infon634, inst_of, [ind:id132, class:man], 1, univ, univ)
fact(infon635, isa, [ind:id132, class:person], 1, univ, univ)
fact(id138, import, [agent:id132, theme_aff:id7], 1, tes(f3_dd17), univ)

6.1. Spatiotemporal Locations, Scenario and Inferential Processes

As already mentioned above, some inferential process is triggered by a definite singular NP which causes the system to activate a search in the external knowledge of the world available in WordNet. This search determines the conditions for a scenario effect or a meronimic part_of relation or other such semantic inferential processes. In particular, the description of these relation is assumed to be very simple and straightforward. If we refer back to the "Restaurant" text presented in the previous chapter we may well notice the scenario effect. What really matters is the way in which the system computes the meronymy inclusion relations that we list here below:

Meronymy Relations
included(door,house).
included(window,house).
included(corner,restaurant).

Social Role Meronymy
included(waiter,restaurant).
included(menu,restaurant).

As to the first two inclusion relations, they are used to introduce a part_of relation, as the texts of the three little pigs commented further on will show. The remaining three inclusion relations are taken by the system as a restriction on the spatial location of the singular definite NP. Then in case it is classified as a social role, a further inference causes the semantic module to assert a property which is a role in that location, or scenery. To better exemplify the behaviour of the system we report again here below the complete updating of the DM, utterance by utterance as well as the final hierarchical reordering of all properties and relations on the basis of the entities they belong to.

```
r01.obj [john, went, into, a, restaurant]
loc(infon4, id1, [arg:main_sloc, arg:restaurant])
ind(infon5, id2)
fact(infon6, inst_of, [ind:id2, class:man], 1, univ, univ)
fact(infon7, name, [john, id2], 1, univ, univ)
fact(infon8, inst_of, [ind:id1, class:place], 1, univ, univ)
fact(infon9, isa, [ind:id1, class:restaurant], 1, univ, id1)
fact(id3, go, [agente:id2, locat:id1], 1, tes(restaur_1), id1)
fact(infon12, isa, [arg:id3, arg:ev], 1, tes(restaur_1), id1)
fact(infon13, isa, [arg:id4, arg:tloc], 1, tes(restaur_1), id1)
fact(infon14, pres, [arg:id4], 1, tes(restaur_1), id1)
fact(infon15, time, [arg:id3, arg:id4], 1, tes(restaur_1), id1)
undef(tes(restaur_1), tes(f1_r01))
after(tes(restaur_1), tes(f1_r01))

r02.obj [there, was, a, table, in, the, corner]
ind(infon20, id6)
fact(infon21, inst_of, [ind:id6, class:place], 1, univ, univ)
fact(infon22, isa, [ind:id6, class:table], 1, id5, id1)
in(infon23, id6, id1)
fact(id7, sit, [actor:id2, locat:id6], 1, tes(f1_id7), id1)
```

```
fact(infon24, isa, [arg:id7, arg:ev], 1, tes(f1_id7), id1)
fact(infon25, isa, [arg:id8, arg:tloc], 1, tes(f1_id7), id1)
fact(infon26, isa, [arg:id8], 1, tes(f1_id7), id1)
ind(infon27, id9)
fact(infon28, inst_of, [ind:id9, class:place], 1, univ, univ)
fact(infon29, isa, [ind:id9, class:corner], 1, id5, id1)
fact(infon30, part_of, [restaurant, id9, id1], 1, id5, id1)
fact(infon31, isa, [arg:id10, arg:vbl], 1, id5, id1)
fact(infon32, has, [nil:id10], 1, id5, id1)
fact(id11, there_be, [prop:id6], 1, tes(restaur_2), id1)
fact(infon34, isa, [arg:id11, arg:st], 1, tes(restaur_2), id1)
fact(infon35, isa, [arg:id12, arg:tloc], 1, tes(restaur_2), id1)
fact(infon36, pres, [arg:id12], 1, tes(restaur_2), id1)
fact(infon37, time, [arg:id11, arg:id12], 1, tes(restaur_2), id1)
includes(tr(restaur_2), id1)
during(tes(restaur_2), tes(f1_r01))

r03.obj [the, waiter, took, the, order]
ind(infon44, id13)
fact(infon45, inst_of, [ind:id13, class:social_role], 1, univ, univ)
fact(infon46, isa, [ind:id13, class:waiter], 1, id5, id1)
fact(infon47, role, [waiter, id1, id13], 1, id5, id1)
fact(infon49, isa, [arg:id14, arg:exist], 1, id5, id1)
fact(id15, take_order, [agente:id13, goal:id14], 1, tes(restaur_3), id1)
fact(infon50, isa, [arg:id15, arg:pr], 1, tes(restaur_3), id1)
fact(infon51, isa, [arg:id16, arg:tloc], 1, tes(restaur_3), id1)
fact(infon52, pres, [arg:id16], 1, tes(restaur_3), id1)
fact(infon53, time, [arg:id15, arg:id16], 1, tes(restaur_3), id1)
includes(tr(restaur_3), id1)
after(tes(restaur_3), tes(f1_r01))

r04.obj [the, atmosphere, was, warm, and, friendly]
ind(infon57, id17)
fact(infon58, atmosphere, [ind:id17], 1, id5, id1)
fact(infon59, inst_of, [ind:id17, class:substance], 1, univ, univ)
fact(infon60, isa, [ind:id17, class:atmosphere], 1, id5, id1)
fact(infon63, isa, [arg:id18, arg:warm], 1, id5, id1)
fact(infon65, isa, [arg:id19, arg:friendly], 1, id5, id1)
in(infon76, id18, id20)
in(infon77, id19, id20)
fact(id21, be, [tema_bound:id17, tema_bound:id20], 1, tes(restaur_4), id1)
fact(infon66, isa, [arg:id21, arg:st], 1, tes(restaur_4), id1)
fact(infon67, isa, [arg:id22, arg:tloc], 1, tes(restaur_4), id1)
fact(infon68, pres, [arg:id22], 1, tes(restaur_4), id1)
fact(infon69, time, [arg:id21, arg:id22], 1, tes(restaur_4), id1)
includes(tr(restaur_4), id1)
```

during(tes(restaur_4), tes(f1_r01))
r05.obj [he, began, to, read, his, book]
fact(infon79, poss, [john, id2, id23], 1, id5, id1)
ind(infon80, id23)
fact(infon81, inst_of, [ind:id23, class:thing], 1, univ, univ)
fact(infon82, isa, [ind:id23, class:book], 1, id5, id1)
fact(id24, read, [agente:id2, actor:id23], 1, tes(finf1_restaur_5), id1)
fact(infon86, isa, [arg:id24, arg:ev], 1, tes(finf1_restaur_5), id1)
fact(infon87, isa, [arg:id25, arg:tloc], 1, tes(finf1_restaur_5), id1)
fact(infon88, pres, [arg:id25], 1, tes(finf1_restaur_5), id1)
fact(infon89, time, [arg:id24, arg:id25], 1, tes(finf1_restaur_5), id1)
fact(id26, begin, [actor:id2, prop:id24], 1, tes(restaur_5), id1)
fact(infon90, isa, [arg:id26, arg:ev], 1, tes(restaur_5), id1)
fact(infon91, isa, [arg:id27, arg:tloc], 1, tes(restaur_5), id1)
fact(infon92, past, [arg:id27], 1, tes(restaur_5), id1)
fact(infon93, time, [arg:id26, arg:id27], 1, tes(restaur_5), id1)
includes(tr(restaur_5), id1)
after(tes(restaur_5), tes(f1_r01))

Entities of the World

INDIVIDUAL: id3 RELEVANCE SCORE: 14
ind(infon5, id3)
fact(infon6, inst_of, [ind:id3, class:man], 1, univ, univ)
fact(infon7, name, [john, id3], 1, univ, univ)
fact(id4, go, [agent:id3, locat:id2], 1, tes(f5_r01), id2)
fact(infon77, poss, [arg:id19, poss:id3], 1, id15, id2)
fact(id20, read, [agent:id3, theme_aff:id19], 1, tes(finf1_free_a1), id2)
fact(id22, begin, [agent:id3, prop:id20], 1, tes(f3_free_a1), id2)

INDIVIDUAL: id11 RELEVANCE SCORE: 6
ind(infon42, id11)
fact(infon43, inst_of, [ind:id11, class:[social_role]], 1, univ, univ)
fact(infon44, isa, [ind:id11, class:waiter], 1, id1, id2)
fact(id13, take, [agent:id11, theme_aff:id12], 1, tes(f5_r03), id2)

INDIVIDUAL: id6 RELEVANCE SCORE: 2
ind(infon21, id6)
fact(infon25, in, [arg:id6, locativo:id7], 1, id1, id2)
fact(infon26, isa, [ind:id6, class:table], 1, id1, id2)
fact(infon27, inst_of, [ind:id6, class:thing], 1, univ, univ)
fact(infon30, in, [arg:id6, locat:id8], 1, id1, id2)
fact(id9, there_be, [theme_unaff:id6], 1, tes(f4_free_r02), id2)

INDIVIDUAL: id7 RELEVANCE SCORE: 0
ind(infon22, id7)
fact(infon23, inst_of, [ind:id7, class:thing], 1, univ, univ)

fact(infon24, isa, [ind:id7, class:corner], 1, id1, id2)
fact(infon25, in, [arg:id6, locativo:id7], 1, id1, id2)

7. The Stories

We shall now discuss in more detail what the Interpreter does in each utterance of the texts analyzed. However we shall not include information from the DM which is irrelevant to the problem we are now tackling: in particular, we shall not comment on DM representations related to utterance which do not add any new entity to the model nor do require any special inferential process to be understood. In each story we have divided up relations from entities, in turn relations may show up as either fact, sit(uation), and conc(ept). Locations are used by the semantic interpreter to assign the Main Spatial Location Index to each term. Time intervals are used to assign the Main Temporal Location index. Facts and sits characterize objects or entities in the model.

7.1. Story 1

[ci erano una volta tre fratelli porcellini che vivevano felici nella campagna]
loc(infon3, id1, [arg:main_tloc, arg:volta])
loc(infon4, id2, [arg:main_sloc, arg:campagna])
set(infon5, id3)
card(infon6, id3, 3)
fact(infon7, fratello, [ind:id3], 1, id1, id2)
fact(infon8, isa, [ind:id3, class:porcellino], 1, id1, id2)
fact(infon9, inst_of, [ind:id3, class:animale_cibo], 1, univ, univ)
fact(infon13, isa, [arg:id2, arg:campagna], 1, id1, id2)
fact(id4, vivere, [actor:id3, locat:id2], 1, tes(f6_po1), id2)
fact(infon18, felice, [arg:id4], 1, tes(f6_po1), id2)
fact(id6, esserci, [theme_unaff:id3], 1, tes(f7_po1), id2)
fact(infon23, isa, [arg:id1, arg:volta], 1, tes(f7_po1), id2)
fact(infon24, nil, [arg:id6, non_punct:id1], 1, tes(f7_po1), id2)

In the first utterance we have a set of three little pigs and a property "fratello"/brother which are asserted as facts, two main relations "essere"/be and "vivere"/live which are also facts and a number of sits associated to these facts. All the entities have positive polarity and are located in space and time.

[nello stesso luogo però viveva anche un terribile lupo che si nutriva proprio di porcellini grassi e teneri]
loc(infon36, id8, [arg:main_tloc, arg:tes(f7_po1)])
ind(infon37, id9)
fact(infon38, terribile, [ind:id9], 1, id8, id2)
fact(infon39, isa, [ind:id9, class:lupo], 1, id8, id2)

fact(infon40, inst_of, [ind:id9, class:animale_feroce], 1, univ, univ)
class(infon41, id10)
fact(infon42, grasso, [ind:id10], 1, id8, id2)
fact(infon43, tenero, [ind:id10], 1, id8, id2)
in(infon44, id3, id10)
fact(infon45, inst_of, [ind:id10, class:animale_cibo], 1, univ, univ)
fact(infon46, isa, [ind:id10, class:porcellino], 1, id8, id2)
fact(id11, nutrire, [experiencer:id9, theme_unaff:id9, cibo:id10], 1, tes(f5_po2), id2)
fact(infon48, isa, [arg:id13, arg:luogo], 1, id8, id2)
fact(id14, vivere, [actor:id9, locat:id13], 1, tes(f6_po2), id2)
fact(infon53, pero_, [arg:id14], 1, tes(f6_po2), id2)
fact(infon54, anche, [arg:id14], 1, tes(f6_po2), id2)

In the second utterance the spatial location remains the same because the locative adjunct is constructed with a deictic "stesso"/same; the main temporal location also has the same index. The model is updated with a new individual, the wolf. The relations show how the static interpreter computes the argument "porcellini" for the predicate "nutrire". This is taken as a sit owing to the fact that it is a plural naked NP, in other words, an intensional object. This NP will be exploited for inferring the meaning of a metaphor, "pasto"/meal, as corresponding to little pigs, being the meal of the wolf.

[questi allora, per proteggersi dal lupo, decisero di costruirsi ciascuno una casetta]
set(infon79, id16)
card(infon80, id16, 3)
fact(infon81, piccolo, [ind:id16], 1, id8, id2)
sit(infon82, isa, [ind:id16, class:casa], 1, id8, id2)
fact(infon83, inst_of, [ind:id16, class:cosa], 1, univ, univ)
sit(id17, costruire_si, [agent:id3, theme_eff:id16], 1, tes(finf4_po3), id2)
fact(id19, decidere, [actor:id3, prop:id17], 1, tes(f5_po3), id2)
fact(infon97, allora, [arg:id19], 1, tes(f5_po3), id2)
fact(id21, proteggere, [agente:id3, esperiente:id3, malef:id9], 1, tes(finf1_po3), id2)
fact(infon103, per, [arg:id19, purpose:id21], 1, tes(f5_po3), id2)

When we get to third utterance a deictic pronoun is used to indicate the persistence of the same individual in the discourse; there is an indefinite NP which is computed as a set of sits by means of quantifier scoping detected in logical form, and owing to the fact that the NP is itself contained in a proposition which is computed as a sit, not a fact, with the relation "costruire". The cardinality of the set of houses is derived from the abstract possessor built in the NP via the benefactive enclitic "si", and the scope assignment wrought on it by the floating quantifier "ciascuno"/each. This in turn is computed in f-structure as an open adjunct which is controlled by the subject NP "questi"/these, a deictic whose resolvant is the set of three little pigs already present in the model.

[il maggiore, jimmi, che era saggio, lavorava di buona lena e costruì la sua casetta con solidi mattoni e cemento]
loc(infon128, id23, [arg:main_tloc, arg:tes(f8_po4)])

```
ind(infon129, id24)
fact(infon130, name, [jimmi, id24], 1, id23, id2)
fact(infon131, saggio, [nil:id24], 1, id23, id2)
in(infon132, id24, id3)
ind(infon133, id25)
in(infon134, id25, id16)
fact(infon135, isa, [ind:id25, class:casa], 1, id23, id2)
fact(infon136, poss, [jimmi, id24, id25], 1, id23, id2)
fact(infon137, isa, [ind:id25, class:mattone], 1, id23, id2)
fact(infon138, isa, [ind:id25, class:cemento], 1, id23, id2)
fact(id26, lavorare, [agent:id24], 1, tes(f6_po4), id2)
fact(infon145, isa, [arg:id28, arg:lena], 1, tes(f6_po4), id2)
fact(infon146, di, [arg:id26, nil:id28], 1, tes(f6_po4), id2)
fact(id30, costruire, [agent:id24, theme_eff:id25], 1, tes(f8_po4), id2)
fact(infon156, [cemento, mattone], [arg:id29], 1, tes(f8_po4), id2)
fact(infon157, con, [arg:id30, nil:id25, prop:infon156], 1, tes(f8_po4), id2)
```

At this point, a name is associated to the elder of the three little pigs and other properties are predicated. We also know he is the possessor of a house made of bricks and cement, both universally located properties of the house. However, the house is now introduced as a definite NP and not as an indefinite NP owing to the fact that the discourse strategy already presented a set of houses, as a sit in the previous portion of text: thus a sit has now supported a fact, the two houses being now computed as a subset of the previous set made up of three members.

```
[gli altri , timmy e tommy, pigri e oziosi se la sbrigarono in fretta costruendo le loro
    casette con la paglia e con pezzetti di legno]
set(infon171, id32)
card(infon172, id32, 2)
ind(infon173, id33)
in(infon174, id33, id32)
fact(infon175, name, [timmy, id33], 1, id23, id2)
ind(infon176, id34)
in(infon177, id34, id32)
fact(infon178, name, [tommy, id34], 1, univ, univ)
in(infon179, id32, id3)
fact(infon180, ozioso, [ind:id32], 1, id23, id2)
fact(infon181, pigro, [ind:id32], 1, id23, id2)
fact(infon182, poss, [porcellino, id32, id35], 1, id23, id2)
set(infon183, id35)
card(infon184, id35, 2)
fact(infon185, piccolo, [ind:id35], 1, id23, id2)
fact(infon186, isa, [ind:id35, class:paglia], 1, id23, id2)
fact(infon187, isa, [ind:id35, class:legno], 1, id23, id2)
in(infon188, id35, id16)
fact(infon189, isa, [ind:id35, class:casa], 1, id23, id2)
```

fact(infon190, isa, [arg:id36, arg:fretta], 1, id23, id2)
fact(id37, sbrigarsi, [agent:id32, modal:id36], 1, tes(f5_po5), id2)
fact(infon197, [legno, paglia], [arg:id39], 1, tes(f5_po5), id2)
fact(id40, costruire, [agent:id32, theme_eff:id35], 1, tes(fgerund1047_po5), id2)
fact(infon203, [legno, paglia], [arg:id39], 1, tes(fgerund1047_po5), id2)
fact(infon204, con, [arg:id40, nil:id35, prop:infon203], 1, tes(fgerund1047_po5), id2)
fact(infon205, coincide, [arg:id37, arg:id40], 1, tes(f5_po5), id2)

In this utterance, the subset of two little pigs is coreferred by a nominal substitute, "gli altri"/the others, which we must compute as two in number, and names are associated to these two little pigs. They are assigned evaluative properties, and they are individuated as possessors of two little houses, which however are introduced as previously happened, with a possessive and no cardinality. The possessor relation is built accordingly on the subset of two houses by accessing one of the most recent properties being assigned to the set of possessors, which in this case is "ozioso"/lazy. Notice that the possession is not specified for each individual house but for the set, and the following text should make this fact persistent, even though we will see that this is not the case. An open adjunct is then used to predicate a property of these houses, the fact that they have been built of "paglia"/straw: this property is computed by accessing the controller of the open adjunct, i.e. the houses.

[i due porcellini pigri passavano le loro giornate suonando e cantando una canzone che diceva: chi ha paura del lupo cattivo]
loc(infon219, id42, [arg:main_tloc, arg:tes(f5_po5)])
ind(infon220, id43)
fact(infon221, isa, [ind:id43, class:canzone], 1, id42, id2)
fact(infon222, inst_of, [ind:id43, class:[astratto, informa]], 1, univ, univ)
fact(infon225, isa, [arg:id44, arg:giornata], 1, id42, id2)
fact(infon226, poss, [arg:id44, poss:id32], 1, id42, id2)
fact(id45, suonare, [experiencer:id32], 1, tes(fgerund1051_po6), id2)
fact(id47, passare, [theme_unaff:id32, theme:id44, gerund:id45], 1, tes(f8_po6), id2)
fact(infon240, focus, [arg:id49], 1, id42, id2)
fact(infon241, isa, [arg:id49, arg:chi], 1, id42, id2)
fact(infon242, paura, [nil:id49], 1, id42, id2)
sit(id50, avere, [arg:id49, prop:infon242], 1, tes(f6_po6), id2)
fact(id52, dire, [agent:id43, propq:id50], 1, tes(f7_po6), id2)
fact(id54, cantare, [experiencer:id32, theme_unaff:id43], 1, tes(fgerund1052_po6), id2)
fact(id47, passare, [tema_unaff:id32, theme:id44, gerund:id45], 1, tes(f8_po6), id2)

At this point, the set of two little pigs is specifically indicated. However we make coreference work in the model due to the previous inference on "the others" which made us build a set of little pigs with cardinality two. Notice that we have two class entities, which translate the implicit locative argument of "passare"/spend, and the subject wh- word of "avere"/have: the restriction on the class is constituted by a semantic feature. However, if it is true that the use of definite article points to the existence of some entity in the model that matches the required reference, it might also be the case that the appropriate reference must be recovered from the presence of the attribute "pigri"/lazy. This property has been associate to one set in the previous DM and this corresponds to the most recently built set of little pigs, with id32 semantic constant associated.

[ma ecco che improvvisamente il lupo apparve alle loro spalle]
fact(infon286, inst_of, [ind:id56, class:cosa], 1, univ, univ)
fact(infon287, isa, [ind:id56, class:spalla], 1, id42, id2)
fact(infon288, part_of, [spalla, id56, id32], 1, id42, id2)
fact(id56, apparire, [actor:id9], 1, tes(f1_po7), id2)
fact(infon289, a, [arg:id56, nil:id35], 1, tes(f1_po7), id2)

No entity is introduced in this and the following utterance, which is not included here.

[questo intanto si leccava già i baffi pensando al suo prossimo pasto così invitante e saporito]
loc(infon332, id66, [arg:main_tloc, arg:tes(f6_po8)])
ind(infon333, id67)
in(infon334, id67, id32)
sit(infon335, isa, [ind:id67, class:pasto], 1, id66, id2)
sit(infon335, kind_of, [ind:id32, class:pasto], 1, id66, id2)
fact(id70, leccare_baffo, [experiencer:id9], 1, tes(f5_po9), id2)
fact(id72, pensare, [actor:id9, theme:id32], 1, tes(fgerund1064_po9), id2)
fact(infon346, isa, [arg:id72, arg:st], 1, tes(fgerund1064_po9), id2)
fact(infon350, coincide, [arg:id70, arg:id72], 1, tes(f5_po9), id2)

In this utterance "pasto" has been computed as an individual included in the set of two little pigs by means of the semantic features associated to it [edible,event], where "edible" is a feature associated to the semantic role "food" and this in turn appears in a relation "think/pensare" where the subject/experiencer is the wolf, and the complement, the metaphoric intensional "food", refers to the "little pigs". The knowledge base is tapped in order to compute fully the inference from selectional restrictions and a further sit is added by means of the "kind_of" relation. Note that the main sentence is constituted by an idiomatic expression whose predicate "leccare"/lick has an OBJect NP which is computed as a FORM. This causes the relation to be treated as a sit rather than a fact with a single argument. Also notice that the predicate has been reinterpreted from "leccare" into the semantic concept "leccare_baffo" by means of the same procedure that has transformed "costruire" into "costruire_si" in a previous utterance. Here below we give the full f-structure of the current utterance.

index:f4
pred:leccare
lex_form:[np/subj/agent/[animate,human], np/obj/theme_aff/[object, body_part], pp/obj2/benef/a/ [animate, human], idioms/obj/form/[baffo], idioms/obj2/form/[si]]
mood:ind
tense:imp
cat:subjective
subj/experiencer:index:sn1

```
            cat:[animate, human]
            pred:questo:[pers:3,gen:mas ,num:sing,case:nom]
            spec:def:+
            tab_ref:[+ ref, + pro, - ana, + class]
            antecedent:external
            interpretation:specific
    obj/form:index:sn148
          cat:[object, body_part]
          pred:baffo:[pers:3,gen:mas ,num:plur]
          spec:def:+
          subj/poss:index:sn149
                cat:[object, body_part]
                pred:pPro
                spec:def:+
                controller:sn146
                tab_ref:[+ ref, + pro, + ana, - me]
          tab_ref:[+ ref, - pro, - ana, + class]
    obj2/form:index:sn146
          cat:[]
          pred:si:[pers:3,gen:_ ,num:_,case:dat]
          spec:def:+
          tab_ref:[- ref, - pro, + ana, + me, - subj]
          antecedent:sn1
          interpretation:specific
    adjs:adv:pred_adv:intanto
          tipo:temp
          duraz:non_punt
          config:[td=tr]
       adv:pred_adv:già
          tipo:temp
          duraz:non_punt
          config:[td=tr]
       adj/gerund:index:fgerund6
             pred:pensare
             lex_form:[np/subj/actor/[human, animate], pp/obl/theme/a/[event|_]]
             mood:ger
             tense:pres
             cat:mental_activ
             subj/actor:index:sn153
                    cat:[human, animate]
                    pred:pPro
                    tab_ref:[+ ref, + pro, + ana, - me]
                    antecedent:sn1
                    interpretation:specific
             obl/theme:index:sn151
                   cat:[event, object]
```

```
                    pred:pasto:[pers:3,gen:mas ,num:sing]
                    spec:def:+
                    subj/poss:index:sn152
                         cat:[]
                         pred:suo:[pers:3,gen:mas ,num:sing]
                         spec:def:+
                         tab_ref:[+ ref, + pro, - ana, + me]
                         antecedent:sn1
                         interpretation:specific
                    mods:mod_r:index:saa14
                          cat:[evaluative]
                          coord:head:coordination
                               coord:index:saa12
                                  cat:[evaluative]
                                  pred:invitante:[gen:mas ,num:sing]
                                  adjs:int:cosi_
                               coord:index:saa13
                                  cat:[evaluative]
                                  pred:saporito:[gen:mas ,num:sing]
                       mod_a:index:sa6
                          cat:[tempor]
                          pred:prossimo:[gen:mas ,num:sing]
                    tab_ref:[+ ref, - pro, - ana, + class]
               aspect:activity
     aspect:state
```

[finalmente i porcellini riuscirono a raggiungere la loro casetta e vi si chiusero dentro sbarrando la porta]
loc(infon369, id74, [arg:main_tloc, arg:tes(f8_po10)])
ind(infon370, id76)
fact(infon371, isa, [ind:id76, class:porta], 1, id74, id35)
fact(infon372, part_of, [casa, id35, id76], 1, id74, id35)
sit(id77, raggiungere, [actor:id32, goal:id35], 1, tes(finf1_po10), id35)
fact(id79, riuscire, [agent:id32, prop:id77], 1, tes(f6_po10), id35)
fact(id81, chiudere, [agent:id32, theme_aff:id32], 1, tes(f8_po10), id35)
fact(infon389, isa, [arg:id83, arg:dentro], 1, tes(f8_po10), id35)
fact(infon390, in, [arg:id81, locat:id83], 1, tes(f8_po10), id35)
fact(id84, sbarrare, [agent:id32, theme_aff:id76], 1, tes(fgerund1072_po10), id35)
fact(infon396, coincide, [arg:id81, arg:id84], 1, tes(f8_po10), id35)

No new entity is introduced in this utterance. However, notice that the house being talked about is the set of two houses already existing in the world, even though the actual NP used in this utterance is a singular one. This coreference is worked out on the basis of definiteness and the possessive which is bound to the subject NP. This NP is clearly ambiguous between a distributive and a collective reading: in the second case, only one house should appear, and since no single individual house exists in the DM belonging to the two lazy little pigs a new entity should have been added. However, the system prefers a distributive reading and looks for inds or sets belonging to a possessor if there is one, and picks up the entity in the DM which fits the current description.

[dalla finestra cominciarono a deridere il lupo cantando la solita canzoncina: chi ha paura del lupo cattivo]
ind(infon417, id86)
fact(infon418, isa, [ind:id86, class:finestra], 1, id74, id35)
fact(infon419, part_of, [casa, id35, id86], 1, id74, id35)
sit(id87, deridere, [actor:id32, theme_unaff:id9], 1, tes(finf1_po11), id35)
fact(id89, cominciare, [agent:id32, prop:id87], 1, tes(f5_po11), id35)
fact(infon433, da, [arg:id89, nil:id32, loc_origin:id86], 1, tes(f5_po11), id35)
fact(infon437, focus, [arg:id91], 1, tes(f5_po11), id35)
fact(infon438, isa, [arg:id91, arg:chi], 1, tes(f5_po11), id35)
fact(infon439, paura, [nil:id91], 1, tes(f5_po11), id35)
fact(id92, avere, [arg:id91, prop:infon439], 1, tes(f5_po11), id35)
fact(id94, cantare, [experiencer:id32, theme_unaff:id43], 1, tes(fgerund1076_po11), id35)
fact(infon448, coincide, [arg:id89, arg:id94], 1, tes(f5_po11), id35)

In this utterance we have a property associated to the individual "canzone"/song, which is interpreted as its subject, "paura"/fear: owing to its definiteness, this song is taken to be the same as the one mentioned previously in discourse. No new entity is introduced in the following utterance.

[il lupo stava intanto pensando al modo di penetrare nella casa]
loc(infon468, id96, [arg:main_tloc, arg:tes(f5_po11)])
sit(id97, penetrare, [actor:id9, locat:id35], 1, tes(finf1_po12), id2)
fact(id99, pensare, [actor:id9, prop:id97], 1, tes(f5_po12), id2)

In this utterance the story becomes inconsistent: the reference to the set of two houses where the two little pigs are hiding has now become a reference to "la casa"/the house, singular definite. There are two possibilities now: either the system might look for individual satisfying the description and find the house belonging to the elder brother, Jimmy; or it might take the most recent set satisfying the description. And this is what it does.

[esso si mise ad osservare attentamente la casetta e notò che non era davvero molto solida]
loc(infon497, id101, [arg:main_tloc, arg:tes(f8_po13)])
sit(id102, osservare, [experiencer:id9, theme_unaff:id35], 1, tes(finf1_po13), id2)
sit(infon501, isa, [arg:id102, arg:st], 1, tes(finf1_po13), id2)
sit(infon505, attentamente, [arg:id102], 1, tes(finf1_po13), id2)
fact(id104, mettersi, [actor:id9, prop:id102], 1, tes(f5_po13), id2)
fact(infon510, solido, [nil:id35], 0, id101, id2)
fact(id106, essere, [prop:infon510], 0, tes(f7_po13), id2)
fact(id108, notare, [experiencer:id9, prop:id106], 1, tes(f8_po13), id2)

The attribute "solido"/solid is now predicated rightly of the two little houses. Moreover, in the following utterance, the (set) of (two) little house(s) gets destroyed by the wolf's powerful blow. No new entity is being introduced in the following utterance.

```
[spaventatissimi i due porcellini corsero a perdifiato verso la casetta del fratello]
fact(id117, correre, [agent:id32, loc_direct:id25], 1, tes(f5_po15), id2)
fact(infon575, isa, [arg:id119, arg:perdifiato], 1, tes(f5_po15), id2)
fact(infon576, a, [arg:id117, nil:id119], 1, tes(f5_po15), id2)
fact(infon577, spaventatissimo, [arg:id117], 1, tes(f5_po15), id2)
included(tr(f5_po15), id110)
```

In order to understand that the little house being referred to is the one belonging to Jimmy, the system looks for an individual, which is a house, and has a possessor, which is again an individual and is a brother: it captures the related identifier, id24. However, the Main Location has not changed yet, owing to the fact that a semantic role like Loc_direct, i.e. a directional location, is not taken as a valid main location.

```
["presto, fratellino, aprici! abbiamo il lupo alle calcagna"]
loc(infon584, id120, [arg:main_tloc, arg:tes(f5_po15)])
fact(infon585, inst_of, [ind:id24, class:animale], 1, univ, univ)
fact(id121, avere, [experiencer:id32, theme_bound:id9], 1, tes(f4_po16), id2)
fact(id123, aprire, [agent:id24, goal:id32], 1, tes(f2_po16), id2)
```

The appearance of direct speech within the story requires the system to compute the reference of first and second person pronouns to previous participants in the story, which however were introduced by third person. Further problems are constituted by the reference to a singular little brother as "fratellino", which should be understood as the wise little pig Jimmy: this is computed by the existence of an individual in the world associated to Jimmy, as opposed to the presence of a set associated to the remaining two little pigs, as discussed above.

```
[fecero appena in tempo ad entrare e tirare il chiavistello]
ind(infon602, id125)
fact(infon603, isa, [ind:id125, class:chiavistello], 1, id120, id25)
fact(infon604, part_of, [casa, id25, id125], 1, id120, id25)
fact(id126, entrare, [agent:id32], 1, tes(finf1_po17), id25)
fact(id128, fare_tempo, [agent:id32, prop:id126], 1, tes(f9_po17), id25)
fact(id130, tirare, [agent:id32, theme_aff:id125], 1, tes(finf4_po17), id25)
fact(id128, fare_tempo, [agent:id32, prop:id126], 1, tes(f9_po17), id25)
```

It is interesting to notice the appearance of the part_of relation as the singular definite NP "il chiavistello" is computed as being a part of the house: the inference is based on a constraint based on the spatial location of the situation in which the definite NP is contained. Also notice that semantic interpretation transforms a coordinate structure into a double relation holding in the DM; the main predicate has also undergone a semantic transformation, from "fare" into "fare_tempo". The same happens in the following utterance where the singular definite NP "pranzetto" is computed by an inference as coreferring to any of the little pigs, since it corefers with "pasto" above.

[il lupo stava già arrivando deciso a non rinunciare al suo pranzetto]
fact(id132, arrivare, [tema_aff:id9], 1, tes(f5_po18), id2)
sit(id135, rinunciare, [actor:id9, theme_aff:id67], 1, tes(finf1_po18), id2)
fact(infon655, not, [prop:id135], 1, tes(f5_po18), id2)
fact(infon656, deciso, [arg:id132, nil:id9, prop:infon655], 1, tes(f5_po18), id2)

In the previous utterance no new individual was introduced and the wolf was the main character being in focus. In the following utterance [non ci fu niente da fare], an impersonal sentence, the wolf is still taken to be the focussed character binding the big PRO subject of the infinitival "fare".

[i tre porcellini si sentivano al sicuro nella solida casetta di mattoni]
loc(infon815, id165, [arg:main_tloc, arg:tes(f6_po22)])
fact(infon817, sicuro, [nil:id3], 1, id165, id25)
fact(id166, sentirsi, [experiencer:id3, prop:infon817], 1, tes(f6_po23), id25)
fact(infon818, isa, [arg:id167, arg:mattone], 1, tes(f6_po23), id25)
fact(infon819, di, [arg:id25, matter:id167], 1, tes(f6_po23), id25)
fact(infon820, in, [arg:id165, nil:id25], 1, tes(f6_po23), id25)

Notice that at this point of the story coreference with the three little pigs is reestablished explicitely by indicating cardinality: in this way the system is able to extract the right ID. Problems arise with the definite singular NP "la solida casetta di mattoni": of course we know that it has been built "con"/with, by means of "mattoni"/bricks and "cemento"/cement. An inference is fired in order to ascertain whether these two properties can have the same meaning.

[riconoscenti i due porcellini oziosi promisero al fratello che da quel giorno anche essi avrebbero lavorato sodo]
sit(id169, lavorare, [agent:id32], 1, tes(f246_po24), id25)
sit(infon841, anche, [arg:id169], 1, tes(f246_po24), id25)
sit(infon842, sodo, [arg:id169], 1, tes(f246_po24), id25)
fact(infon843, isa, [arg:id171, arg:giorno], 1, tes(f246_po24), id25)
sit(infon844, da, [arg:id169, nil:id171], 1, tes(f246_po24), id25)
fact(id172, promettere, [actor:id32, theme_unaff:id24, propint:id169], 1, tes(f247_po24), id25)
fact(infon849, riconoscente, [arg:id172], 1, tes(f247_po24), id25)

However, the final utterance of the story mentions the set of lazy little pigs again by indicating explicitly its cardinality. As we already said, at the end of the computation the discourse model algorithm automatically generates the rank list of the entities of the model or world of the story according to the relevance score: we compute this score by taking into account the topicality of each entity, i.e. the type of Topic it represents in the story and the times it is so treated by the system. There is a separate entry for each SET, INDIVIDUAL or

CLASS where hierarchically all properties and relations the story has ascribed to it are inherited.

7.2. Story 2

As said in the introduction, this story is just a small excerpt from a newspaper article which deals with politics, and in particular with a man called Avveduti who was implied in a number of political scandals. The first sentence of the story has been added in order to provide the rest of it with some context, which otherwise would have been lacking. The portion of the text that we chose is remarkable as far as textual cohesion mechanisms are concerned: the use of pronouns is very extended and the discourse module captures all the relevant passages in the right way. The model representation is enriched here as to relations, in that it assigns a restriction to them in terms of event or state. This information is important for the temporal interpretation which however is not represented in the book.

```
[fino a tre anni fa franco avveduti non si era mai immischiato col mondo della pubblica
amministrazione]
loc(infon3, id1, [arg:main_tloc, arg:anno])
ind(infon4, id2)
fact(infon5, surname, [franco, id2], 1, id1, univ)
fact(infon6, inst_of, [ind:id2, class:uomo], 1, univ, univ)
fact(infon7, name, [avveduti, id2], 1, univ, univ)
fact(infon22, isa, [arg:id3, arg:mondo], 1, id1, univ)
fact(infon23, isa, [arg:id4, arg:amministrazione], 1, id1, univ)
fact(infon24, pubblico, [arg:id4], 1, id1, univ)
fact(infon25, di, [arg:id3, specific:id4], 1, id1, univ)
fact(id5, immischiare, [agent:id2, theme_aff:id2, comitat:id3], 0, tes(f3_avv01), univ)
fact(infon30, isa, [arg:id1, arg:anno], 1, tes(f3_avv01), univ)
fact(infon31, fino_fa, [arg:id5, nil:id1], 1, tes(f3_avv01), univ)

[come burocrate, era un immigrato che veniva dal di fuori]
loc(infon42, id7, [arg:main_tloc, arg:tes(f3_avv01)])
loc(infon43, id8, [arg:main_sloc, arg:fuori])
ind(infon44, id9)
fact(infon45, burocrate, [ind:id9], 1, id7, id8)
fact(infon46, role, [immigrato, id9, id2], 1, id7, id8)
fact(infon47, inst_of, [ind:id9, class:[ind, real, soc, role]], 1, univ, univ)
fact(infon48, isa, [ind:id9, class:immigrato], 1, id7, id8)
fact(infon49, immigrato, [nil:id2], 1, id7, id8)
class(infon50, id10)
fact(infon51, inst_of, [ind:id10, class:uomo], 1, univ, univ)
fact(infon52, isa, [ind:id10, class:uomo], 1, univ, univ)
fact(id11, essere, [prop:infon49], 1, tes(f4_avv02), id8)
```

[figlio di buona famiglia, a venti anni decise di iscriversi alla accademia militare di cavalleria]
loc(infon71, id13, [arg:main_tloc, arg:anno])
loc(infon72, id14, [arg:main_sloc, arg:accademia])
fact(infon74, isa, [arg:id14, arg:accademia], 1, id13, id14)
fact(infon75, militare, [arg:id14], 1, id13, id14)
fact(infon76, isa, [arg:id15, arg:cavalleria], 1, id13, id14)
fact(infon77, di, [arg:id14, specific:id15], 1, id13, id14)
fact(id16, iscrivere, [actor:id2, theme_unaff:id2, goal:id14], 1, tes(finf1_free_avv03), id14)
fact(id18, decidere, [actor:id2, prop:id16], 1, tes(f3_free_avv03), id14)

[era un buon allievo con ottime qualifiche]
loc(infon97, id20, [arg:main_tloc, arg:tes(f3_free_avv03)])
fact(infon98, allievo, [nil:id2], 1, id20, id14)
fact(infon99, buon, [ind:id2], 1, id20, id14)
fact(id21, essere, [prop:infon98], 1, tes(f3_avv04), id14)

[più tardi fu un ufficiale di,successo]
loc(infon113, id23, [arg:main_tloc, arg:più_tardi])
ind(infon114, id24)
ind(infon115, id25)
fact(infon116, inst_of, [ind:id25, class:[ind, abst, soc, state]], 1, univ, univ)
fact(infon117, isa, [ind:id25, class:successo], 1, id23, id14)
fact(infon118, di, [arg:id24, specif:id25], 1, id23, id14)
fact(infon119, role, [ufficiale, id24, id2], 1, id23, id14)
fact(infon120, inst_of, [ind:id24, class:militare], 1, univ, univ)
fact(infon121, isa, [ind:id24, class:ufficiale], 1, id23, id14)
fact(infon122, ufficiale, [nil:id2], 1, id23, id14)
fact(id26, essere, [prop:infon122], 1, tes(f3_avv05), id14)

At this point of the story we have a certain number of properties and relation being predicated of the main character Franco Avveduti, who has been assigned the semantic constant identifier id2. It is important now to notice that in the latest utterance we learn that he was also an officer. This new property however is indirectly negated in the following utterance, where we are told that Avveduti "si dimise"/resigned "dall'esercito"/from the army. No indication is directly made to the role of officer which must be indirectly inferred. A number of interesting inferences are realized in the following utterances and are all based on the collective noun "esercito"/army. They are all discussed in the text above.

[poi nel 1945 avveduti si dimise dallo esercito]
loc(infon136, id28, [arg:main_tloc, arg:tes(f3_free_avv03)])
loc(infon137, id29, [arg:main_sloc, arg:esercito])
set(infon138, id30)
card(infon139, id30, >100)
fact(infon140, inst_of, [ind:id30, class:militare], 1, univ, univ)

```
fact(infon141, isa, [ind:id30, class:esercito], 1, id28, id29)
in(infon142, id24, id30)
fact(infon143, role, [ufficiale, id24, id2], 0, id28, id29)
fact(id31, dimettere, [actor:id2, actee:id2, locat:id30], 1, tes(f4_avv06), id29)
fact(infon150, isa, [arg:id33, arg:1945], 1, tes(f4_avv06), id29)
fact(infon151, in, [arg:id31, nil:id33], 1, tes(f4_avv06), id29)
fact(infon152, adj, [temp_seq:id31], 1, id28, id29)
fact(infon153, poi, [prop:infon152], 1, id28, id29)
```

In the following utterance "i militari" a plural definite NP is equalled to the "army" seen that the latter is made up of "militari", as the default class inclusion clearly testifies. So no new entity is asserted in the DM.

```
[i militari lo avevano deluso]
loc(infon163, id34, [arg:main_tloc, arg:tes(f4_avv06)])
fact(id35, deludere, [causer_emot:id30, experiencer:id2], 1, tes(f3_avv07), id29)
```

In the following utterance, however a metonimic coreference is realized: "divisa"/uniform is made to refer to the "army", where such clothes are used by "militari". The solution we chose is thus to fire a part_of assertion holding between "uniform" and "army".

```
[avveduti, deposta la divisa, si iscrisse alla università]
class(infon173, id37)
fact(infon174, inst_of, [ind:id37, class:cosa], 1, univ, univ)
fact(infon175, isa, [ind:id37, class:divisa], 1, id34, id29)
fact(infon176, part_of, [divisa, id37, id30], 1, id34, id29)
fact(infon178, isa, [arg:id38, arg:universita_], 1, id34, id29)
fact(id39, iscrivere, [actor:id2, theme_unaff:id2, goal:id38], 1, tes(f3_avv08), id29)
```

```
[nel 1947 era laureato e nel 1948 era procuratore legale]
ind(infon201, id43)
fact(infon202, role, [laureato, id43, id2], 1, id34, id29)
fact(infon203, inst_of, [ind:id43, class:[ind, real, soc, role]], 1, univ, univ)
fact(infon204, isa, [ind:id43, class:laureato], 1, id34, id29)
fact(infon205, laureato, [nil:id2], 1, id34, id29)
ind(infon206, id44)
fact(infon207, legale, [ind:id44], 1, id34, id29)
fact(infon208, role, [procuratore, id44, id2], 1, id34, id29)
fact(infon209, inst_of, [ind:id44, class:[ind, real, soc, role]], 1, univ, univ)
fact(infon210, isa, [ind:id44, class:procuratore], 1, id34, id29)
fact(infon211, procuratore, [nil:id2], 1, id34, id29)
fact(id45, essere, [prop:infon205], 1, tes(f3_avv09), id29)
fact(infon218, isa, [arg:id47, arg:1947], 1, tes(f3_avv09), id29)
fact(infon219, in, [arg:id45, nil:id47], 1, tes(f3_avv09), id29)
fact(id48, essere, [prop:infon211], 1, tes(f5_avv09), id29)
fact(infon225, isa, [arg:id50, arg:1948], 1, tes(f5_avv09), id29)
```

fact(infon226, in, [arg:id48, nil:id50], 1, tes(f5_avv09), id29)

New properties are introduced in the previous and the following utterance. However, the most interesting ones are the latter properties because they allow the system to realize the meaning postulate associated to "father-in-law". In the following utterance we are told that Avveduti met and married Paola, daughter of Antonio Alberti, important senator belonging to the political party of the Christian Democrats. All these information are needed in the following text to derive the coreference for the definite singular NP "il suocero"/the father-in-law.

[intanto a verona aveva conosciuto paola, figlia di antonio alberti, potente senatore democristiano, e la aveva sposata]
loc(infon239, id51, [arg:main_sloc, arg:verona])
ind(infon240, id52)
ind(infon241, id53)
fact(infon242, surname, [antonio, id53], 1, id34, id51)
fact(infon243, inst_of, [ind:id53, class:uomo], 1, univ, univ)
fact(infon244, name, [alberti, id53], 1, univ, univ)
fact(infon245, relat, [figlia, id52, id53], 1, id34, id51)
fact(infon246, inst_of, [ind:id52, class:[ind, real, nat, relat]], 1, univ, univ)
fact(infon247, isa, [ind:id52, class:figlia], 1, id34, id51)
fact(infon248, inst_of, [ind:id52, class:[ind, real, nat, hum]], 1, univ, univ)
fact(infon249, name, [paola, id52], 1, univ, univ)
fact(infon252, isa, [ind:id53, class:senatore], 1, id34, id51)
fact(infon253, democristiano, [ind:id53], 1, id34, id51)
fact(infon254, potente, [ind:id53], 1, id34, id51)
ind(infon257, id55)
fact(infon258, inst_of, [ind:id55, class:[luogo]], 1, univ, univ)
fact(infon259, name, [verona, id55], 1, univ, univ)
fact(id56, conoscere, [experiencer:id2, theme_emot:id52], 1, tes(f3_avv10), id51)
fact(infon268, a, [arg:id56, nil:id55], 1, tes(f3_avv10), id51)
fact(id58, sposare, [agent:id2, theme_aff:id52], 1, tes(f5_avv10), id51)

A number of utterances follow which however do not modify the DM. The following utterance of the text introduces "suocero"/father-in-law which is computed as such by means of inferential processes based on previous knowledge available in the DM.

[gli piaceva parlare del suocero come di una facile occasione mancata che chiunque altro avrebbe sfruttato ma che lui, avveduti, preferiva lasciare perdere]
fact(infon379, isa, [ind:id53, class:suocero], 1, id1, nil)
fact(infon380, relat, [suocero, id53, id2], 1, id1, nil)
ind(infon383, id81)
fact(infon384, facile, [ind:id81], 1, id80, id14)
fact(infon385, mancato, [ind:id81], 1, id80, id14)
fact(infon386, isa, [ind:id81, class:occasione], 1, id80, id14)
fact(infon387, inst_of, [ind:id81, class:[evento]], 1, univ, univ)

class(infon388, id82)
fact(infon389, inst_of, [ind:id82, class:uomo], 1, univ, univ)
fact(infon390, isa, [ind:id82, class:uomo], 1, univ, univ)
fact(id83, sfruttare, [agent:id82, theme_aff:id81], 1, tes(f3_p01), id14)
fact(id87, perdere, [actor:id2, theme_unaff:id81], 1, tes(finf3_p01), id14)
fact(id89, lasciare, [actor:id2, prop:id87], 1, tes(finf2_p01), id14)
fact(id91, preferire, [actor:id2, prop:id89], 1, tes(f4_p01), id14)
fact(id93, parlare, [actor:id2, subj_dis:id53], 1, tes(finf1_p01), id14)
fact(id95, piacere, [propint:id93, experiencer:id2], 1, tes(f5_p01), id14)

In the third utterance a new individual is created, which is a "posto"/position and is treated as a sit rather than a fact because it is the argument of a [-tense] predicate in turn an open complement of a higher predicate "decidere"/decide which produces opacity for its arguments.

[solo verso il 1950 decise di accettare un posto nella organizzazione della fiera di verona]
loc(infon448, id97, [arg:main_tloc, arg:1950])
loc(infon449, id98, [arg:main_sloc, arg:verona])
ind(infon450, id99)
ind(infon451, id100)
ind(infon452, id101)
ind(infon453, id102)
fact(infon454, inst_of, [ind:id102, class:[luogo]], 1, univ, univ)
fact(infon455, isa, [ind:id102, class:verona], 1, id97, id98)
fact(infon456, di, [arg:id101, specif:id102], 1, id97, id98)
fact(infon457, inst_of, [ind:id101, class:[coll, real, soc, event]], 1, univ, univ)
fact(infon458, isa, [ind:id101, class:fiera], 1, id97, id98)
fact(infon459, has, [arg:id100, tema:id101], 1, id97, id98)
fact(infon460, inst_of, [ind:id100, class:istituzione], 1, univ, univ)
fact(infon461, isa, [ind:id100, class:organizzazione], 1, id97, id98)
fact(infon462, in, [arg:id99, locativo:id100], 1, id97, id98)
sit(infon463, isa, [ind:id99, class:posto], 1, id97, id98)
fact(infon464, inst_of, [ind:id99, class:[attivita, luogo, stato]], 1, univ, univ)
fact(id103, accettare, [actor:id2, theme_unaff:id99], 1, tes(finf1_p02), id98)
fact(id105, decidere, [actor:id2, prop:id103], 1, tes(f3_p02), id98)
fact(infon480, verso, [arg:id105, nil:id107], 1, tes(f3_p02), id98)

In the fourth utterance there is a long list of predicates and arguments which however do not constitute legal IDs, being either plural or singular NPs with no coreferent in the world of the model nor in the external knowledge network. We only know now that a number of properties are associated to the main topic with a number of restrictions.

[lo nominarono delegato cioè una specie di funzionario viaggiante con incarichi diplomatici di tenere i rapporti con le delegazioni commerciali, curare i produttori stranieri, le grandi ditte, la stampa]
loc(infon493, id108, [arg:main_tloc, arg:tes(f3_p02)])

ind(infon494, id109)
fact(infon495, role, [delegato, id109, id2], 1, id108, id98)
fact(infon496, inst_of, [ind:id109, class:uomo], 1, univ, univ)
fact(infon497, isa, [ind:id109, class:delegato], 1, id108, id98)
fact(infon498, delegato, [nil:id2], 1, id108, id98)
class(infon499, id110)
fact(infon510, viaggiante, [ind:id110], 1, id108, id98)
fact(infon512, inst_of, [ind:id112, class:uomo], 1, univ, univ)
sit(infon513, isa, [ind:id112, class:funzionario], 1, id108, id98)
sit(infon514, kind_of, [ind:id109, class:funzionario], 1, id108, id98)
fact(id113, nominare, [agent:id100, prop:infon498], 1, tes(f4_avv15), id98)

No new ID is created in this utterance and in the following one. However, we should note the special function devoted to the indefinite NP "un compito/a task" in a predicative function, which is translated by the system as a property ascribed to an entity coreferred by the deictic "this/questo" subject of the predication. The entity is recovered by means of the special semantic restriction associated to the noun "task", which is classified as "activity" in the lexicon. Now the semantic interpreter understands an activity to be coreferrable to a "social role": and the one available in the previous portion of text is the "delegato/delegate", which is picked up as coreferent for "this".

[questo era un compito che corrispondeva bene alla sua vocazione e nel quale avveduti sapeva giostrare con, notevole agilità]
loc(infon530, id115, [arg:main_tloc, arg:tes(f6_p03)])
ind(infon531, id116)
fact(infon532, questo, [nil:id116], 1, id115, id98)
fact(infon533, isa, [ind:id116, class:compito], 1, id115, id98)
fact(infon534, isa, [compito, id109], 1, id115, id98)
fact(infon535, isa, [arg:id117, arg:vocazione], 1, id115, id98)
fact(infon536, poss, [arg:id117, poss:id2], 1, id115, id98)
fact(id118, corrispondere, [theme_bound:id116, theme_unaff:id117], 1, tes(f5_p04), id98)
fact(infon538, bene, [arg:id118], 1, tes(f5_p04), id98)
sit(id120, giostrare, [agent:id2, modal:id122], 1, tes(finf1_p04), id98)
fact(infon540, isa, [arg:id122, arg:agilità], 1, tes(finf1_p04), id98)
fact(infon541, notevole, [arg:id122], 1, tes(finf1_p04), id98)
sit(infon542, con, [arg:id120, nil:id122], 1, tes(finf1_p04), id98)
fact(id123, sapere, [actor:id2, prop:id120], 1, tes(f6_p04), id98)
fact(id125, essere, [prop:infon532], 1, tes(f7_p04), id98)

In this utterance there is a new ID which is created and a number of individuals are also referred to by proper names. However no coreferent exists in the world so that they are simply dropped. In case we computed the whole of the story, that we would have known which person the proper name "Alberti" corefers to.

[a verona il collegio di alberti lo aveva ereditato trabucchi e col collegio aveva ereditato la presidenza della fiera]
loc(infon585, id123, [arg:main_tloc, arg:tes(f6_p05)])
ind(infon586, id124)
fact(infon587, inst_of, [ind:id124, class:uomo], 1, univ, univ)
fact(infon588, name, [trabucchi, id124], 1, univ, univ)
fact(infon590, isa, [arg:id125, arg:collegio], 1, id123, id98)
fact(id126, ereditare, [receiver:id124, theme_unaff:id125], 1, tes(f3_p06), id98)
fact(infon596, a, [arg:id126, nil:id55], 1, tes(f3_p06), id98)
fact(infon597, isa, [arg:id129, arg:collegio], 1, id123, id98)
fact(infon598, con, [arg:id128, nil:id124, comitat:id129], 1, id123, id98)
fact(infon599, isa, [arg:id130, arg:presidenza], 1, id123, id98)
fact(id131, ereditare, [receiver:id124, theme_unaff:id130], 1, tes(f5_p06), id98)
fact(infon604, isa, [arg:id129, arg:collegio], 1, tes(f5_p06), id98)
fact(infon605, con, [arg:id131, nil:id124, comitat:id129], 1, tes(f5_p06), id98)

No new entity is introduced in this utterance: rather, the story now has two protagonists which are continually coreferred by the use of pronouns.

[trabucchi continuò a valersi della collaborazione di avveduti]
fact(infon625, isa, [arg:id133, arg:collaborazione], 1, id123, id98)
fact(id134, valersi, [experiencer:id124, theme_unaff:id133], 1, tes(finf1_p07), id98)
fact(id136, continuare, [agent:id124, prop:id134], 1, tes(f3_p07), id98)

In this utterance a reference to the main topic, Avveduti, is realized by means of a compound noun, "ex-ufficiale"/ex-officer, where the prefix indicates that the property of being an officer no longer holds for the referent, Avveduti. To compute the meaning of this noun, a complex inferential process has been activated: in particular we know at the beginning of the story that Avveduti gets enlisted as officer of cavalry. Then in the following text we also know that he decides to quit the army to become a lawyer. Reasoning processes analysed these events in such a way as to produce an interpretation for the prefix "ex", indicating explicitly that the property denoted by the noun was previously predicated of the individual but that at a certain moment in time, preceding the actual time indicated by the discourse has been suspended.

[lo ex ufficiale del novara_cavalleria gli era simpatico]
loc(infon643, id138, [arg:main_tloc, arg:tes(f3_p07)])
fact(infon644, simpatico, [nil:id2], 1, id138, id98)
fact(infon649, isa, [arg:id140, arg:novara_cavalleria], 1, id138, id98)
fact(infon650, di, [arg:id2, specif:id140], 1, id138, id98)
fact(id141, essere, [prop:infon644], 1, tes(f3_avv20), id98)

In this utterance and the following one no new ID is created.

[la sua distinzione lo impressionava]
fact(infon665, isa, [arg:id143, arg:distinzione], 1, id138, id98)

```
fact(infon667, poss, [arg:id143, poss:id2], 1, id138, id98)
fact(id144, impressionare, [causer_emot:id143, theme_emot:id124], 1, tes(f3_p09), id98)
```

Consider now the inference required to maintain the same location: we are faced with a property, "fiera/fair" which is also a location, however we do not want to assert a new location since the fair we are talking about is just a place in Verona. Inferences are activated on the model on the basis of a specification role associated with the id of the fair.

```
[lo confermò nello incarico alla fiera]
ind(infon681, id146)
fact(infon682, isa, [ind:id146, class:incarico], 1, id138, id98)
fact(infon345, isa, [incarico, id109], 1, id138, id98)
fact(id148, confermare, [experiencer:id124, prop:id2], 1, tes(f6_p10), id98)
```

In this utterance we know that Avveduti was working as special secretary of the ministry Trabucchi, something which did not appear in the previous text.

```
[avveduti funzionava benissimo come segretario particolare]
loc(infon697, id150, [arg:main_tloc, arg:tes(f4_p10)])
ind(infon698, id151)
fact(infon699, particolare, [ind:id151], 1, id150, id98)
fact(infon700, role, [segretario, id151, id2], 1, id150, id98)
fact(infon701, inst_of, [ind:id151, class:uomo], 1, univ, univ)
fact(infon702, isa, [ind:id151, class:segretario], 1, id150, id98)
fact(infon703, segretario, [nil:id2], 1, id150, id98)
fact(id153, funzionare, [prop:infon703], 1, tes(f3_p11), id98)
fact(infon714, bene, [arg:id153], 1, tes(f3_p11), id98)
```

In this utterance we are informed about Avveduti's skill to contact important people which however are introduced in the plural as bare generic NPs. In the model, the relation interpreter creates a set of individuals which includes both reference to classes. Also notice that default properties are augmented by the additional information that they can be referred as "uomo"/man.

```
[sapeva mobilitare prefetti e questori]
class(infon725, id155)
fact(infon728, isa, [ind:id155, class:questore], 1, id150, id98)
fact(infon730, inst_of, [ind:id155, class:uomo], 1, univ, univ)
fact(infon731, isa, [ind:id155, class:uomo], 1, univ, univ)
class(infon732, id156)
fact(infon735, isa, [ind:id156, class:prefetto], 1, id150, id98)
fact(infon737, inst_of, [ind:id156, class:uomo], 1, univ, univ)
fact(infon738, isa, [ind:id156, class:uomo], 1, univ, univ)
set(infon733, id159)
card(infon734, id159, >10)
in(infon736, id156, id159)
```

in(infon739, id155, id159)
fact(infon740, [questore, prefetto], [arg:id159], 1, id150, id98)
fact(id160, mobilitare, [agent:id2, prop:infon740], 1, tes(finfl_p12), id98)
fact(id162, sapere, [actor:id2, prop:id160], 1, tes(f3_p12), id98)

Finally, the last sentence is rather tricky because the reference to Avveduti is recovered via the property "segretario"/secretary which makes it possible to assign the right coreferent to the clitic pronoun "gli"/him and the possessor "suo"/his, i.e. Trabucchi.

[tutti gli invidiavano il suo segretario particolare]
class(infon757, id164)
card(infon758, id164, all)
fact(infon759, isa, [arg:id164, class:umano], 1,id150, id98)
fact(id165, invidiare, [experiencer:id164, theme_unaff:id2, actor:id124], 1, tes(f5_p13), id98)

7.3. Story 3

We come now to the semantic analysis of the last bit of story which is taken from the original version of the story of the three little pigs: however, only the first 24 utterances are commented here, because they contain quite a number of new and interesting phenomena from the point of view of discourse structure. The first sentence introduces the story of the three little pigs, by means of an inverted copular structure which is very common in texts like these. The deictic pronoun is now bound to the referential element, the story, which however is not taken as the argument of discourse, being the inverted structure a rhetorical means for introducing a new entity in the adjunct modifier of the noun "story" itself. The story of "X" is computed as a SUBJ_DISC by the grammar and the story itself constitutes a [+info] piece of information which is demoted from its relevance by being assigned the semantic role theme_bound, a non semantically independent role, even though syntactically SUBJ_FOC, i.e. an inverted subject focalized by the syntactic construction. This information causes the interpreter to reject the story as a new individual to be asserted in the world, and the three little pigs as the new ID. Here below is the DM which has been filtered out from event/state time infos.

[questa è la storia di tre porcellini che andarono per il mondo a cercare fortuna]
loc(infon0, id8, [arg:main_tloc, arg:tr(f7_pig01)])
loc(infon1, id1, [arg:main_sloc, arg:mondo])
set(infon2, id2)
card(infon3, id2, 3)
fact(infon4, isa, [ind:id2, class:porcellino], 1, id8, id1)
fact(infon5, inst_of, [ind:id2, class:animale_cibo], 1, id8, id1)
fact(infon8, isa, [arg:id3, arg:storia], 1, id8, id1)
fact(infon10, isa, [arg:id4, arg:fortuna], 1, id8, id1)
sit(id5, cercare, [agent:id2, theme_unaff:id4], 1, tes(finfl_pig01), id1)
fact(infon15, isa, [arg:id1, arg:mondo], 1, id8, id1)

fact(id7, andare, [agent:id2, arg:id5, locat:id1], 1, tes(f7_pig01), id1)
fact(infon20, poss, [arg:id3, poss:id2], 1, id8, id1)
fact(infon21, questa, [nil:id3], 1, id8, id1)
fact(id9, essere, [prop:infon21], 1, tes(f6_pig01), id1)

In the second utterance, the names of the three little pigs are assigned and they start to be individuated by some attribute. Names are assigned appropriately by the discourse module which binds the possessive pronoun "loro" to the argument of discourse, id1. However, assigning names to members of a set constitutes a means for individuating each member as a separate individual thus existing in the world in its own right. This is what the interpreter does, when the coordination of proper names is met and is found as pertaining to a set: each name is thus associated to a new individual in the world which in turn is included as such in the set of the little pigs. As in the previous stories, names are treated as permanent properties, as far as the partial model is concerned, i.e. they are constants which cannot be modified in time or space. The relation interpreter computes the static information contained in the proposition, i.e. the fact that the set of three names is an open proposition which is an argument of the predicate BE. Notice that the properties associated to each name are not computed by the interpreter, due to the fact that they are expressed by means of naked NPs.

[i loro nomi erano timmy, suonatore di flauto, tommy, violinista e, jimmy, grande lavoratore]
ind(infon36, id12)
in(infon37, id12, id2)
fact(infon38, name, [tommy, id12], 1, univ, univ)
ind(infon39, id13)
in(infon40, id13, id2)
fact(infon41, name, [jimmy, id13], 1, univ, univ)
ind(infon42, id14)
in(infon43, id14, id2)
fact(infon44, name, [timmy, id14], 1, univ, univ)
fact(infon45, isa, [ind:id14, class:animale], 1, id8, id1)
fact(infon46, isa, [violinista:id12], 1,id8, id1)
fact(infon47, isa, [lavoratore:id13], 1, id8, id1)
fact(infon60, [tommy, timmy, jimmy], [arg:id15], 1, id8, id1)
fact(infon61, nome, [nil:id15], 1, nil, id1)
fact(id16, essere, [prop:infon60, prop:infon61], 1, tes(f6_pig02), id1)

The following utterance repeats more or less the contents of a similar utterance used in the previous story, but there is one detail missing from this construction, and that is the clitic "si" benefactive has been omitted in this case. In this way there is no direct indication that the singular indefinite NP has to be constructed as a plural NP with an ID made up of a set with cardinality equal to 3. The only hint comes from the floating quantifier which has the indefinite in its scope, and is functionally bound to the subject NP: thus the module for Quantifier Raising tells the Interpreter to build the indefinite as a plural rather than as a singular, and the functional structure indicates the cardinality, which in turn must be recovered from the discourse where the coreferent of the empty little pro can be found.

Consider then that the interpreter assigns the ID of the little house to sits rather than to facts due to semantic reasoning: the NP is the argument of a relation "costruire" which is also computed as a sit. In other words, an opaque relations turns its arguments into opaque arguments even if they are indefinite NPs, which is regarded as the usual structure for introducing a new entity in the world.

```
[giunti in un bel bosco, decisero di costruire ognuno una comoda casetta]
loc(infon66, id19, [arg:main_sloc, arg:bosco])
ind(infon68, id19)
fact(infon69, bel, [ind:id19], 1, id24, id19)
fact(infon70, isa, [ind:id19, class:bosco], 1, id24, id19)
fact(infon71, inst_of, [ind:id19, class:luogo], 1, id24, id19)
set(infon72, id20)
card(infon73, id20, 3)
fact(infon74, piccolo, [ind:id20], 1, id24, id19)
fact(infon75, comodo, [ind:id20], 1, id24, id19)
sit(infon76, isa, [ind:id20, class:casa], 1, id24, id19)
fact(infon77, inst_of, [ind:id20, class:cosa], 1, id24, id19)
sit(id21, costruire, [agente:id2, tema_eff:id20], 1, tes(finf1_pig03), id19)
fact(id25, giungere, [actor:id2, goal:id19], 1, tes(fpart_pass1_pig03), id19)
```

In the following utterance, however, the text turns to "capanna"/hut rather than little house. This metaphor requires an ad hoc inference which however is not required at the moment. As with the previous utterance, the indefinite NP is not asserted as a fact due to the opacity of its governing relation. Being opaque, no possession relation is being built by the interpreter, which would have been available by the presence of the usual SI benefactive, which binds an abstract possessor in the object NP: the clitic SI is in turn bound by the binding module to the subject NP.

```
[a timmy non piaceva per niente lavorare così pensò di costruirsi rapidamente una
    capanna di paglia]
fact(infon119, poss, [timmy, id14, id27], 1, id37, id19)
ind(infon120, id27)
fact(infon121, paglia, [ind:id27], 1, id37, id19)
fact(infon122, isa, [ind:id27, class:capanna], 1, id37, id19)
fact(infon123, inst_of, [ind:id27, class:cosa], 1, id37, id19)
fact(id28, lavorare, [agent:id14], 1, tes(finf1_pig04), id19)
fact(id30, piacere, [propint:id28, experiencer:id14], 0, tes(f6_pig04), id19)
fact(infon158, isa, [arg:id32, arg:niente], 1, tes(f6_pig04), id19)
fact(infon159, per, [arg:id30, nil:id32], 1, tes(f6_pig04), id19)
fact(infon162, isa, [arg:id33, arg:paglia], 1, tes(f6_pig04), id19)
fact(infon163, di, [arg:id27, matter:id33], 1, tes(f6_pig04), id19)
sit(id34, costruire, [agent:id14, theme_eff:id27], 1, tes(finf4_pig04), id19)
sit(infon168, rapidamente, [arg:id34], 1, tes(finf4_pig04), id19)
fact(id36, pensare, [experiencer:id14, arg:id34], 1, tes(f9_pig04), id19)
fact(infon173, così, [arg:id30, result:id36], 1, tes(f6_pig04), id19)
```

As we predicted before, in this utterance the "hut" has been turned into a little house, and the inference is fired by the fact that there is a singular definite NP and in the most recent segment of text there is also an NP as far as semantic features are concerned, which the actual NP can cospecify. And in fact, since the previous reference to the hut was introduced as a sit, it takes a singular definite NP in a transparent extensional context to turn the sit into a fact. Consider the role of the adjective "pronto"/ready which is classified as [+telic] in our lexicon: it indicates that a certain process has ended, and the sentence as a whole is computed as an event even though the verb BE, a stative, is present. As a result of the computation, "ready" is assigned as an attribute of the hut, this in turn is also a "house" and is subsumed under the previous set of houses. In this utterance we also learn that the three little pigs are actually also little brothers: by stating that one of them "timmy" is the possessors of "fratellini"/little brothers, we understand that all of them are little brothers. The relation property of brotherhood is in fact a reflexive property.

[in breve la casetta fu pronta e timmy decise allora di andare a vedere che cosa stavano facendo i suoi fratellini]
fact(infon189, isa, [ind:id2, class:fratello], 1, id40, id19)
fact(infon190, relat, [fratello, id14, id2], 1, id40, id19)
fact(infon203, pronto, [nil:id27], 1, id40, id19)
fact(id39, essere, [prop:infon203], 1, tes(f6_pig05), id19)
fact(infon208, isa, [arg:id41, arg:breve], 1, tes(f6_pig05), id19)
fact(infon209, in, [arg:id39, nil:id41], 1, tes(f6_pig05), id19)
fact(infon214, focus, [arg:id42], 1, id40, id19)
fact(infon215, isa, [arg:id42, arg:cosa], 1, id40, id19)
sit(id43, fare, [agent:id38, arg:id42], 1, tes(f10_pig05), id19)
sit(id45, vedere, [perceiver:id14, propq:id43], 1, tes(finf2_pig05), id19)
sit(id47, andare, [agent:id14, prop:id45], 1, tes(finf1_pig05), id19)
sit(infon224, isa, [arg:id47, arg:ev], 1, tes(finf1_pig05), id19)
fact(infon225, isa, [arg:id48, arg:tloc], 1, tes(finf1_pig05), id19)
fact(infon226, pres, [arg:id48], 1, tes(finf1_pig05), id19)
sit(infon227, time, [arg:id47, arg:id48], 1, tes(finf1_pig05), id19)
fact(id49, decidere, [actor:id14, prop:id47], 1, tes(f9_pig05), id19)
fact(infon232, allora, [arg:id49], 1, tes(f9_pig05), id19)

In this utterance Tommy reappears, and his role is now introduced with a definite NP: this causes the interpreter to set up a new individual in the world associated to the role: this simply means that social or institutional roles, like these ones, corresponding to activities or jobs of a participant in a story may become relevant at a certain point of a story and if that happens, differently from what we did at the beginning of the story, they may live a life of their own in a separate ID.

[incontrò dapprima tommy il violinista]
ind(infon247, id51)
fact(infon248, violinista, [theme:id51], 1, id53, id19)
fact(infon249, role, [violinista, id12, id51], 1, id53, id19)
fact(id52, incontrare, [experiencer:id14, actor:id12], 1, tes(f6_pig06), id19)

fact(infon261, dapprima, [arg:id52], 1, tes(f6_pig06), id19)

Here again we have a new little house which is introduced with an indefinite NP, and is computed as being included in the previous set of houses. Notice that the material of which the house is made is also interpreted as an attribute. Even though we agree with the fact that it should live a life of its own, with possibly different attributes and properties from the ones of the final artifact, the house, it makes up, we find it difficult not to admit to the fact that there must be a very strict relationship between material and artifact. In other words, in case the wood which made up the little house was soaked wet or rotten, the final result is that the little house it makes up is also soaked wet and rotten.

[anche lui non aveva molta voglia di faticare così costruiva con dei pezzi di legno una semplice casetta]
ind(infon265, id54)
fact(infon266, piccolo, [ind:id54], 1, id60, id19)
fact(infon267, semplice, [ind:id54], 1, id60, id19)
fact(infon268, isa, [ind:id54, class:casa], 1, id60, id19)
fact(infon269, inst_of, [ind:id54, class:cosa], 1, id60, id19)
class(infon270, id55)
card(infon271, id55, some)
fact(infon272, pezzo, [ind:id55], 1, id60, id19)
sit(infon273, isa, [ind:id55, class:legno], 1, id60, id19)
class(infon274, id56)
card(infon275, id56, a_lot)
fact(infon276, isa, [ind:id56, class:voglia], 1, id60, id19)
fact(infon277, inst_of, [ind:id56, class:[stato, emotivo]], 1, id60, id19)
fact(infon300, voglia, [nil:id12], 1, id60, id19)
fact(id57, avere, [experiencer:id12, prop:infon300], 0, tes(f7_pig07), id19)
fact(infon305, anche, [arg:id57], 1, tes(f7_pig07), id19)
fact(id59, costruire, [agent:id12, theme_eff:id54], 1, tes(f10_pig07), id19)
fact(infon318, con, [arg:id59, nil:id54, matter:id55], 1, tes(f10_pig07), id19)
fact(infon319, così, [arg:id57, result:id59], 1, tes(f7_pig07), id19)

Also this little house is now ready.

[ben presto anche la casa di legno fu pronta]
fact(infon336, isa, [arg:id61, arg:legno], 1, id63, id19)
fact(infon337, di, [arg:id54, matter:id61], 1, id63, id19)
fact(infon338, pronto, [nil:id54], 1, id63, id19)
fact(id62, essere, [prop:infon338], 1, tes(f7_pig08), id19)

However, in this utterance a comparison is set up in order to assert the same attribute in the negative, to both little houses being built so far.

[come quella di paglia, non era certo molto resistente]
fact(infon347, resistente, [nil:id27], 0, id65, id19)

fact(infon348, resistente, [nil:id54], 0, id65, id19)
fact(id64, essere, [prop:infon348], 1, tes(f6_pig09), id19)

At this point of the story we know that two little pigs, who are lazy, have built their little house hastily and carelessly: the story now indicates their identity as a set, which being members now of the same set, share some if not many properties together. In turn, this set must be subsumed under the one made up of three little pigs which we encountered at the beginning of the story. This is all done as has been explained in the previous chapter, in the Discourse Module: however, a great part is also due to the interpretation of the plural definite NP with cardinality two. Notice that the two little pigs are never referred together in the previous portion of text and are now three or four utterances far back. So knowledge of the world is called for to individuate the two components of the set by means of an inference on the property "scansafatiche"/lazy-bones. Since the only information available is the one that comes from the previous text and has been stored in the DM, we want to express it in order to both clarify the word sense of "scansafatiche" but also in order to set the two individual entities apart. Thus the meaning associated with this property is included in the inferential trigger and roughly says that to be lazy-bones corresponds to not having pleasure in working hard or simply not liking to work. We see here the importance to express polarity within a meaning denotation.

infer_trig(scansafatiche, [avere(voglia,(faticare,1),0), piacere(_,(lavorare,1),0)]).

[ma i due porcellini scansafatiche se la erano sbrigata in poco tempo ed ora potevano tranquillamente divertirsi]
set(infon358, id66)
card(infon359, id66, 2)
fact(infon360, scansafatiche, [ind:id66], 1, id70, id19)
in(infon361, id66, id2)
fact(infon362, isa, [ind:id66, class:porcellino], 1, id70, id19)
in(infon363, id12, id66)
in(infon364, id14, id66)
fact(id67, sbrigarsi, [agent:id66], 1, tes(f8_pig10), id19)
fact(id69, divertirsi, [experiencer:id66], 1, tes(f11_pig10), id19)

It would seem that in order to make things clear, the two little pigs had to be recalled by their names, which is what happens in this very complex utterance. Notice that the empty little pro subject of the coordinate with the predicate "spassarsi", has been bound to split antecedents with the syntactic indices associated to the two subjects expressed as proper nouns in the previous simplex sentences. However, the interpreter looks for a set available in the previous text to corefer the split pronoun, by identifying their referents with the names expressed locally.

[mentre timmy suonava il suo flauto, tommy lo accompagnava con il suo violino e insieme se la spassavano allegramente]
fact(infon453, isa, [arg:id71, arg:violino], 1, id75, id19)
fact(infon454, poss, [arg:id71, poss:id12], 1, id75, id19)

fact(id72, accompagnare, [agent:id12, instrument:id71, tema_nonaff:id14], 1, tes(f9_pig11), id19)
fact(id76, suonare, [experiencer:id14, theme_unaff:id27], 1, tes(f6_pig11), id19)
fact(infon474, mentre, [prop:id72, temp_coinc:id76], 1, nil, id19)
fact(id74, spassarsi, [experiencer:id66], 1, tes(f11_pig11), id19)
fact(infon463, insieme, [arg:id74], 1, tes(f11_pig11), id19)
fact(infon464, allegramente, [arg:id74], 1, tes(f11_pig11), id19)
fact(id76, suonare, [experiencer:id14, theme_unaff:id27], 1, tes(f6_pig11), id19)
fact(infon474, mentre, [prop:id72, temp_coinc:id76], 1, nil, id19)

Now consider the following utterance where the two lazy little pigs are coreferred as set and the remaining little pig, Jimmy, wise and hard-working is coreferred al "fratellino"/little brother. In order to recover this information we need to find out who is the individual entity which is referentially disjunct from the other referring expression present in the same utterance which however is coreferred as a set and not as individual.

[poi stanchi di fare baldoria decisero di andare a vedere che cosa stava facendo il loro fratellino]
fact(infon490, stanco, [emotivo:id66], 1, id86, id19)
fact(infon499, isa, [ind:id13, class:fratello], 1, id86, id19))
fact(infon500, relat, [fratello, id66, id13], 1, id86, id19))
sit(id79, fare, [theme_unaff:id13], 1, tes(f10_pig12), id19)
sit(id81, vedere, [perceiver:id66, propq:id79], 1, tes(finf5_pig12), id19)
sit(id83, andare, [agent:id66, prop:id81], 1, tes(finf4_pig12), id19)
fact(id85, decidere, [actor:id66, prop:id83], 1, tes(f9_pig12), id19)
fact(infon524, isa, [arg:id87, arg:baldoria], 1, tes(f9_pig12), id19)
sit(id88, fare, [agent:id66, theme_unaff:id87], 1, tes(finf1_pig12), id19)
fact(infon529, stanco, [arg:id85, nil:id66, prop:id88], 1, tes(f9_pig12), id19)
fact(infon530, adj, [temp_seq:id85], 1, id86, id19)
fact(infon531, poi, [prop:infon530], 1, id86, id19)

And in the following utterance the little brother is coreferred by its name to make sure that everybody has understood it correctly:

[si misero in cammino e ben presto raggiunsero jimmy]
fact(infon558, isa, [arg:id90, arg:cammino], 1, id94, id19)
fact(id91, mettersi, [agent:id66, modal:id90], 1, tes(f6_pig13), id19)
fact(id93, raggiungere, [actor:id66, goal:id13], 1, tes(f9_pig13), id19)

The story introduces the last little house by a singular definite NP which however has the possessive "suo" explicitly expressed: this would be needed in any case for discourse wellformedness reasons. However, at this point of the story, we are faced with the problem of a singular definite NP cospecifying rather than coreferring a referent in the world. There is no little house belonging to Jimmy in the world at the moment, which is something that could also be gathered from the progressive construed with the verb "build", an accomplishment, thus indicating that the building process has not come to an end yet. But without resorting to such reasoning, which would however be available from conceptual representation and temporal interpretation, we simply assert that the little house is an individual in the world but not yet a fact.

[il bravo porcellino stava costruendo anche lui la sua casetta]
ind(infon574, id95)
in(infon575, id95, id20)
sit(infon576, isa, [ind:id95, class:casa], 1, id97, id19)
sit(infon577, poss, [jimmy, id13, id95], 1, id97, id19)
sit(id96, costruire, [agent:id13, theme_eff:id95], 1, tes(f6_pig14), id19)
fact(infon597, anche, [arg:id95], 1, tes(f6_pig14), id19)

At this point of the story it would seem that the Main Topic of discourse is clearly individuated: however, the name Jimmy is used instead of a pronoun or a property to continue. The new utterance is very interesting from a semantic point of view: it introduces the wolf as a definite NP and also discusses the properties of the house Jimmy is building as an intensional object. Jimmy "wanted/wished" a robust house: this use of an indefinite NP has been already discussed in the previous sections: the house now being referred to is the one Jimmy is wishing should be the outcome of the one he is currently building. So the net result of the interpretation process is that the house in Jimmy's intentions should be "sturdy". In other words, no new entity for the indefinite NP should be generated: the only addition to the model is a new property which however is a sit.

[jimmy voleva una casa robusta perché sapeva che il lupo cattivo viveva nel bosco vicino]
sit(infon655, robusto, [ind:id95], 1, id109, id19)
ind(infon656, id107)
fact(infon657, cattivo, [ind:id107], 1, id109, id19)
sit(infon658, isa, [ind:id107, class:lupo], 1, id109, id19)
fact(infon659, inst_of, [ind:id107, class:animale_feroce], 1, id109, id19)
fact(id108, volere, [agent:id13, theme_unaff:id106], 1, tes(f3_pig16), id19)
fact(id110, vivere, [actor:id107, locat:id19], 1, tes(f21_pig16), id19)
fact(id112, sapere, [actor:id13, prop:id110], 1, tes(f18_pig16), id19)
fact(infon713, perché, [arg:id108, cause:id112], 1, tes(f3_pig16), id19)

Utterance number 20 has a quantification on the event expressed by the main predicate "tornare/go back": we decided to interpret this fact by asserting the existence of a set of two houses here being referred to belonging to the two little pigs: the distributive reading is computed on the relation "tornare/go back" by the usual function, which in this case is a many_to_many.

[i due porcellini, sempre suonando e ballando, tornarono ciascuno alla propria fragile casetta]
loc(infon714, id134, [arg:main_sloc, arg:casa])
set(infon849, id134)
card(infon850, id134, 2)

in(infon859, id27, id134)
in(infon860, id54, id134)
fact(infon861, isa, [ind:id134, class:casa], 1, id136, id134)
fact(infon862, poss, [porcellini, id66, id134], 1, id136, id134)
fact(id135, tornare, [agent:id66, goal:id134], 1, tes(f5_pig20), id134)

In this way we are able to recover the reference to the little house which is however only indirectly coreferred in the following utterance by the referring expression "porta"/door, and explicitely in the next utterances:

[ma appena timmy aprì la porta, sbucò fuori dal bosco il lupo cattivo]
fact(infon878, part_of, [casa, id27, id141], 1, id139, id19)
fact(id138, sbucare, [agent:id107, locat:id19], 1, tes(f11_pig21), id19)
fact(infon886, isa, [arg:id140, arg:fuori], 1, tes(f11_pig21), id19)
fact(infon887, in, [arg:id138, locat:id140], 1, tes(f11_pig21), id19)
fact(infon890, isa, [arg:id141, arg:porta], 1, id139, id19)
fact(infon897, ma, [prop:id138, advers:id143], 1, id139, id19)

[il porcellino lo vide e tremante di paura si chiuse immediatamente in casa]
loc(infon918, id27, [arg:main_sloc, arg:casa])
fact(id146, vedere, [perceiver:id14, tema_nonaff:id107], 1, tes(f6_pig22), id27)
fact(infon923, isa, [arg:id145, arg:casa], 1, nil, id27)
fact(id148, chiudersi, [agent:id14, locat:id27], 1, tes(f11_pig22), id27)
fact(infon929, isa, [arg:id151, arg:paura], 1, tes(f11_pig22), id27)
fact(infon930, tremante, [arg:id148, nil:id14, cause:id151], 1, tes(f11_pig22), id27)

[il lupo cattivo cominciò a chiamarlo]
sit(id152, chiamare, [actor:id107, theme_unaff:id14], 1, tes(finf1_pig23), id19)
fact(id154, cominciare, [agent:id107, prop:id152], 1, tes(f6_pig23), id19)

[“apri la porta e fammi entrare nella tua casetta di paglia“]
sit(id158, entrare, [agent:id107, goal:id27], 1, tes(finf1_pig24), id19)
fact(id160, fare, [agent:id14, patient:id107, prop:id158], 1, tes(f5_pig24), id19)
fact(id162, aprire, [agent:id14, theme_aff:id141], 1, tes(f2_pig24), id19)

Chapter 3

INTERPRETING SPATIOTEMPORAL LOCATIONS

1. INTRODUCTION

In our model all entities and relations are assigned a spatiotemporal location which is made up of two indices: a temporal and a location index. In case of temporal index, we operate a bipartition and distinguish two types of temporal locations: in the case of individuals, the index is bound to the main temporal location. As to relations and modifiers of the main relation, the index for the time location is derived from the event/state time, i.e. TES. In turn, this index is in a given logical relation with the TES of the previous text span, the discourse focus: it may be BEFORE, AFTER, MEETS, OVERLAP etc. with it. The reference of the current TES is furthermore asserted to be included in some main temporal location which could be present in the previous text span. Thus, individuals receive directly a time index which bind their existence in the world and their properties, such as roles, or attributes, to some main temporal location; in case of names associated to individuals, we assign them to a universal location, in other words, we assume that in the domain specified by the text that name is used as a constant, and unambiguously refers to a single well defined individual. This bipartition is quite natural and intuitive: entities such as individuals or sets are assumed to be in a given location for a longer stretch of time than the actual relation in which they are currently involved. The latter might be a punctual event, thus having a very short duration in time. Event properties are thus different from entity properties as to their temporal location proper.

Temporal interpretation is computed compositionally from local features associated to verb tense and the static lexical label associated to aspect, plus a number of relevant information like definiteness of Subject NP, and of Object NP, plus their number. These features contribute to assigning a first dynamic aspectual label to the sentence in which the verbal predicate is analysed. This allows the system to compute local temporal relation intersententially, taking into adequate account all elements which can contribute to the definition of temporal relations, which are essentially taken from Reichenbach's proposal. This computation is added to the f-structure of each clause - we follow LFG theoretical framework, where it will have to face the complexity arising from the presence of subordinate, coordinate and complement clauses. Finally, the result of utterance temporal computation is passed on to the discourse module for temporal reasoning which is based on Allen's proposal (Allen, 1983). At this level, temporal intervals are generated and are attached at nodes in a cluster. The logical notation introduced by Allen is perspicuous enough to allow for the overall representation of discourse structure, where reference intervals are generated by taking into account local logical relations.

In the following sections, we discuss the relation intervening between distributivity and the participants in an event. We argue that there is a strict dependency between aspectual features and the quantificational properties of each participants in a given situation; we also argue for a distinction of events in terms of their polyadicity, or their number of arguments. In more general terms, we propose a principled way to deal with the problem of representing the structure of events and their relation with the situation and the participants in that situation.

At first we introduce a "static" description of predicates as conceptual representations in a computational lexicon, where event structure is expressed in terms of a combination of time "t" and event "e" which may assume a variable or a constant value according to aspectual class and to number and type of arguments of the governing predicate. We hypothesize internal quantification on the event-time only whenever a variable is associated with "t", and external quantification on the number of events only when a variable is associated with "e" in the static description.

Then we deal with "dynamic" quantificational properties of events which derive from syntactic and semantic properties of the utterance or situation in which they are contextualized. In this case we propose two main notions: "Global" and "Internal", that apply to event structure and establish a point of view by means of which to decide whether temporal interpretation affects the overall event, or only portions of it; the two notions are also related to factuality of the event, and to its perfectivity or telicity. Finally, we discuss the introduction of a function that relates participants in the event according to their quantificational nature and event structure. With respect to the subdivision of quantification into distributive and collective operators, we establish an inward and outward mapping from participants into the event.

2. Lexical Representation

At first we shall focus our attention on a particular problem pertaining to lexical semantics: the one of defining a lexical encoding adequate for the representation of event structure for event and state predicates. The lexical representation is regarded the static starting point to enable a text understanding system to compute final meaning representation where event or states may be assigned a dynamic interpretation according to syntactic and semantic properties of current utterance.

In our attempt we want to link features like aspectual and semantic inherent features belonging to a given predicate,, and quantification properties of event structure. This is however dealt with in a much deeper way in Book I – Chapt. 3. The concepts we will be tackling are ideas and theories put forward basically by Vendler (1967) and Jackendoff (1992), among others.

2.1. Conceptual Representations

The examples reported here are representatives of the various types of event structures generated in our computational lexicon:

derubare[CAUSE(<receiv>(GO(<possesn>(FROM<ex_owner>)))){(e1,tn),(e2,t2)]/rob
dimostrare[LET(<agent>(GO(REP(<theme_unaff>(TO<perciv_a>))))){(e1,tn)}]/show
contrastare[CAUSE(<agent>(GO(AGAINST<theme_aff><instr_con>))){(e1,t1)(e2,tn)}]/thw
art
costruire[CAUSE(<agent>(GO(TO[exist]<theme_eff>))){(e1,t1),e1,tn,(e2,t2)}]/build
esistere[BE(<theme_unaff>(STAYposit(AT))){(en,tn)}]/exist
bussare[CAUSE-iter(<agent>(GOtouch(TO[<theme_a>))){(en,t1)}]/knock
chiedere[LET(<address>(GO(REP(<informtn>(FROM<goal_a>)))){(e1,t1)}]/ask_for_inform
ation

The event structure is automatically generated from aspectual information and is made up of two basic components: "e" stands for "event" and may be a single constant identifier, for instance "e1"; a variable like "en"; or a split value, where the event is partitioned into more than one subevent ordered sequentially in time, "e1... e2".

The other component is "t", time, which can be represented again either as a single constant value, as a variable or as a split value. In all such cases we understand time to be made up of intervals as Allen(1983) proposes; we also assume that events must be spatiotemporally located or anchored as is usual in Situation Semantics(see references to Barwise, Cooper). Finally we end up with seven such structures in occurrence of some aspectual well defined characteristic which will be commented in the following section:

1. {(e1,tn),(e2,t2)} for achievements (with a preparatory phase)
2. {(e1,tn)} for activities
3. {(e1,t1),(e2,tn)} for ingressive accomplishments
4. {(e1,t1),(e1,tn),(e2,t2)} for accomplishments
5. {(en,tn)} for states
6. {(en,t1)} for iterable achievements
7. {(e1,t1)} for achievements (with focus on result) or result_state

In what follows we will try to motivate this kind of classification and to verify its validity in actual contexts of use.

3. Aspect and Lexical Features

The first topic we shall tackle is the procedure that assigns default classification to predicates in aspectual classes on the basis of syntactic classes. The main idea is a simple one: a transitive verb argument structure possesses an Agent as SUBJect an Affected Theme as OBJect and will be classified as an Accomplishment; the presence of an Unaffected Theme as Subject or as Object causes the verb to be classified as Stative. Unergatives are classified as

Activities since they lack an OBJect argument and unaccusatives as Achievements. In addition, reflexives are assigned the same class as their corresponding transitive base form and inherent reflexives are computed as Achievements with an Affected Theme as Subject. Ergatives and passives derive directly from transitive verbs, and have an Affected Theme as Subject. However, default classification is not enough to account for a more fine grained subdivision of lexical entries. For instance, transitives may be computed as Statives, Activities or Achievements according to the kind of event denoted by the predicate, as happens with perceptive verbs. In turn Achievements have been subdivided into subclasses in order to capture temporal inferences: one subclass, which may be called iterable achievement, overlaps with activities, and is used to account for predicates like: hiccup, sob, which does not result in a change of state, since, after a momentary change the subject recovers its previous state. Transitive verbs may then be computed as transformative irreversible achievement which require a complete irreversible change in the theme, as for instance with a verb like "kill": in this case, the role Effected Theme might be instantiated, as happens with verbs of creation like build, create, or perceptual verbs like notice which do not simply indicate a change of state, possession, position or perception or information but introduce a new entity in the world. Finally, Accomplishments which denote a single event protracted in time, a preparatory phase and a culmination, have also been subdivided into two subclasses one of which denotes an Eventuality, i.e. a set of identical events, rather than a single event. In case the Theme be expressed as a mass noun or as a plural NP, the eventuality is completed via a number of successive iteration of the same action, in order to affect the whole object: these are verbs like “accumulate books”, “wash the dishes”, “taste or cook something”, beat someone, screw, accompany, use, slice, help, feed, exercise, grow, water, drink, burn, follow, drive and so on.

Finally, we have the following combinations between syntactic and aspectual classes:

a. transitives: Ingressive Accomplishments;
b. transitives, unaccusatives: Irreversible Transformative Achievements;
c. unergatives: Iterable Achievements;
d. process verbs: Abortives; Continuatives; Completives; Iteratives.

These are the event representations proposed in Pustejovsky(1988), who subclassifies events as State, Process and Transition:

1. STATE(S): sick, love, know [S e]S
2. PROCESS(S): run, push, drag [P e1 ... en]P
3. SIMPLE TRANSITION: give, open, close [T e1 ... en]T
4. LOGICAL TRANSITION: build, draw, destroy [T [P* e1 ... en]P* e]T
5. CULMINATING TRANSITION: die, lose, win, arrive [T [P e1 ... en]P e*]T
6. PROCESS TRANSITION: throw, drop, mail, send [T [P e1 ... en]P e]T

Another interesting proposal is the one made by L. Talmy (2000: Vol.2, p.68), where he recognizes six types of aspectual types:

i. one-way nonresettable (for verbs like “die”)
ii. one-way resettable (for verbs like “fall”, “rise”)

iii. full cycle (flashing)
iv. multiplex (sets of full cycle events like processes)
v. steady states (for states)
vi. gradient (gradable changes like “widen”)

Our representation presented above is made up of seven subclasses rather than six, and captures the fundamental features underlying Pustejovsky's and Talmy’s argument, while organizing event structures in relation to temporal computation. Inferences can now be drawn as follows:

a. accomplishments give rise to inferences which view the affected theme in two different states, e1 at t1 when the Object existed in its primary unchanged state, and e2 at t2 after the action denoted by the predicate has been fully carried out, and the Object undergoes a change of state. Temporal interval is bounded both ends – at the beginning of the changing event and at the end. Intermediate events have no relevance even though they may have some, in case the action or the process is abruptly interrupted and the accomplishment is not carried out, so that the event “en” suddenly becomes relevant in the sense that if realized, it prevents e2 to be accomplished;
b. states, possess no internal structure – are temporally unbounded, even though they may be stopped;
c. achievements are made out of a indefinite number of preparatory events which however have no relevance: the "head" event is the final one, when something is actually achieved – so it is bounded at the end but not at the beginning;
d. activities have internal structure only from a temporal point of view in the sense that they possess the subinterval property: in case the activity is interrupted, say at tn=t3, the inference we draw is that the event has already taken place: they are internally homogenous. Temporally speaking the "head" event is at the beginning. In addition, we also want to infer that at an intermediate time, tn=t2<t3, the subject was engaged in that activity;
e. achievements-iterable, are just punctual achievements with no preparatory phase, which introduce no change of state in the world, in that the subject returns to its previous state every time the achievement is realized;
f. accomplishments-ingressive, whose "head" event is at the beginning. They have an eventuality structure which is usually an iteration of the same process but which, either does not imply that the change of state in the Object will actually take place, or it applies to a mass noun or a plural noun – they are gradable but not internally homogenous;
g. achievements with focus on result which present a new entity in the world and require that the final state has actually taken place at the interpretive level.
h. finally, accomplishments which do not only introduce a change of state but also introduce a new entity in the world, like "build, draw, create...", they make it to come into existence. They are the socalled “creation/destruction” predicates.

Inferences on spatio-temporal locations of the participants in the situation are computed after all syntactic and semantic computations have been successfully carried out.

4. Event Structure and Quantification

There is a further semantic dimension that must be highlighted in the process of interpreting the meaning of an event and this is strictly interrelated with its internal structure and with temporal interpretation. In the preceding section, we saw how tense specification may alter the import of aspect on the interpretation of the event constituted by the main verbal predicate: we analyzed each aspectual class and related it to properties like perfectivity and the subinterval property, which should belong only to events which have some internal structure, i.e. accomplishments and activities. However, we were forced to admit that in order to compute the overall meaning of a given event there is a number of elements like tense, definiteness of the NP Object, temporal adverbial adjuncts which contribute to modify semantic properties associated to the static lexical meaning of the main verbal predicate.

Event structure is used for quantifications on the event (see Delmonte,1994) which may affect either the time "t" or the event "e" in case they have "n" as index. Thus activities allow quantification on temporal extension, whereas iterable achievements on the number of events; quantification on achievements implies a repetition of the event at a different time location, or in case of achievements on the preparatory phase; accomplishments only allow quantification on the internal process. States allow quantification both on the number of events and on time extension. For instance an adverb like "little, much, enough" may quantify on time extension with activities, but it quantifies on events with iterable achievements:

1 i. Gino ha dormito poco/John has slept little
ii. Gino dorme spesso supino/John often sleeps supine
2 i. Gino ha tossito poco/John coughed little
ii. Gino tossisce spesso/John coughs often
3 i. Gino ha raggiunto in fretta/*abbastanza l'ufficio/John reached the office in a hurry/*enough
ii. Gino raggiunge spesso l'ufficio in fretta/John ofter reaches the office in a hurry
4 i. Gino ha scritto in fretta/*abbastanza l'avviso/John wrote in a hurry/*enough
ii. Gino scrive spesso l'avviso in fretta/John often writes the notice in a hurry
5 i. A Gino piace poco/spesso/John likes (it) little

Generally speaking, we assume that states and activities are distributive if not specified otherwise by some collective operator like "together"(see Lasersohn,1990). Generic statements with an explicit distributive marker, "each" indicate that there is a one to one mapping between its participants, for all occurrences of that relation in a given spatial location and for all temporal locations. As Lasersohn comments, the operator "together" may contribute in assigning a collectivizing interpretation to the relation, thus meaning that the participants are to be regarded as a group: our function will then be an "all-to-one". On the contrary, if we consider states such as "sit", and a sentence as "John and Mary were sitting", we want to infer that both John and Mary were in a given state, independently of one another. Motion predicates usually also must be understood as distributive in meaning: thus the sentence "John and Mary are running together", should be interpreted with the operator "together" indicating spatial or local proximity, i.e. as a function on spatial location rather than as a function on the main relation. Anyhow, both achievements and accomplishments require some knowledge to understand what is going on. Notice that the same selective import that "together" has, might be achieved by using comitative "with", as Lasersohn clearly shows.

Similar problems are discussed by Roberts C.(1990), where the distributive-group distinction is also viewed from the point of view of verb classes. The definition he gives is interesting and we report it below,

"The distributive reading may be triggered either by a quantificational determiner in the subject NP or by the presence of an explicit or implicit adverbial distributivity operator on the predicate. If a plural subject is nonquantificational (doesn't contain a quantificational determiner), we say that it is group denoting. A group reading arises when neither a group-denoting subject nor an adverbial element of its predicate contributes the quantificational force underlying distributivity."(ibid, 80).

In the following text, when dealing with a verb like GIVE which has a double object structure, Roberts notes how we are faced with fuzziness in case we want to specify the internal structure of an event, and there seems to be no fixed criteria to "denote an event", which makes it difficult to find a direct correlation between "truth conditions of such sentences and the number of events involved"(ibid.,81). Nonetheless we think it possible to divide up verbal predicates into classes denoting group/distributive readings, in lack of explicit quantified markers. These classes usually correspond to aspectual classes, as we already said above, with the exceptions of predicates containing lexical information as to their nature. Talking about this class of predicates R. mentions verbs like "walk, eat, talk, know, own, have, be" as inherently distributive predicates,, which he assumes to be distributive since they are "related to personal identity of individual will"(ibid., 88). However consider the case of

6. John and Mary own/have a beautiful car.

in case they are married, the coordination can only be understood as group. Clearly R. is not personally in favour of indicating specifically the semantic nature of a given predicate "since it will follow from the sense of the predicate itself", in this case following Dowty(ibid., 94). However, we believe that lexical classification is required and may help to reach an automatic classification of situations. In trying to find a theory for the group/distributive distinction on the properties of predicates, we surely need to take into account the contribution of adverbial modifiers and quantifiers, as well as of generic interpretations. As R. comments(ibid., 94), in case we are dealing with states and actions (in our terms, activities and processes), we understand a distributive predication simply because they deal with one single individual at a time. Some predicates are only understandable with a group reading: for instance a predication about a team, like winning a rally race are group predicates, and these might as well be encoded in the lexicon, contrary to what R. assumes, and thus derive directly from our knowledge of selectional restrictions on their use as in the case of simple predicates. In the same way we understand predicates like "disperse, walk together, be among" which require groups rather than individuals, and reciprocals which have also an additional number of semantic restrictions. Further on, we see that achievements and accomplishments with definite plural NP subjects, have a preferred group reading: they are "bring, carry, lift, leave, give, take, build". However, some have rather a distributive preferred reading: "ask, get up, wake up, vote". As said above, they require some knowledge on the nature of the participants in the events.

4.1. Events and Participants' Number

We might divide up utterances into two kinds, according to whether their subject is singular or plural; in addition, singular number might be overrun by quantified interpretation, in case we are dealing with a generic assertion. In order to decide whether we are in presence of a single event or multiple event, we then compositionally look for a second argument or participant in the event. In case there is none, we have a monadic predicate which receives its information directly from number specification: in a language like Italian, number might be only specified on verbal morphology and from there copied on to an empty pronominal subject. So in lack of information to the contrary, i.e. genericity or habituality, which could ensue from the presence of temporal adverbials, the event is interpreted as a "single_event" for singular number, or as a "multiple_event" for plural number, according to aspectual features - as we shall discuss below in more detail. The problem has been treated extensively in Stirling(1985), where distributive interpretation of individuals or events has however always been connected to the presence of some quantifier.

Also consider the contribution of tense which might be dubbed as follows:

i. the present progressive refers to an event that is part of/internal to an ongoing activity and so it is only computable with those events that have internal structure;
ii. ii. the simple present refers to and individual state of affairs that holds at a definite or indefinite point in time, so it is computable with those events like states; as for activities and accomplishments, these are also computable whenever they are construed as states, thus receiving a habitual, arbitrary or generic reading/interpretation.
iii. past tense refers to an event fully completed in the past, hence factual;
iv. future tense refers to an event yet to take place, hence non-factual.

Monadic predicates are verbs belonging to syntactic classes unaccusative, unergative, ergative, passive, reflexives, reciprocals, inherent_reflexives, impersonal: with these syntactic classes, the event is interpreted as single or as multiple according to subject NP number: singular NP subject induce a single event reading, while plural NP subject do the opposite. The distributive-group dichotomy is easily solved in favour of the distributive reading - with the only exception of reciprocals, as can be shown by the following examples:

7.a. John and Mary arrived at ten
b. John and Mary run all morning
c. The two boats sunk slowly / The two boys died yesterday
d. The two boys have been killed intentionally
e. The two houses have been built together
f. John and Mary are staring at themselves in the mirror
g. John and Mary are kissing each other
h. John and Mary got angry at the birthday party

i. John and Mary are easy to bribe

In case we add "together" at the end of each sentence we get different interpretations according to whether they are punctual or not: examples d. and h. might be understood as meaning a single "killing" event, or a single "getting angry" event. The reason lies in the fact that in both cases, the subject semantic role is interpreted as an Affected Theme and the focus is on the Change brought about by the existence of an unexpressed indefinite Agent implied by the event meaning and implicit in the lexical representation of the corresponding predicate argument structure. On the contrary, with ergative and inherent_reflexive (or inchoative) predicates, there is no Agent involved and we are focussing on the result_state itself and the introduction of "together" will contribute an interpretation by which the adverbial meaning quantifies over a spatial location, though lexically implied. Now consider a group quantification over the temporal location like "at the same time, contemporarily": only in the case of punctual predicates we get the right interpretation, which is also available with "together". The group interpretation is automatically produced in the case of the reciprocal g.

However, monadic predicates are only one possible type of predicates, and we can safely say that the great majority of verbal predicates are dyadic ones. In that case, determining the nature of the event requires control of each participants' number: in particular, we would like to state what is the relation existing between the two participants in the event, and the object NP with its semantic role are relevant in the determination of distributivity.

As the following examples show, unless there is some special marker for cumulative or collective reading, plural Objects contribute a distributive event reading with predicates allowing quantification on time “tn”, belonging to achievement (with preparatory phase), accomplishment, activity and ingressive accomplishment classes:

8.a. John killed three pigs this morning
b. John reached the top of three mountains last year
c. John built/painted three houses last year
d. John ate three sandwiches this morning
e. John read three pages this morning/three newspapers this morning
f. John washed three cups this morning
g. John ran five times around the house

Plural objects contribute a collective reading with stative and with iterable achievement predicates:

9.a. John loved three women
b. John knocked twice at the door

Perceptual predicates are a subclass of stative predicates which however induce an ambiguous reading very much like result_states:

c. John saw three girls this morning/three flowers in his garden
d. John heard three sonatas this morning/three people talk in his neighbour's flat

Finally, they contribute an ambiguous reading with result_state achievements:

10.a. John met three friends this morning
b. John noticed three Mayan books this morning/at Dillon's this morning
c. John found three pencils this morning/ three pencils in his pocket this morning

We use simple past tense which has a unifying import on the predicate event meaning; in case we used progressive and simple present – substituting "now" with "last year"-, all examples under 8) and 9) remain the same, but those under 10) disambiguate their meanings according to factual conditions determined by our knowledge of the world. In any case, the result we get is to force the collective reading, where possible: notice that real punctual predicates like "find, see, notice" don't allow internal views, i.e. progressive tense.

With dyadic predicates, this information is combined with the one deriving from the interpretation of the object NP and aspectual classes of the predicate. Consider now what happens when the object is a singular definite NP:

11.a. Three bandits killed John this morning
b. Three climbers reached the top of the mountain last summer
c. Three friends woke John this morning
d. Three friends built that house last year
e. Three friends love that woman

With temporally bounded predicates, achievements (with preparatory phase) and accomplishment only one event is understood; in particular with accomplishment, the global view implies a collective reading of the "building of the house" event, even though the process of building itself might have been distributed among the three friends. The same applies to stative predicades: the loving event can only be interpreted collectively as a single identical state in which three friends found themselves.

On the contrary, ingressive accomplishments have a different preferred reading, even though they finally must be computed as one single event. In other words, we understand that: there is one single accomplishment - in turn, the house painted, the one sandwich eaten, the one beer drunk, the one page read, the one cup washed - but also that the process has been partitioned, divided up among the three agents at different times:

12.a. Three friends painted that house last year
b. Three friends ate one sandwich this morning
c. Three friends drank one beer this morning
d. Three friends read one page this morning/one newspaper this morning
e. Three friends washed one cup this morning

Finally, punctual achievements or result_states as we call them, induce distributive reading, in line with our representation that does not allow quantification internally but only globally:

13.a. Three friends noticed that book this morning/at Dillon's this morning
b. Three friends found that pencil this morning/in their pocket this morning
c. Three friends saw that girl this morning/that flower in the garden
d. Three friends heard the sonata this morning/the man talk in the neighbour's flat

As before, we comment on the possibility to interpret the examples under 11), 12) and 13) with progressive and simple present, and the temporal adjunct substitution. The unit of time in the "now" induces collective readings for all predicates that allow these tenses.

More examples could be made up with indefinite NPs: however, we take examples with indefinite NPs in subject position to be equivalent to the ones we already commented with a definite NP, simply because we tend to compute indefinite subject NPs as specific, but then for some classes of predicate the event may be quantified on. So we shall only present examples with indefinite NPs as OBJect.

14.a. Three bandits killed a man this morning
  b. Three climbers reached the top of a mountain last summer
  c. Three boys saw a girl this morning/a flower in the garden
  d. Three boys heard a sonata this morning/a man talk in the neighbour's flat
  e. Three boys washed a cup this morning
  f. Three boys met a man this morning
  g. Three boys noticed a book this morning/a book at Dillon's this morning
  h. Three friends painted/built a house last year
  i. Three friends read a page this morning/a newspaper this morning

The previous examples have all ambiguous interpretations. However in the following example, related to stative, again we only get one possible meaning: they are all in the same loving state, with the same woman, at the same time, a necessarily collective interpretation:

15.a. Three men love a woman

On the contrary, with result_states we get a distributive interpretation as preferred reading:

16.a. Three friends ate a sandwich this morning
  b. Three friends drank a beer this morning
  c. Three men found a pencil this morning/in the pocket this morning

Also, notice that since the indefinite NP is not spatially linked, there is always a different reading available, due to the simultaneous happening of the event reported. Thus punctual and stative predicates are all distributionally readable with different individuals of the same class in different locations, though. The same reasonings can be made in case we change tenses from simple past to simple present and present progressive. In this case, the Quantized NP internal argument or OBJect interacts more closely with scoping of the plural cardinal NP "three men" overriding the static interpretation afforded by lexical representations.

Procedurally speaking, distributivity is added in the model as a function, which should be built up compositionally. Starting from the first argument, we may have the following encoding:

17.a. "all" for plural/or mass NP with collective reading;
  b. "many" for plural NP with distributive reading;
  c. "one" for singular NP and for generic reading.

As a result we might end up with the following typology:

18. distributive reading
    1. many_to_one
    2. many_to_all
    3. one_to_many
    4. many_to_many
19. collective reading
    1. all_to_one
    2. all_to_many
    3. one_to_all
    4. one_to_one
    5. all_to_all

It is reasonable to assume at this point, that the interaction between our two parameters, Global and Internal, may be filtered by this mapping, and that the interpretation may result from the interaction with the proposals put forward above. The typology we created, represents a much finer-grained distinction of the mapping between participants and event which may be ascribed to quantificational properties of the external argument, the Subject, plus properties of the Object argument and may possibly be extended to properties of Indirect Object, Obliques and locative and temporal Adjuncts. Since these properties are already encoded and realize one kind of mapping, the interpretative process is much more straightforward.

4.2. Global vs Internal: Two Features for Event Structure

The interaction of the syntactic realization of arguments of a predicate with its aspectual properties must then be filtered through the additional contribution made by tense. Constraints coming from aspectual classes interact with tense specifications and with the syntactic realization of arguments to give as a final result a bipartition into two main interpretive classes for the whole utterance: these classes have been traditionally discussed in the literature as the perfective/imperfective opposition. We shall reformulate this subdivision in the following section by two different but related features, global vs internal view. We shall now discuss the nature of this bipartition from a traditional perspective.

The perfective/imperfective opposition can be considered a universal linguistic principle, which can find different realizations in the verb or lexical case systems of particular languages. Perfectivity indicates the view of a situation as a single whole, without distinction of the various separate phases that make up that situation, while the imperfective pays essential attention to the internal structure of the situation.

This conceptual distinction obviously applies to any situation described in any natural language, regardless of how or if a particular linguistic code may express it morphologically, syntactically or lexically. Dahl incorporates the concept of boundedness in that of perfectivity:

"... a perfective verb will typically denote a single event, seen as an unanalyzed whole, with a well-defined result or end-state, located in the past. More often than not, the event will be punctual or, at least, it will be seen as a single transition from one state to its opposite, the duration of which can be disregarded..."(1984:13).

As appears from the context, Dahl applies perfectivity to past situations. It stems from the observation that virtually all the languages screened in the survey have both perfective and imperfective forms to refer to the past but use mainly the imperfective ones to refer to the present. This is a direct consequence of the fact that a situation described in a perfective form is perceived as bounded, that is to say as having a definite result or endpoint. Present situations have not reached an end when they are communicated and consequently cannot normally be considered as bounded. Only momentary actions may be taken to have already reached an endpoint when they are described, and thus a number of languages express them in the perfective. For the same reason, it is also quite common to use perfective forms for performative verbs and for descriptions in the so-called historical present.

The property of boundedness associated with perfective descriptions allows far-reaching generalizations. Only accomplishments and achievements, in fact, express by definition bounded actions, since they represent events that bring about a specific result or that have a definite end. Thanks to this property, they are often labelled aspectually as [+telic]. Activities and states, on the other hand, are [-telic], since they specify no goal to be reached. Thus, predicates belonging to the latter two verb classes are expected to behave differently from accomplishments and achievements when they are in a perfective form (if they can appear in such a form at all). We shall check this prediction by means of a few examples. In English, the perfective/imperfective opposition is realized mainly in the verb system. The Simple Past Tense, for instance, is aspectually marked as [+perfective], while the Past Progressive is imperfective, that is to say [-perfective]. Thus, a sentence like:

20. Helen wrote a letter at 11 o'clock

conveys a perfective view of the accomplishment, whose internal constituency is not analysed. According to the definition of perfectivity given above, the duration of a perfective event is disregarded. This stands out clearly in 20, since the process of writing a letter has intrinsic duration and Helen was presumably still engaged in it at some time after 11 o'clock; however, the perfective form of the verb is compatible with a punctual temporal expression, which proves that the accomplishment is perceived as having virtually no duration.

The same accomplishment can be described by using an imperfective form, as in:

21. Helen was writing a letter at 11 o'clock.

Here the process is considered without any reference to the attainment of its endpoint. The imperfective aspect can then be exploited to emphasize the duration of an event, forcing the hearer to concentrate on its internal structure rather than on its result.

The examples considered confirm that an accomplishment can be described either in a perfective or in an imperfective form without any special restriction. The aspect actually used therefore corresponds to a choice operated by the speaker. Achievements are also [+telic] and are consequently expected to behave in a similar way with respect to the aspectual category of perfectivity. However, while iterable achievements can be viewed internally - like "knock" -, real achievements can't. Achievements capture either the inception - like "find, lose" - or the climax of an act with some preparatory phase, and therefore have no duration at all. If an achievement is instantaneous, its beginning virtually coincides with its end. This implies that an achievement entails its result and therefore, from a linguistic point of view, its internal constituency is irrelevant.

The only way in which achievements can be considered as imperfective, that is to say as having no completion, is either to take into consideration a sequence of them or to focus on the time immediately preceding their realization. Thus:

22. The bus was stopping

can be paraphrased as: "The bus was about to stop". In this case, the achievement is the endpoint, the final instant of the time interval considered. Something may still occur at RT or between RT and the achievement time that prevents the achievement from happening.

It is difficult to see how an activity, which is [-telic] since it describes an event that involves no culmination or specific result, can be considered as "an unanalyzed whole, with a well-defined result or end-state". The acceptability of sentences like:

23. John ran at 11 o'clock,

however, forces us to conclude that also activities can appear in perfective forms. It must be noticed that the perfective form somehow limits the activity: in 23., the invited inference is that John participated in a particular running-event at 11 o'clock. The sentence would also be appropriate if it were the case that John ran for some time at about 11 o'clock. The run is then seen as a temporally limited event whose duration is not important, so that it can be conceived as contemporaneous with the punctual RT expressed by the temporal adverbial. Nevertheless, not all activity verbs can appear in the same context, as exemplified by:

24. *Helen wrote at 11 o'clock.

The parallel imperfective sentences, on the other hand, are perfectly normal, as proved by:

25. Helen was writing at 11 o'clock.
26. John was running at 11 o'clock.

This is not exceptional, since nothing prevents an activity from being expressed in an imperfective form. It is in fact an essential feature of imperfectivity that it does not entail the completion of the event described.

Sentences like 26, however, prove that activities can occur in the Simple Past, which we defined as a perfective tense. One may want to dismiss 23. as an accomplishment use of an activity verb (especially if it is taken to mean that John took part in a sports event), but sentences like the following can only express genuine activities:

27. (What did you do at the party?) We danced.

The English Simple Past can also convey an imperfective meaning for the occasion: 27. refers to a single activity, located in the past and seen as an unanalysed whole, whose duration is disregarded. The PP "at the party", and perhaps the perfective form itself, specifies that the activity corresponds to a particular, bounded situation. All the requirements of perfectivity are therefore met, since, even though there is no defined result of the action, its endpoint is implicit in the utterance. In fact, if it is assumed that a situation is a state, an activity, an accomplishment or an achievement not because of its ontology but simply because language describes it as belonging to one of these four categories, then situations are not in themselves perfective or imperfective: they are described by our linguistic codes as such, and different codes may present conspicuous dissimilarities.

State verbs are similar to those describing activities in that they are [-telic] and may be expected to display a similar behaviour when they are in a tense aspectually marked as [+perfective] such as the Simple Past. However, while it is clear that not all activities can appear in a perfective form, stative verbs generate perfectly acceptable sentences when they appear in the Simple Past, as exemplified by:

28. John was young
29. John was in London
30. John had a cat
31. Methuselah lived 969 years.

Yet, not all the sentences 28-31 are undoubtedly perfective. In fact, only the verb in 31. is unequivocally [+perfective], since it expresses a past state with a well-defined duration, seen as an unanalysed whole. Examples 28-30 describe past states whose internal constituency is not analysed either, but lack the boundedness of 31. Thus, it is impossible to say whether these sentences are perfective or imperfective, as they present properties of both aspectual categories. They can then be assumed to be ambiguous between a perfective and an imperfective interpretation.

Coming now to temporal adverbials, we see that frequency adverbials yield unacceptable sentences if they modify permanent states, i.e. states that in the natural course of things cannot end before the death or disintegration of the subject, or irreversibly transformative achievements, as shown by,

32. *John is tall every day.
33. *John often kills Mary.

As various verbs can express either activities or accomplishments in different contexts, several tests have been worked out to separate the former from the latter. They all show that ADJuncts are an essential component of the temporal-aspectual representation and of the inferential processes.

34.a. ?John painted a picture for an hour.
b. John painted a picture in an hour.
c. It took John an hour to paint a picture (accomplishment).
35.a. John walked for an hour.
b. *John walked in an hour.
c. ?It took John an hour to walk (activity).

Even though 34a and 34b can be accepted in some contexts, their meaning is very different from that of their more common counterparts. 34a can in fact be roughly paraphrased as: "John painted at a picture for an hour", meaning that John did not paint a whole picture; while 34b means that John did paint the picture. Analogously, 35a implies that John had a walk, while 35b could only mean that it took him an hour to start walking. The paraphrases in c. with "take an hour to.." apply then naturally to the grammatical and most acceptable examples, i.e. 34b. and 35a. This test brings to the light a peculiarity of accomplishments, since stative verbs cannot appear in this construction and achievements are interpreted semantically like activities:

36. *It took John an hour to know the answer.
37. It took John an hour to notice the painting.

Another interesting case is the use of "interrupt" which fits naturally with activities and accomplishment, giving however different inferences. In,

38. John was walking when he was interrupted.

we imply that "John walked"; while from:

39. John was painting a picture when he was interrupted.

it is inferred that: "John did not paint a picture". As achievements capture either the inception or the climax of an event, they are represented by language as having virtually no duration. This is the basic concept that underlies the tests for achievement verbs:

40. John noticed the painting in ten minutes.

entails: "Ten minutes elapsed before John noticed the painting", rather than:" *John was noticing the painting during ten minutes".

5. Factuality and the Structure of Events

Factuality can be regarded as the main features that contribute to the meaning conveyed by an event. In other words we want to ascertain whether a given event has actually taken place in a given spatiotemporal location, and whether it has come to an end or not. This is clearly orthogonal to the interpretation of the participants in the event: in case the event is not factual, then some of its internal arguments may not be factual themselves. Also, in case the event is not completed, we may have to assume that some of its internal arguments are not "completed", or are entities not fully realized in the world. In particular, both states and activities may point to bounded spatiotemporal locations, and their events are thus fully completed in the past, for instance. As to achievements we saw that they might be viewed from the moment immediately preceding their realization, thus indicating that some goal may not have taken place. Also accomplishments, having clear internal structure, may indicate events which have begun, or are in the course of realization but are not completed: in this case, some entity may be in completion and being not fully realized does not constitute a factual individual. A number of inferences should be drawn in the model whenever some of these event structures are realized: in particular, an event may continue a previous ingressive event, in case it is an accomplishment; an event may complete a previous incomplete event; states and activities may have an end and a change of state/activity may take place with an egressive or completive process verb like "end, finish". In addition, all four classes may constitute habitual and/or iterated events, or even generic events, which however are non factual.

In line with the subdivision of predicates into perfective and non perfective discussed in the section above, we make the hypothesis that there are two features by which events contribute to the interpretation of the clause in which they are contained: Internal vs Global. The internal view only allows us to see one interval of the global event, whereas the global view gives us a complete view of the whole event. In turn, the internal view may be specified as Internal-Ingressive in case the event has just begun, or Internal-Egressive in case it is almost finishing. In addition, we need an Internal-Iterated, for iterable events when viewed from an internal view; and a Global-Iterated for iterated events viewed globally. Finally, Global-Nonfactual for all generic and habitual events, but also for intensional predicates, conditionals, and those expressing some modality. We also need an Internal-Nonfactual for all accomplishments which express and event that has not come to an end, thus implying that its internal argument cannot be computed as a factual entity in the world. Finally we need a Global-Egressive and a Global-Process for characterizing the type of event where a process verb governs a semantic lexical predicate, modifying its meaning concurrently.

Thus, we ended up with ten possible classes of events which should allow us to express all possible combinations of meaning compositionally built from tense, aspect, temporal adverbs and other elements of the proposition under analysis. We shall now illustrate with examples how the classification captures the relevant features of event structure.

A. Internal-Egressive -> Only with achievements with a preparatory phase

41a. The bus was stopping. - b. L'autobus si stava fermando / *L'autobus stava fermando

c. John is killing a woman.

d. John is dying.

e. When I arrived at the station, my friends were leaving. - f. Quanto il treno partì, Gino stava arrivando.

In Italian, the inchoative inherent reflexive class of the same underlying verb should be chosen. "Fermare" does not possess an ergative alternation, which could allow the required egressive reading.

B. Internal -> Only process verbs

42a. John is running.

b. John was being a fool.

c. John was walking when he was interrupted.

d. John was painting a picture when he was interrupted.

e. John was running at 11 o'clock.

f. John is drinking (a beer).
g. John is loading hay on the truck.
h. John loves Mary.

As we noted above, with the exception of b. which is only allowed in English - and marginally - the remaining cases regard verbs with time as a variable (tn), i.e., we are viewing always activities and accomplishments. States, since do not have temporal boundaries always allow internal views: however the examples has at least two possible interpretations: 1. John loves Mary now; John is involved in a loving state with Mary and this lasts for an unbounded time period.

C. Global -> All classes are allowed

43a. The bus has been stopping all the time.
b. John painted a picture (in an hour /at 11 o'clock.).
c. John walked (for an hour / at 11 o'clock).
d It took John an hour to notice the painting.
e. John hit a woman.
f. John knocked at the door (at 11 o'clock).
g. (What did you do at the party?) We danced.
h. John was young / in London.
i. John has/had a cat.
l. John lived 969 years.
m. John loved Mary.
n. John sang (Hey Jude)/ for hours.
o. John read stop on the traffic lights.

Notice that the use of simple past may override static specification for lexical entries like stative "love", or activity "sing" and generate a bounded reading of the event.

D. Global-Iterative -> Only temporally bounded events

44a. John discovered quaint little villages for years.
b. John hit every woman/(all) the women.
c. John ran every morning last week.

Activities may be included but not stative verbs.

E. Internal-Iterative -> Only with iterable achievements

45a. The light is flashing
b. John was knocking at the door at 11 o'clock.
c. John is hitting a woman

F. Internal-Ingressive -> All classes allowed except for punctual achievements

46a. The two little pigs began to run as fast as they could.
b. John started to love music when he was a child.
c. Le patate hanno iniziato a bollire./The potatoes have started to boil.
d. John started to collect his books.
e. John started writing a book this morning.

f. John started to understand what she said.

G. Internal-Nonfactual -> Only with accomplishments (non-gradual).

47a. John is building a house.
b. John is loading a truck with hay.
c. Jimmy began to build his little house.

H. Global-Nonfactual -> All classes

48a. John will love Mary.
b. John wants (to buy) a car.
c. John plays football every weekend.

I. Global-Egressive -> Only for (ingressive) accomplishment

49a. John finished reading his book
b. John finished washing the dishes

L. Global-Process -> All process verbs

50a. John stopped/continued loving Mary
b. John stopped/continued reading
c. John stopped/continued building his house
d. John stopped/continued washing the dishes

Stopping the process involved in an accomplishment implies the denial of the factual realization of the event; on the contrary, continuing a process in an accomplishment instantiates a new starting point in time. As to activities and statives, an end point or a lower boundary in the time interval related to the predicate meaning is imposed at the current reference time.

From a cursory view at each classification, we may conclude that there is a strong relationship between broad aspectual classes and factuality. Thus we may group the above classes into two subgroups: 1. Global-Nonfactual, Internal-NonFactual, Global-Process, on the basis of which Factuality depends; the remaining classes, which determine features of the interpretation. The question we pose ourselves now, is the following one: what are the interpretive properties of these classes, and are the two basic parameters semantically founded?

Krifka (1992),proposes to define general interpretive conditions for event structures from the similarity in semantic behaviour between nominal and verbal predicates. He postulates the existence of two reference classes, Cumulative and Quantized, by which verbal and nominal expressions are assigned a denotation: this is achieved by a purported semantic similarity of their underlying concepts. Thus, Cumulative concepts have an interpretation by which no set terminal point may be assumed for events; in the same way, if we assume a spatial mapping for objects, we may say that there is no set border for Cumulative objects. The same reasoning, in reverse, may be applied to Quantized concepts related to events and to objects. A number of properties may then be associated with these two classes and a number of restrictions will apply to event types from the interpretation of objects: for instance, Uniqueness of Object requires Uniqueness of Event, i.e. if I drink a glass of wine, there will only be one drinking event, even though the drinking event may be characterized internally by a number of subevents which however must have the same Set Terminal Point, and these are all interpretable as part of the overall Unique event of drinking. However, if I drink wine, there will be no Uniqueness of Object and consequently no Uniqueness of event. In the former case a Quantized Object restricts the interpretation of the event as being Quantized; in the latter case a Cumulative Object restricts the interpretation of the event as being Cumulative. The core of the interpretative scheme is thus the part-of relation which can be postulated for Quantized concepts, as opposed to Cumulative concepts, in relation to the notion of temporal and spatial constitution of an Object which is qualifiable as possessing a Set border, and for an Event a Set terminal point in case it belongs to Quantized concepts.

The two notions introduced by Krifka are important, but are not sufficient in our view to interpret all the features present in event structures of a given context or situation. A number of theoretical consequences will then carry over to a mapping of the internal or patient participant of the event in terms of Thematic Relations, which will have to specify Graduality, Summativity and Uniqueness of event in order to attain the final labelling. In this case, we may notice that information must be supplied by the lexical representation of each verbal predicate: in particular in order to differentiate stative perception verbs like SEE from achievements like TOUCH which will classify their internal argument as STIMULUS and as AFFECTED OBJECT respectively in the former and the latter case.

Even though we believe Krifka's paper has quite a number of important insights into the relation between events and objects, we take it to be only a preliminary and insufficient treatment of the questions to be solved which are listed in our classification above. We shall now turn to Cooper's paper, which is cast into situation semantics and is much closer to our framework than Krifka's. In Cooper's paper there is a first subdivision of Eventuality, a superconcept, into States and Events

i. An eventuality E is a history where there is some f_l in E such that for all f'_l in E, l' is temporally included in l.
ii. An eventuality is a state if its facts contain only unlocated individuals; it is an event if its facts contain only located individuals
iii. An event is an activity if it contains more than one fact; it is an accomplishment otherwise.
iv. An accomplishment with member f_l is an achievement in a history h, if there is no other fact f'_l in h where l' is temporally included in l.

As it may be seen, he ties his definitions to broad aspectual classes: however, stativity is derivable from the interaction of factuality, aspectual classes, verb typology and tense, in particular when progressive tense is used. Then he introduces a hierarchy of concepts related to event structure, where the higher concept, the History is recursively defined as eventuality in case some internal lower condition applies. In turn, states and events are defined in terms of spatiotemporal location. He formulates a condition on statives which is partially extended to activities in a second axiom,

v. **Conditions on statives: Independence of space**
If r is a stative relation then any realized history which contains the fact
$(l, r, x_1, ..., x_n, 1)$

also contains the fact
$(l',r, x'_1, ..., x'_n, 1)$
where l' is the spatial extension of l to include all space.

vi. **Temporal ungroundedness**
If r is a stative or activity relation then any realized history which contains the fact
$(l,r, x_1, ..., x_n, 1)$
also contains the fact
$(l',r, x'_1, ..., x'_n, 1)$
for some l' properly temporally included in l.

The basic logical mechanism is the inclusion relation, which may apply to spatial and/or temporal locations between two realizations of the same relation in different spatiotemporal location within a history. From these two first definitions, we may note that stativity possess two distinguishing properties, i.e. independence of space and temporal ungroundedness, whereas activities only possess one property, i.e. temporal ungroundedness. Events or non stative relations have distinguishing properties partly derivable from the previously defined conditions and partly depending on their peculiar status: in particular, histories may not contain two contradictory facts,

vii. **Spatial extendability**
If r is a non stative relation then any realized history which contains the fact
$(l,r, x_1, ..., x_n, 1)$
does NOT also contain the fact
$(l',r, x'_1, ..., x'_n, 0)$
for any l' properly temporally including l'.

Then, achievements and accomplishments are differentiated according to the internal structure of the event, with properties that partially overlap, as follows,

viii. **Conditions on achievements: Punctuality**
If r is an achievement relation then any realized history which contains the fact
$(l,r, x_1, ..., x_n, 1)$
does not contain ANY fact with any l' properly temporally contained in l.

ix. **Temporal groundedness**
If r is an accomplishment relation then any realized history which contains the fact
$(l,r, x_1, ..., x_n, 1)$
does NOT also contain the fact
$(l',r, x'_1, ..., x'_n, 1)$
where l' is properly temporally contained in l.

As a final comment on the properties of states and events, he gives the following definitions:

x. If something is an activity, then it is neither an accomplishment nor an achievement
xi. If something is an accomplishment, then it is not an activity (though it may be an achievement)
xii. If something is an achievement, then it is an accomplishment (but not an activity)

6. Inferring Spatial Locations

As said at the beginning of this chapter, spatial locations in narrative texts and newspaper articles might vary according to the presence of one or more participants. In our stories both situations may be found: Avveduti's story is all located in Verona, even though more than one participant is present. On the contrary, the story of the three little pigs has a very high number of locations which may change according to what each character is doing in the story. Consider again the translated text which we report here below and where we highlight spatial locations:

Once upon a time there were three little pigs who lived happily *in the countryside*. But **in** *the same place* lived a wicked wolf who fed precisely on plump and tender pigs. The little pigs therefore decided to build a small house each, to protect themselves from the wolf. The oldest one, Jimmy who was wise, worked hard and built his house with solid bricks and cement. The other two, Timmy and Tommy, who were lazy settled the matter hastily and built their houses with straw and pieces of wood. The lazy pigs spent their days playing and singing a song that said, "Who is afraid of the big bad wolf?" And one day, lo and behold, the wolf appeared suddenly behind their backs. "Help! Help!", shouted the pigs and started running as fast as they could to escape the terrible wolf. He was already licking his lips thinking of such an inviting and tasty meal. The little pigs eventually managed to reach *their small house* and shut themselves in, barring the door. They started mocking the wolf from the window singing the same song, "Who is afraid of the big bad wolf?" In the meantime *the wolf* was thinking a way of getting into the house. He began to observe the house very carefully and noticed it was not very solid. He huffed and puffed a couple of times and the house fell down completely. Frightened out of their wits, the two little pigs ran at breakneck speed towards their brother's house. "Fast, brother, open the door! The wolf is chasing us!" They got **in** just in time and pulled the bolt. Within seconds *the wolf* was arriving, determined not to give up his meal. Convinced that he could also blow the little brick house down, he filled his lungs with air and huffed and puffed a few times. There was nothing he could do. The house didn't move an inch. In the end he was so exhausted that he fell *to the ground*. The three little pigs felt safe *inside the solid brick house*. Grateful to their brother, the two lazy pigs promised him that from that day on they too would work hard.

The story sets the main spatial location right at the beginning, in the "countryside". In the second utterance the story introduces a new character which not necessarily is in the same location: however, this is explicitly stated. Thus, the same location is asserted and maintained up to the point in the story in which houses have been built and they can become suitable locations for the little pigs. At first the current location for the set of two lazy little pigs is their little house. When the perspective moves to the wolf, the spatial location returns to the previous one in which the wolf was located in preceding stretch of text, and we highlighted this by italicizing the wolf. Then again a change in perspective, and the two lazy little pigs are the current topics of discourse: no location is actually expressed and the system assumes that the current location is the one that they share with other character in focus, the wolf. Suddenly, they manage to "get in" somewhere. We understand that they entered their little brother's little house, even though this is not explicitly stated in the text. In order to infer the current location, we recover some previous relation in which the two lazy little pigs where involved as subject/actor directing themselves towards some location: this is the "running" event in one of the previous utterances. In this way, we may safely infer that now they entered the house they were running towards, i.e. their brother's little house. Again, a change of perspective and the wolf is highlighted: he is not in the same location as the little pigs, and no explicit location is present in the current utterance. Thus we assume that the wolf is again in the same location he was before. Notice now that a location is expressed, "to the ground": but this is not to be computed as a new location, in as far as the ground is included as part of the main current location, "the countryside". This clearly constitutes external world knowledge, which is present in our domain knowledge. Finally, the perspective moves again to the three little pigs which are in the solid brick house: this is the location previously associated to the two lazy little pigs. Recency, is activated in order to compute the right association.

At this point we might state the following rule for spatial locations:

6.1. Inferential Rule for Spatial Locations

Topic-consistency: A location should be consistent with the current topic

A. Old Locations : there is a previous main location to be asserted.

CASE 1 - No location is explicitly expressed in the current utterance

- The current location is topic-inconsistent, an old location should be recovered
- Infer a suitable location for the current topic from the previous stretch of text
- The topic changes but the previous location is deictically assigned to the new topic

CASE 2 - There is a location explicitly expressed in the current utterance

- The new location has already been associated with the current topic in the previous stretch of text
- The new location is inferentially included in the current main location
- The new location is inferentially a suitable location which came into existence in the previous stretch of text

B. New Locations : a new main location is asserted

1. Assert a new location whenever it is explicitly stated in the current utterance.

7. The Algorithm for Temporal Interpretation

In our model all entities and relations are assigned a spatiotemporal location which is made up of two indices: one index is bound to the main temporal location in the case of individuals. As to relations and modifiers of the main relation, the index for the time location is derived from the event/state time, i.e. TES. In turn, this index is in a given logical relation with the TR(Reference Time) of the previous text span, which is related to the discourse focus TF: it may be BEFORE, AFTER, MEETS, OVERLAP etc. with it. The reference of the current TR is furthermore asserted to be included in some main temporal location which could be present in the previous text span. Thus, individuals receive directly a time index which bind their existence in the world and their properties, such as roles, or attributes, to some main temporal location; in case of names associated to individuals, we assign them to a universal location, in other words, we assume that in the domain specified by the text that name is used unambiguously to refer to a single well defined individual. This bipartition is quite natural: entities such as individuals or sets are assumed to be in a given time location for a longer stretch than the actual relation in which they are currently involved. The latter might be a punctual event, thus having a very short duration in time. Event properties are thus different from entities properties as to their temporal location. As we shall see in this chapter, event properties are basically derived from the aspectual classification associate to the predicate, and only partly from the semantic role associated to the arguments of the predicate.

Temporal interpretation is computed compositionally from the local features associated to the verb tense and the static lexical label associated to aspect, plus a number of relevant information like definiteness of the subject NP, and of the Object NP, plus their number. These features contribute to assigning a first dynamic aspectual label to the sentence in which the verbal predicate is analysed. This allows the system to compute local temporal relation intersententially, taking into adequate account all the elements which contribute to the definition of temporal relations; these elements are essentially taken from Reichenbach's proposal. This computation is added to the f-structure of each clause, where it will have to face the complexity arising from the presence of subordinate, coordinate and complement clauses. Finally, the result of the utterance temporal computation is passed on to the discourse module for temporal reasoning which is based on Allen's proposal. At this level, temporal intervals are generated and are attached at nodes in a cluster. The logical notation introduced by Allen is perspicuous enough to allow for the overall representation of discourse structure, where reference intervals are generated by taking into account local logical relations.

The following is a text adapted from Webber(1988), where we see that the second utterance expresses an activity which is presumably ended by the time Mario arrives: in this case, we want the system to understand the relationship intervening between someone waiting for somebody else which has now arrived, a FINISHED-BY relation, which is computed by means of semantic control. A more generic temporal logical relation would be CONTAIN, where the "waiting" time interval CONTAINS the "running home" event.

51.a. Mario ieri corse a casa/Yesterday Mario ran home
b. Maria lo aspettava/Maria was waiting for him
c. Lei lo insultò/She insulted him

7.1. Tense and Aspect: Two Separate Relations with Time Reference

We shall concentrate on f-structures representing temporal interpretation at sentence level. The algorithm for temporal interpretation is called in order to compute the role of arguments, adverbs and other adjuncts. These are accessed in order to establish whether some additional interpretation is available. We use the tripartite Reichenbachian structure made up of TR=reference time, TD=speech time, and TES=event/state time, which may be equivalent, may be included into one another, may precede or follow one another.

The computation is worked out into two separate relations, Rel1, and Rel2: Rel1 works according to tense information, Rel2 according to aspectual information. At first we compute Rel1 by matching mood and tense information in a table loookup as follows,

```
calc1(F,pres,td(F)=tr(F)).
calc1(F,pres_progr,td(F)=tr(F)).
calc1(F,pass_pross,tr(F)<td(F)).
calc1(F,imperfect,tr(F)<td(F)).
calc1(F,imp_progr,tr(F)<td(F)).
calc1(F,trap_pross,tr(F)<td(F)).
calc1(F,pass_rem,tr(F)<td(F)).
calc1(F,past,tr(F)<td(F)).
calc1(F,past_perf,tr(F)<td(F)).
calc1(F,perf,tr(F)≤td(F)).
calc1(F,trap_rem,tr(F)<td(F)).
calc1(F,future,td(F)<tr(F)).
calc1(F,fut_progr,td(F)<tr(F)).
calc1(F,fut_ant,td(F)<tr(F)).
```

where we see the Italian and the English set of tenses: pass_pross translates sometimes the English Perfect and sometimes the Simple Past; "imperfetto" has no English correspondence; we have Present Perfect and Past Perfect with their actual English value; pass_rem translates Past Tense; fut_ant translates future in the past. This Relation is passed on to "calc2" which computes Rel2 taking aspect into account. Then temporal modifiers are accessed and some further changes may take place. As can be seen from the following table, Progressive tense together with aspect set on Achievements contributes an interpretation "prec_imm", i.e. precedes immediately:

```
calc2(F,pres_progr,achiev_tr,event,_,prec_imm(tr(F),tes(F))).
calc2(F,imp_progr,achiev_tr,event,_,prec_imm(tr(F),tes(F))).
calc2(F,pres,_,td(F)=tr(F),included(tr(F),tes(F))).
calc2(F,pres_progr,event,_,included(tr(F),tes(F))).
calc2(F,pass_pross,_,tr(F)<td(F),tr(F)=tes(F)).
calc2(F,imp,_,_,included(tr(F),tes(F))).
calc2(F,imp_progr,event,_,included(tr(F),tes(F))).
calc2(F,trap_pross,_,_,tes(F)<tr(F)).
calc2(F,pass_rem,_,_,tr(F)=tes(F)).
calc2(F,future,_,_,tr(F)=tes(F)).
calc2(F,future,state,_,included(tr(F),tes(F))).
calc2(F,fut_progr,event,_,included(tr(F),tes(F))).
calc2(F,fut_ant,_,_,tes(F)<tr(F)).
```

Adverbs or adjuncts may specify the internal structure of temporal location, and this information be explicitly stated in the final output. In our parser, temporal adverbs are lexically assigned a configuration, a type and a duration if any: these parameters are passed to the routine that interprets Rel1 and Rel2. There are two main calls to adverbs and temporal adjuncts: one is just a table lookup which taps directly lexical information; the other one computes the contents of the adverbial phrase or prepositional phrase first, and then passes this information to a table lookup.

```
adverb(F,Type,Config,Durat,Rel1x,Rel2x,Rel1,Rel2):-
    tab_adv(Type,Config,Durat,Rel1x,Rel2x,Rel1,Rel2).
adverb(F,Head,Type,Duration,RelAdv).

adverb(F,Head,deictic,punct,tr(F)=Head).
adverb(F,Head,deictic,non_punct,included(tr(F),Head)).
adverb(F,Head,clock_cal,punct,tr(F)=Head).
adverb(F,Head,clock_cal,non_punct,included(tr(F),Head)).
adverb(F,Head,duration,non_punct,durat(tr(F),Head)).
adverb(F,Head,temporal,non_punct,durat(tr(F),Head)).
adverb(F,Head,frequency,iterate,iterate(te(F),Head)).
adverb(F,Head,frequency,intervalled,intervalled(te(F),Head)).

tab_adv(deictic,[td<tr],_,td(F)<tr(F),tes(F)<tr(F),td(F)<tr(F),included(tes(F),tr(F))).
tab_adv(deictic,[td=tr],non_punct,tr(F)<td(F),tes(F)<tr(F),tr(F)<td(F),tr(F)=tes(F)).
tab_adv(temporal,[td=tr],non_punct,td(F)=tr(F),tes(F)<tr(F),tr(F)<td(F),tr(F)=tes(F)).
tab_adv(clock_cal,[tr<td],_,tr(F)<td(F),Rel2,tr(F)<td(F),Rel2).
```

More or less the same procedure is used to compute the overlapping of tenses in sentential complements and subordinate clauses, which however in addition have a semantic marker as subordinator. The Rels of two sentences at first are computed separately and then together, where "reltr" and "reltes" attributes appear. The subordinate clause is a transformative achievement and has a TR = reference time which is included in the TD = discourse time and is equal to the TES = event/state time. In the case of the main clause, we have an activity where the TD is included in the TR and the TES includes the TR. It is temporally specific and has as referential interval the label f4_sub2. The comparison of the two separate clauses gives as a result the following: the TR relation is expressed as an equality between the two - main and subordinate - TRs. In turn the TES are in an inclusion relation, the subordinate TES being included in the main one.

Consider now a simple example,

52. [mario telefonò a luigi perché voleva delle informazioni]/Mario called Luigi because he wanted some piece of information

```
aspect:state
        rel1:[tr(f8_sub1)<td(f8_sub1)]
        rel2:[included(tr(f8_sub1), tes(f8_sub1))]
        specificity:+
        reltr:[tr(f4_sub1)=tr(f8_sub1)]
```

```
        reltes:[included(tes(f4_sub1), tes(f8_sub1))]
aspect:activity
rel1:[tr(f4_sub1)<td(f4_sub1)]
rel2:[tr(f4_sub1)=tes(f4_sub1)]
specificity:+
ref_int:[td(f4_sub1)]
```

As can be easily understood from the representations, the information now available is that the subordinate is a state and the main clause is an activity and the relations intervening between the two are now different: in particular the two TRs are now in an equality relationship. This computation allows the semantic module to assign spatio-temporal locations to participants in an event/state. More examples can be studied, and we think it important to give a sequence of utterances which can then be analysed in discourse by means of Allen's module.

Going back to our three sentences making up our text, the following temporal computations are taken from the f-structures included above:

```
a. adjs:adv:pred_adv:yesterday
        type:deictic
        durat:non_punct
        config:[tr<td]
   aspect:accomp
   rel1:[tr(f4_ta)<td(f4_ta)]
   rel2:[tr(f4_ta)=tes(f4_ta)]
   specificity:+
   ref_int:[tr(f4_ta)]
b. aspect:activity
   rel1:[tr(f4_tb)<td(f4_tb)]
   rel2:[included(tr(f4_tb), tes(f4_tb))]
   specificity:+
   ref_int:[tr(f4_tb)]
c. aspect:achiev_tr
   rel1:[tr(f4_td)<td(f4_td)]
   rel2:[tr(f4_td)=tes(f4_td)]
   specificity:+
   ref_int:[tr(f4_td)]
```

In a. we have a temporal main location(MTL), "yesterday", which is assumed as encompassing the main temporal streamline of narration: in turn, tense moves reference times TR of each main proposition forward and backward on this streamline, until a new MTL is asserted in the narration.

In a. we have the information that the TR precedes the TD and that it coincides with the TES; in addition we know that it is "specific", hence not generic, and that a given time interval is assigned a given label. In b. TR always precedes TD but this time it includes the TES. Finally, in c. we know that the TR precedes the TD as before but there is coincidence between the TR and the TES.

These information are then passed on at text level to the further level of computation which is explained below.

7.2. Implementing Allen's Algorithm

In Allen's paper(1983) an interval-based temporal logic is introduced, together with a computationally effective reasoning algorithm. The temporal representation takes the notion of temporal interval as primitive; a notion of reference intervals is also introduced which is used to control the amount of deduction performed automatically by the system. By using reference intervals, the amount of computation involved when adding a fact in the temporal knowledge base can be controlled in a predictable manner, comments the author(ibid.,833). In our algorithm we also use Allen's explicit notation to express all the possible relations that can hold between two intervals by means of 13 relations.

Our implementation of Allen's algorithm takes as input Reichenbach's relations as they are independently computed at f-structure level. However, one of the main component's of the overall computation is the relation intervening between Time Focus and the Time Reference of the current utterance. Time Focus is a notion introduced by Webber(1985) which captures temporal information relevant for discourse and text analysis: it can be viewed as a stack which has on top the TR on which the discourse is currently focussing for any given utterance. The main call of our version of Allen's algorithm is the following,

```
anaphor_temp(SNo, Asp, S_id,tr(S_id)<td(S_id),tr(S_id)=tes(S_id)) :-
   one time_focus(_, tes(TF_id)),
   !, Asp\=state,
   allen_1(S_id,tr(S_id)),
   relation(tr(TF_id),tes(TF_id),R1),
   constraints([bf],R1,R),
   create_interval(tr(TF_id),tr(S_id)),
   add_rel(tr(TF_id),tr(S_id),R),
   asserta(time_focus(NoFr, tes(S_id))),

anaphor_temp(SNo, Asp, S_id,tr(S_id)<td(S_id),tr(S_id)=tes(S_id)) :-
   one time_focus(_, tes(TF_id)),
   !, Asp=state,
   allen_1(S_id,tr(S_id)),
   relation(tr(TF_id),tes(TF_id),R1),
   constraints([dr],R1,R),
   create_interval(tr(TF_id),tr(S_id)),
   add_rel(tr(TF_id),tr(S_id),R).
```

It instantiates the current TF on top of the stack and determines the relation intervening between the TF and the TR of the current utterance. Subsequently, it determines the relation intervening between the TRs and it is asserted in the graph or cluster of relations and TRs computed so far. In order to do this, constraints are checked on whether two adjacent nodes may be included or not in the same Reference Interval. Finally the TF is updated if necessary.

The following is the main call for utterances in which the TR precedes the TD, and equals the TES. We have sentence number and identifier, aspect and the relations inherited from f-structure. We recover the TF and we check that aspect be different from State: for temporal representation with a State aspect the call is the following one, where TF is not updated. The call to allen_1 looks for temporal relations of sentences which have that TR as Reference Interval in the graph and memorizes them. The new intervals created have the current TR as reference interval.

The call to Relation looks for comparable nodes and then for a "direct" or "indirect" connection between TR and the TES in the sentence which has fixed the TF,

```
relation(I,J,R) :-
  comparable(I,J),
  direct_relation(I,J,R), !.
```

Finally, it tries an intersection with the set of 13 logical relations and then passes the output to the following call on Constraints, which however has already a logical relation as internal constraint; then, the algorithm looks at a transitivity table for each pair of labels and returns the union of all the answers.

```
indirect_relation(I,J,R) :-
  bagof(Rel,path_rel(I,J,Rel),ListRel),
  rix(ListRel,R).
path_rel(I,J,R) :- go_to(J,I,Path),
    onstraints_along_path(Path,R).
```

We then take the intersection of these constraints with the previously known constraint, very much in the line of what Allen suggests (ibid.,837). In this way, we are ready to add_rel, or to add a new relation to the network which has the current TR as time reference. In this way a Reference Interval is created with all relations which fall along the path. Finally we assert the current TES as new TF.

```
add_rel(I,J,R) :-
   subset(R,[bf,af,dr,cn,ov,ob,me,mb,st,sb,fn,fb,eq]),
   !, (direct_relation(I,J,N),
   !, intersection(R,N,X),
   (subset(X,N),
   !, write_rel(I,J,X),
   assertz(todo(I,J)),
   update
   ;
   write_rel(I,J,R),
   assertz(todo(I,J)),
   update).
```

7.3. Semantic Representation

The example might be consider an exceptional case: there is a past progressive (in Italian "imperfetto") which has to be computed as FINISHED-BY relation with the previous discourse segment. As said above, this requires semantic control to be activated. By semantic control we mean a linguistically based strategy which checks whether the same individual associated with identifier Id1 is a participant of an accomplishment, i.e. is an Agent in the previous portion of text, and is an Unaffected Theme in the current utterance which represents an Activity. This is what actually takes place in the text. Here below we follow Allen's computation at text level:

53. Mario ieri corse a casa/Yesterday Mario ran home
rel_temp(infon6, td, tr(f4_ta), [af])
rel_temp(infon7, tes(f4_ta), tr(f4_ta), [eq])
ref_interval(tr(f4_ta))
time_focus(1, tes(f4_ta))
loc(infon3, id1, [arg:main_tloc, arg:ieri])
included(tr(f4_ta), id1)

We have only two temporal relations, a time focus, and a reference interval; in the model a temporal main location which in this case is represented by the deictic "yesterday". Besides adverbials, we can have any kind of temporal adjunct in the form of a PP. The inclusion relation is expressed every time there is a deictic main location which the reference time of the current event/states may be anchored at. From temporal relations we also know that this reference time is situated before the TD or speech time and that is equal to the event/state time. Finally, from the full semantic representation produced by the model we also know that the actual time is in the past.

54. Maria lo aspettava/Maria was waiting for him
rel_temp(infon20, td, tr(f4_tb), [af])
rel_temp(infon22, tr(f4_ta), tr(f4_tb), [eq])
rel_temp(infon23, tes(f4_ta), tr(f4_tb), [eq])
rel_temp(infon26, tes(f4_ta), tes(f4_tb), [fn])
rel_temp(infon27, tes(f4_tb), tr(f4_ta), [fb])
rel_temp(infon28, tes(f4_tb), tr(f4_tb), [fb])
ref_interval(tr(f4_tb))
finished_by(tes(f4_ta),tes(f4_tb))

In utterance 2 – example 54 - we still know that reference time is situated in the past, and that the two reference times of the current and the previous utterance coincide, but also that there is a finishing relation between the two. There is also a new reference interval which is however abandoned in the following utterance. No new time focus is produced. When we get to utterance no.3 – example 55 - we notice that temporal relations are entertained only with utterance no.1 to which the insulting event is actually connected and not to waiting event expressed in the closely adjacent clause. We also have a new time focus which is the event/state time of the current utterance.

```
55. Lei lo insultò/She insulted him
rel_temp(infon38, td, tr(f4_td), [af])
rel_temp(infon39, tes(f4_td), tr(f4_td), [eq])
rel_temp(infon40, tr(f4_ta), tr(f4_td), [bf])
rel_temp(infon41, tes(f4_td), tr(f4_ta), [af])
time_focus(3, tes(f4_td))
ref_interval(tr(f4_ta), tr(f4_td))
included(tes(f4_td), id1)
```

However, in order to generate that temporal interpretation we need to keep track of Discourse Structure, Discourse Domain and Discourse Relations; in turn, discourse level information is related to temporal information in order to compute the Current Temporal Interval where a certain stretch of discourse can be included. Decisions both at discourse and at temporal level are sensitive to the Time Focus.

The main predicate used to compute Temporal Interval takes as input Preceding Discourse Relation, Change in the World, Factuality, Temporal Relation at sentence level.. The algorithm maps a temporal logical relation from the interplay of all these parameters and the temporal relation assigned by the independent computation of Allen's algorithm.

```
temp_relation(_,Tense,NoFr, Root, TesIndex, PreTesIndex, PreDisRel, Change,Factive,
    TRel) :-
  TesIndex\=PreTesIndex,!,
  temporal_rel(Root,TesIndex, PreTesIndex, PreDisRel, Change, Factive, Rel),
  map_temp_rel(Rel, Rel1),
  TRel=..[Rel1, TesIndex, PrecTesIndex], !.
temp_relation(_,_,_, _, TesIndex, PreTesIndex, _, _, _,undef(TesIndex, PrecTesIndex)) :-
  TesIndex\=PreTesIndex,!.

map_temp_rel('<', before).
map_temp_rel('>', after).
map_temp_rel('=', overlap).
map_temp_rel(different, after).
map_temp_rel(contemporary overlap).
map_temp_rel(included, contains).
map_temp_rel([eq], overlap).
map_temp_rel([af], after).
map_temp_rel([bf], before).
map_temp_rel([dr], during).
map_temp_rel(Rels, finished_by) :- on(fb, Rels).
map_temp_rel(Rels, started_by) :- on(sb, Rels).
map_temp_rel(Rels, contains) :- on(cn, Rels).
map_temp_rel(Rels, after) :- on(bf, Rels).
map_temp_rel(Rels, after) :- on(af, Rels).
map_temp_rel(Rels, during) :- on(dr, Rels).
```

In turn the temporal relation may be inferred by letting Discourse Relation and logical relation as derived from Allen's algorithm interact in a controlled fashion:

```
temporal_rel(_,TesIndex, PreTesIndex, _, _, _, Rel) :-
      rel_temp(_, TesIndex, PreTesIndex, Rel).
     temporal_rel(_,TesIndex, tes(TempIndex), PreDisRel, _, Factivity, Rel1) :-
      rel_temp(_, TesIndex, tr(TempIndex), Rel),
      infer_temp_rel(PreDisRel, TesIndex, tr(TempIndex), Rel, Rel1).
temporal_rel(Root,TesIndex, tes(TempIndex), PreDisRel, _, Factive, Reltr) :-
      node(Root)::reltr::[Rel|_],
      Rel=..[Reltr, _, Td].
temporal_rel(_, tes(TesIndex), tes(TempIndex), PreDisRel, _, Factive, Rel1) :-
      rel_temp(_, tes(TesIndex), tr(TesIndex), Rel),
      Rel\=[eq],
      infer_temp_rel(PreDisRel, tes(TesIndex), tr(TempIndex), Rel, Rel1).
temporal_rel(_,TesIndex, tes(TempIndex), PreDisRel, Change, Factive, Rel) :-
      (Change=null, Rel=[dr]
       ;
       PreDisRel=egression(_-_), Rel=[fb]
       ;
       (Factive=factive;PreDisRel=narration), Rel=[af]
      ;
      Rel=[dr]).
infer_temp_rel(PreDisRel,tes(TesIndex), TrIndex, Rel, Rel1) :-
      rel_temp(_, tes(TesIndex), tr(TempIndex), Rel),
      (PreDisRel=inception,
       (on(sb,Rel), Rel1=[sb])  ;
       (on(af,Rel), Rel1=[af])  ;
       PrecDiscRel\=inception,
       Rel1=Rel).
infer_temp_rel(_,tes(TesIndex), TrIndex, Rel, Rel1) :-
      rel_temp(_, tes(TesIndex), tr(TempIndex), Rel),
      rel_temp(_, tr(TempIndex), tr(TesIndex), Rel1).
```

Chapter 4

Discourse Relations and Rhetorical Structures

1. Introduction

In describing the meaning of a text or discourse there are two main perspectives from which one can impose structure on it: the Informational Perspective and the Intentional Perspective. If we view natural language as a tool that is primarily used to convey information about situations, relying on shared knowledge, as Hobbs suggests(1993) we will end up with the following statements: the Informational Perspective on discourse interpretation tells us how to understand the situations described in a discourse; the Intentional Perspective tells us how to discover the uses to which this information is being put(ibid. 3). Together with Hobbs, we believe that the two are closely knit in case one wants to reach an understanding of coherence relations. In order to do this, if we follow the intentional perspective, we need to do plan recognition, that is to discover the process of reasoning followed by an agent (including intentions, beliefs and goals) in each situation. Coherence will result as an integration of the rhetorical relations intervening between segments of the discourse or text and the underlying plan. However, as Hobbs puts it, to recognize a plan is a problem of abduction: if we encode as axioms beliefs about what kind of actions cause and enable what kinds of events and conditions, then when in presence of complete knowledge of the speaker's goals and beliefs, it is a matter of deduction to prove that the speaker believes a sequence or more complex arrangement of actions will achieve the goals. As Hobbs comments (ibid., 4) unfortunately, we rarely have complete knowledge and we will almost always have to make assumptions. We believe, however, that the problem is different in case we are dealing with narrative texts: in this case, the informational aspect completely overshadows considerations of intentions. In other words, we would need to understand what information the utterance would convey independent of the speaker's intention(ibid.,3). In our case, then, what is the content of an utterance and why the speaker wishes to convey it, or the narrator has used it, is our task.

Hobb's proposal is in our opinion not on the right track: in his perspective, there is no room for linguistic analysis, rather all relations are derived from "commonsense knowledge" as he himself claims(ibid.,24). For a particular set of relations to be validated, it would require showing that a given set of relations, as defined precisely in terms of commonsense knowledge, was adequate for the interpretation of large amount of texts(ibid,24). It is a fact that to prove a causal relations between two assertions, you must make up a certain number of axioms – see the following chapter. But of course, if the example slightly changes, we shall have to change the analysis: "each example, of course, has to be analyzed on its own"(ibid.,18). There is clearly a contradiction here, between what he states in the conclusions and what comes out from the analysis of a single example. We believe that, in order to attain some level of generality, we cannot possibly rely on a set of axioms which might fit into the interpretation of a single example with a given linguistic form. Linguistic knowledge should be used first and that should be integrated with general knowledge about the domain.

Suppose now the domain be "children stories" – as the "Story of the 3 Little Pigs" - where ferocious bad animals seek tender good edible animals in order to eat them, there will be a simple chain of reasoning to follow, in the form of axioms. The primary Goal is established in our stories in the discourse segments marked as Setting; the remaining subgoals are determined by the chains of local cause-effects described in the text and highlighted by discourse relations:

```
A. Plan:- goals([Primary_Goal, Subgoals]):-
     Plan 1. primary_goal([feed_on(w, l_p), Subgoals])
                  subgoals(1,[_, catch(w, l_p)])
                  subgoals(2,[_, destroy(w, h & poss(l_p, h))])
                       subgoal(2.1,[_, blow_down(w, h)])
     Plan 2. primary_goal([protect(l_p, l_p, from(w)), Subgoals])
                  subgoals(1,[_, build(l_p, h) & sturdy(h)])
                       subgoal(1.1,[destroyed(h), escape(l_p, from(wolf))])
                       subgoal(1.2,[_,appear(w) & run(l_p)])
```

In words: there is a plan 1. which assumes that wolves feed on little pigs and they catch them in order to eat them: however to catch little pigs might require to destroy their little houses and to do this the wolf has to blow them down; then a plan 2. which assumes that little pigs build houses which are sturdy in order to protect themselves from the wolf; however, if their little house is destroyed, the little pigs escape from the wolf and to do that when they see it they run. This simple plan might be checked by a Plan-checker by looking up discourse structures, where discourse relations have been built. However, in order to access discourse structure through discourse relations, these must be expressed in a safe and logically relevant way.

The proponents of Rhetorical Structure Theory(RST) (see Mann & Thompson, 1987) assume that coherence in a text can be measured by rhetorical relations to relate each continuous segment of text. However, as Suthers(1993,128) clearly states, the rhetorical characterization of coherence does not account for the source of coherence, nor does it say why the text is coherent since rhetorical relations are merely descriptive tools for coherent text, which might fit into the description of incoherent text as well. We also assume with Suthers, that the task of generating coherent text is different from that of analysing a text and the constraints one has to satisfy might be different in each case. Indeed, we use rhetorical or discourse relations only for analysis and understanding. For sure, we need to deal with multiple descriptions when analyzing a text: however, we also believe it important to differentiate coherence from the point of view of the understander, from coherence from the point of view of the generator(ibid., 130).

Besides, it is a fact that rhetorical relations as they have been defined by their proponents are primarily intended for text analysis. As we know, they constitute neither mandatory nor committal nor certain judgements: from the point of view of the analyst, they are simply deemed as plausible ways to judge the relations intervening between clauses and text spans(ibid., 4). The strange thing about rhetorical relations is however the fact that - even though they are deemed to be "linguistically useful" by their proponents (ibid. in the abstract) - RST analysis has no sound linguistic foundation being based simply on intuitions rather than on the actual semantic or linguistic content of the text analyzed, as their proponents puts it:

> "As a result, an RST analysis always constitutes a plausible account of what the writer wanted to achieve with each part of the text. An RST analysis is thus a functional account of the text as a whole.
>
> This point is important in establishing just how our approach offers a functional account of text structure. RST provides an explicit plausible functional account of a text as a side effect of the analysis, precisely because the definitions are stated in terms of how the text produces an effect on the reader which the writer could reasonably have intended. In applying a relation definition, the analyst affirms the plausibility of each Effect.
>
> The application of a relation definition never depends directly on the form of the text being analyzed; the definitions do not cite conjunctions, tense, or particular words. RST structures are, therefore, structures of functions rather than structures of forms." (ibid.,19).

and further on,

> "For a given relation, one can identify a corresponding assertional form (or proposition).
>
> In reading natural texts, people consistently judge that the text conveys the relational propositions, even in cases where no morphosyntactic signal of the relation exist...
>
> Since the relations need no signal in the text, neither do the relational propositions. Relational propositions are not compositional in the usual sense - the communication effect arises from something other than the composition of interpretations of explicit parts. And they are about as numerous as independent clauses.
>
> Relational propositions, therefore, challenge theories of language that equate the communication effect of a text with the "meanings" of its sentences and compose those meanings from the meanings of its syntactic structures and lexical items."

The intuitional approach and the circularity of the basic backbone on which relation definitions hold is very clear from the above quote.

In this chapter we shall deal briefly with discourse relations as they can be computed from temporal and aspectual interpretation and how access to knowledge of the world may be relevant in some cases. We surmise it important to verify the coherence of a text on the basis of the intentions of its participants, or their plan: however, we think that rhetorical relations, or discourse relations as we understand them, can and should be derived from morphosyntactic, lexical and semantic properties of the underlying text. In other words, all knowledge related to some special property or other of these relations should be encoded basically in the predicate lexical entry. Thus the main lexical item, the central concept or main predicate of each clause, where we intend all possible clauses made exception only for restrictive relative clauses, is the carrier of linguistic information necessary for establishing a given discourse relation. However, in case subordinate clauses are present, the subordinator is the semantic marker which we use to establish local discourse relation intervening between the main and the subordinate clauses. In case it is unambiguous this would be straightforward; otherwise, some kind of disambiguation needs to be carried out.

Do rhetorical relations or discourse relations account for or predict coherence of a text? M & T seem to be convinced that their approach provides a safe tool for establishing coherence between text spans. However, we are again somewhat puzzled by the contradictory nature of RST. On the one hand the proponents say that there is basically no limit to the number of relations, and that they can be made up to suit a particular text organization or genre; on the other hand they assert that when assigning a set of relations, coherence will result. Actually, the import of RST on text coherence is asserted in negative rather than as a positive must.

> "While studying text relations and developing RST, we became aware that the presence of structural relations in a text has consequences that closely resembles the consequences of clausal assertion. The text structure conveys propositions, and propositions conveyed in this way are called relational propositions... The relational propositions are essential to the coherence of their text. Perturbing text to prevent the (implicit or explicit) expression of one of its relational propositions causes the text to become incoherent....
> We find all the relational propositions essential to the coherence of the text. If they can somehow be neutralized, as by explicit contrary assertions, the coherence of the text is broken at the point of the missing relation; it becomes incoherent or takes on some alternate interpretation." (ibid.,21)

This is only part of the story seen that not all propositions need to be coherent in the whole text structure: there are neutral propositions which only look forward, so to say, and have no relation whatsoever with the previous stretch of discourse.

2. Discourse Relations and Temporal Interpretation

The logical relations which can occur between two utterances or text spans are called coherence or discourse relations; coherence relations have such labels as sequence, cause, contrast, etc. For example, in the discourse below taken from Webber(1988,65) hers 8.:

1. John went to the hospital.
2. He had twisted his ankle on a patch of ice.

sentences 1 and 2 stand in a cause relation: the event described in 2 causes the event described in 1; in other words, the latter occurs as a result of the former. In this case the discourse relation might be interpreted on the basis of tense relations and topic persistence between the two adjacent segments of discourse, in addition to knowledge of the world and the fact that both verbs need to be labeled as Causatives in the lexicon. However, this is not always the case. More on this topic in the following chapter.

As said above, coherence relations can be assigned on the basis of lexical and syntactic information, plus an inferential component, based on temporal and aspectual interpretation. In this we follow J.Allen's temporal interpretation system. For example, no lexical or syntactic clues indicate that sentences 1 and 2 in (2) are related in the way we claimed, i.e. a Cause relation; in fact, that relation is assigned from temporal and aspectual interpretation and knowledge of the world. Consider the next discourse, always taken from Webber(1988,71), hers 24,25:

3. John went to the hospital.
4. He took a taxi, because his car was in the shop.

As Webber herself comments, 4. is understood as part of the preparatory phase of 3. and therefore precedes it. In this case, the discourse relations intervening between the two segments of discourse is no longer a Cause relation but simply a Sequence relation, and this can only be captured from external world knowledge.

There are tenses which are typologically determined by the way in which each language encodes tense. For instance, Italian encodes English past tense with the "imperfetto" in case the meaning to convey is a lack of temporal progression, and aspectual class belongs to statives or activities. Imperfetto is a tense lacking in English but present in French even though with some additional meaning. Italian uses "passato remoto" to convey a forward movement of discourse focus, this tense corresponding closely to one of the meanings of English simple past. The following examples are taken from Dowty(1986), his 4, 5, 8:

5. John entered the president's office. The president sat behind a huge desk.
6. John entered the president's office. The clock on the wall ticked loudly.
7. John entered the president's office. The president realized why he had come.

The corresponding Italian sentences will have imperfetto in the second sentence for stative "sit" and activity "tick", and passato remoto for achievement "realize":

5a. Gino entrò nell'ufficio del presidente. Il presidente sedeva dietro un'enorme scrivania ≠ sedette dietro un'enorme scrivania

6a. Gino entrò nell'ufficio del presidente. L'orologio alla parete ticchettava rumorosamente ≠ ticchettò rumorosamente

7a. Gino entrò nell'ufficio del presidente. Il presidente capì perché era venuto ??% capiva perché era venuto

We marked with a ≠ the version with passato_remoto and with ??% the version with imperfetto in 7a. With the exception of 7a, if we use passato remoto we get a different meaning, i.e. after John entered the office and the president was standing, he sat, for 5a.; however, 7a. has only that version in order to preserve coherence, the imperfetto is not interchangeable with the passato remoto! Also note that stative predicates in English may be turned into inceptive achievements, as in the following example again from Dowty, his 9:

8. John sat in his chair going over the day's perplexing events again in his mind. Suddenly, he was asleep.

8a. Gino sedeva sulla sua sedia ripercorrendo nella sua mente gli eventi preoccupanti della giornata. Improvvisamente, si addormentò ??% era addormentato ??% dormiva

There are two main differences to note: in the Italian version of the first segment, the verb "sit" is rendered with imperfetto as before, and not with passato remoto; the second segment can only be rendered with an inceptive or ingressive verb "addormentarsi" meaning "fall asleep", but not with "dormire" an activity verb, nor with "essere addormentato" a stative verb.

The same problems arise with English BE in stative copulative sentences such as the one reported by Lascarides and Asher(1991), which we list here below:

9. Max opened the door. The room was pitch dark.
10. Max switched off the light. The room was pitch dark.
11. Max took an aspirin. He was sick.

In 9 we would like to have a Background relation, whereas in 10 the relation holding between the two discourse segment should be Result. And finally, in 11 we would like Cause or Motivation to hold. However, in English, the main predicate of the second segment is always BE and the tense is always the same, simple past. Thus, it would seem that without tapping external knowledge of the world the meaning underlying the discourse relations cannot possibly be grasped. Look now at the corresponding Italian versions of the three discourses,

9a. Max aprì la porta. Nella stanza c'era buio pesto. ??%Nella stanza ci fu buio pesto
10a. Max spense la luce. Nella stanza fu buio pesto. = Ora nella stanza era buio pesto.
11a. Max prese un'aspirina. Si sentiva male. ??%Si sentì male

At first we must note that the direct translation would be absolutely ungrammatical, "*La stanza era/*fu buia pesto": even though the shortened version "la stanza era/*fu buia" is possible, it does not convey the same meaning as the English counterpart. There is an additional restriction, and that is the passato remoto cannot possibly be used because the meaning conveyed by the sentence is just a state. As said previously, the imperfetto in Italian is not interchangeable with passato remoto, this is why 9 and 11 which should convey Background must be rendered with imperfetto. However, in 10 the Result relation could be expressed both by imperfetto and by passato remoto: in the latter case, no problem would ensue for the interpretation module, since passato remoto overwrites stativity and the final output would always be a Culminated event. As a consequence, a Result could be read out from the Discourse Relation interpreter. Also note that the lexical locative expletive "ci" is absent from the sentence because it would somehow prevent the resultative reading. The version with the imperfetto has a specific deictic temporal indicator "ora"/now which again prevents the stative reading in favour of a punctual reading.

3. Information and Rhetorical Structure

Two notions have been highlighted in the literature on discourse which are particularly relevant to narrative as a genre: foreground and background. The foreground is that part of a discourse which provides the main information; in a narrative, for example, the foreground is the temporal sequence of events; foreground information, then, moves the story forward. The background, on the contrary, provides supportive information, such as elaborations, comments, etc., and does not move the story forward(see Alberti,1992).

To compute foreground and background information, three main rhetorical relations are assigned by the algorithm in the form of attribute-value pairs, or features:

DISCOURSE DOMAIN, CHANGE IN THE WORLD, RELEVANCE.

The Discourse Domain of a sentence may be "subjective", indicating that the event or state takes place in the mind of the participant argument of the predicate and not necessarily in the external world. Then it may be "objective", which indicates that the action described by the verb affects the whole environment. A sentence may also describe a "change in the world", in case we pass from the description of one situation to the description of another situation which precedes or follows the former in time but which is not temporally equivalent to it; we have then the following inventory of changes: null (i.e. no change), gradual, culminated, earlier, negated. The third value, the "relevance" of a sentence, corresponds to the distinction between foreground and background which has been discussed above.

In addition to these, the algorithm checks the structure of each sentence and assigns a fourth feature, i.e. CLAUSE TYPE: if the sentence is made up of just one main clause, it writes main/prop; otherwise, i.e. if the sentence is made up of two or more coordinate clauses, it writes coord/prop for each clause; if the sentence is in direct speech, it writes dir_speech/prop. In case a special explicit cue word is used, we shall have such labels as result, tempor_coinc, cause, and others. These labels are used directly by the interpreter of discourse relations.

We have now to explain the way each utterance receives its set of values: the algorithm relies heavily on grammatical cues, i.e. those linguistic elements encoded in the grammar of a language which allow interpretation without the intervention of pragmatic or non-linguistic elements such as conversational implicatures, presupposition or inferencing. The cues we make use of are chiefly extracted from the verb and are such things as semantic category, polarity, tense, aspect. The procedure is very simple from a theoretical point of view: once the algorithm has recognized a cue, it assigns a value to the sentence. Note that we distinguish between the direct and indirect speech portions of the text, since the perspective is not the same in the two cases.

CLAUSE TYPE: as we have said above, this value is related only to the syntactic structure of the sentence: the algorithm checks the f-structure of the sentence (which is the output of the parsing module) and indicates whether the sentence is made up of a main clause or other. The algorithm looks for subordinate clauses, and recognizes propositional adjuncts - implicit or explicit, i.e. tensed or untensed, like gerundives, participials, infinitives etc.

DISCOURSE DOMAIN: to assign the point of view of a sentence, the algorithm checks the sem(antic)_cat(egory) of the main verb of the sentence and a number of other opacity operators, like the presence of future tense, a question or an exclamative, the presence of modals, etc, as we argued in Book 1, Chapter IV – to be published.

CHANGE IN THE WORLD: to establish whether a clause describes a change or not, and which type of change it describes, the algorithm takes into account four parameters: polarity (i.e. affirmative or negative), domain, tense and aspect of the main verb.

If polarity is set to NO (i.e. if the clause is negative), CHANGE is negated; but if the verb describes a state, CHANGE is null because a stative verb can never express a change, apart from the fact that it is affirmed or negated. Thus, if DISCOURSE DOMAIN is subjective and the verb is stative, CHANGE is null: this captures the fact that, in such a case, the action affects only the subject's mind and has no effects on the outside world. In all other cases the algorithm takes into account tense and aspect of the main verb and obeys the following rules: if tense is simple present, CHANGE is null; if tense is passato remoto or simple past, CHANGE is culminated; if tense is pluperfect or trapassato remoto, CHANGE is earlier; if tense is the imperfetto and describes a state, CHANGE is null, but if it describes an activity, a process, an accomplishment, or if it is a mental activity, CHANGE is gradual.

FACTIVITY: this relation may only assume two values: factive and nonfactive. A factive relation is assigned every time change is non null. Other sources of information may be used to trigger factivity, and that is the presence of a factive predicate, like a presuppositional verb, know.

RELEVANCE: to compute the relevance of a sentence, the algorithm checks CHANGE: if it is null, RELEVANCE is background; in all other cases, RELEVANCE is foreground. In other words, we take a clause to be in foreground if it describes a change in the world; whatever is not in foreground, i.e. whatever does not describe a change in the world, is the background of the text: the background provides supportive information and is always expressed by states.

We now turn to the cues for direct speech. Once the algorithm has recognized a clause to be in direct speech, the CLAUSE TYPE value is dir_speech/prop. The DISCOURSE DOMAIN is also subjective: this is so because direct speech reports the thoughts and perceptions of the characters in the story, so that any intervention of the writer is left out. As far as CHANGE is concerned, the algorithm obeys the following rules: if the main verb is in the imperative mood, CHANGE is null because, although the imperative is used to express commands, there is no certainty that once a command has been imparted it is going to be carried out. If the verb is in the indicative mood, and it is the future, CHANGE is null as well since the action has still to take place; if we have a past tense such as the passato prossimo or the trapassato, CHANGE is culminated or earlier, respectively; if tense is present, the algorithm checks its aspect: if the verb describes a state, CHANGE is null, otherwise (i.e. if the verb describes an activity) CHANGE is gradual. Finally, the RELEVANCE of a sentence in direct speech is computed according to the same rules given above for indirect speech.

Finally, two more attributes are computed: they are TEMPORAL RELATIONS and DISCOURSE FOCUS. Temporal Relations are the output of Allen's algorithm which are documented in Allen(1989), and are commented in previous Chapter. As argued there, the task of this computation is that of building reference intervals in order to relate temporal sequences in the ongoing analysis of a text or discourse. Interval logic, however, is too redundant as it is, i.e. the number of possible relations between two intervals is almost never given deterministically in terms of a single relation. In order to overcome this fuzziness in the original algorithm, we used temporal focus and semantic relations to infer which is the appropriate relation to be instantiated in a given context, from the set of possible relations computed independently by Allen's algorithm.

3.1. Computing Rhetorical Relations

In all the literature on Rhetorical and/or Discourse Relations there is no indication of a procedure or algorithm to derive them automatically from the analysis of a text. M & T in their paper(1987) comment each relation with a somewhat intuitive flavour, assigning it to the analyzer's most plausible interpretation of the current text span. In "Intentional" papers on the topic, of which Hobbs' (1979) and Grosz & Sidner(1986) are the most authoritative representatives, discourse relations are derived directly from logical relations intervening between two adjacent propositions. However, it is a fact, that in the latter case, discourse or text structure would be just a matter of world knowledge without any contribution whatsoever from linguistic knowledge. We assume that discourses are typically different from written texts, in particular narratives, user manuals, newspaper news and so on, because in the former there is a lot more of implicit, background and mutual knowledge which the participants in the conversation should share, and a system should possess, before trying to compute the meaning of what is being said. However, in the latter case we assume that most of what is required to understand the text is explicit stated, with the notable exceptions of common sense knowledge which is covered in part by default properties, as we partly stated them in Chapt. I. Clearly in the process of deriving discourse or rhetorical relations from the ongoing text, a system should have access to inferential chains underlying the main goals participants have, which may intersect or contrast. This would not be requested for the understanding of relations in other textual genres.

Our system relies basically on semantic information, which is made general by the use of semantic classes associated to each predicate in the lexicon or to WordNet. However special inferential processes may be triggered when a Result or a Cause relation has to be computed, in order to check whether, in the particular text we are working, such relation intervenes between the two main predicates under analysis. After topic persistence has been checked, i.e. whether the two segments have the same topic or not, we fire an appropriate inference, in case Change is culminated and the two clauses to be related are factive. More on this in the sections below and in the following chapter.

Dahlgren(1988), reviewing a large corpus of literature on discourse, proposes a set of twenty coherence relations. These relations include: sequence, reported event, enablement, cause, goal, parallel, contrast, evidence, generalization, elaboration, restatement, qualification, evaluation, description, situation-activity, situation-time, situation-place, import, biased comment, unbiased comment. Our set is somehow different in that it incorporates some of M & T's rhetorical relations. We shall list here below the twenty relations that we use in the stories.

SETTING, INCEPTION, CAUSE, PURPOSE, RESULT, CONTRAST_RESULT, CIRCUMSTANCE, CONDITION, ELABORATION, EXPLANATION, EVALUATION, NARRATION, EVIDENCE, CONTRAST, BACKGROUND, CONCESSION, PARALLEL, REQUEST, QUESTION, ALTERNATIVE

Rather than using Dahlgren's SEQUENCE we use NARRATION, always implying that such a relation is assigned because the events in S2 follow the event in S1 in time, but are not otherwise causally related. We also use INCEPTION and SETTING, which are connected with other parameters available to the algorithm. INCEPTION is triggered by the presence of a process verb as main predicate which is interpreted as inceptive from conceptual representations. SETTING is triggered by the discourse module, and translates the state of Shifting which is triggered by the presence of a FOCus in the syntactic structure of the utterance being analysed. A focalized subject is used in a discourse to convey the pragmatic information that a new topic is introduced or presented, usually in inverted subject position. CIRCUMSTANCE indicates a relation in which the temporal relations of the two adjacent segments of discourse overlap and there is a stative predicate. When Change is gradual or when tense is pluperfect, ELABORATION appears. BACKGROUND is used only when there is a nonfactive modality. CONTRAST and EVIDENCE are used with negated propositions, the first in concomitance with foreground, and the second with background; it can also appear when a copulative construction is analyzed, i.e. when Subject has a role Theme_Bound, and the predication is constituted by a non evaluative predicate. EVALUATION is related to the presence of an adjunct which has the semantic category of "subjective_intensional", is in foreground and its Change is Gradual; it can also appear when Subject has a semantic role of Theme_Bound, and the predication is constituted by an evaluative predicate. EXPLANATION is related to the presence of a proposition which introduces a Change which is Null and is otherwise Objective, Factive and its Relevance is Background; it can also appear when Subject has a role Theme_Bound, and the predication is constituted by a stative predicate. CAUSE and RESULT require checking procedure, as we already said, for inferable relations which are defined on the basis of domain and general knowledge about the world – but see Chapter V. Both are activated when Change is Culminated, the proposition is factive and is in foreground: RESULT may follow Cause or Inception in the previous clause, wherever topic persistence allows it. The remaining discourse relations are triggered by the presence of cue words or phrases, i.e. by specific subordinating conjunctions which act as semantic markers of the subordinated proposition. Chains of Inception-Result and Cause-Result constitute the backbone of the inferential chain to be used by the Plan checker.

In a discourse, there are special words and phrases directly indicating the structure of the topic to the hearer; these words and phrases play the role of discourse markers, and are referred to as cue words or discourse markers. As said above, we use cue words only whenever they are unambiguous, and refrain from identifying discourse relations with them whenever they are ambiguous. In particular, coordination with "and" and subordination with "when" can lead to quite different interpretations according to aspectual and temporal interpretation. We will now start presenting the Finite State Discourse Automaton or FSDA for short, which computes automatically discourse relations.

Table 1. Discourse Relations and Semantic Informational Structure

View	ClauseType Func/Role	Relev-ance	Factu-ality	Aspect	Change	State	Predicate	Support	Sem. Cat	Focal-izers	Prec.Disc. Relation	Discourse Relation
						shifting						setting
social_ engagement								shall				obligation
social_ engagement	_/Role											relation_role Relation
social_ engagement								~modal _verb				inception
							Verb inception					inception
	Role\= prop				Change							relation_role
	_/prop		factual	state					hypoth-esis			result
	{adj; coord}/ Role				Change							relation_role
	_/gerund				culminated		~narration verb				egression	result
	_/gerund				culminated		~narration verb				{narration; evidence}	result
										focal-izers		evidence
		back-ground			negated							evidence

Table 1. (Continued)

View	ClauseType Func/Role	Relev-ance	Factu-ality	Aspect	Change	State	Predicate	Support	Sem. Cat	Focal-izers	Prec.Disc. Relation	Discourse Relation
	main/_	back-ground	factual		null	contin-ue			~presup-positive			explanation
	main/_		factual			state	Verb=be					explanation
								be_ going				parallel
internal_ intensional		back-ground			null		evaluation_ verb					evaluation
		fore-ground			negated		~applicat-ive_verb	~modal _verb				contrast
internal_ intensional		f ore-ground			gradual							evaluation
							result_verb					result
external		back-ground	non-factual	state	null			~modal _verb				evaluation
{internal; internal_ intensional}	dir_ speech	back-ground		state	null							evaluation
external	_/gerund				Change\= null		~narration_ verb					elaboration
external	_/prop	fore-ground	factual		gradual							elaboration
	fcomp/_	back-ground		Aspect\= state	{null; gradual}				~presup-positive			elaboration
{internal; internal_ intensional}	report/_	back-ground			null							elaboration

Table 1. (Continued)

View	ClauseType Func/Role	Relev-ance	Factu-ality	Aspect	Change	State	Predicate	Support	Sem. Cat	Focal-izers	Prec.Disc. Relation	Discourse Relation
	_/gerund				culminated						narration	narration
	_/gerund				culminated						egression	narration
					culminated						narration	result
	coord /prop								result_ sequence			result
internal_ extensional												evaluation
external	_/prop	fore-ground	factual	achiev_tr	culminated				result			evidence
external		back-ground	non-factual	state	null			modal_ verb				obligation
		fore-ground			negated		{applica-tive;-definition}					prohibition
		back-ground	non-factual		null			permiss-ive				permission
												narration

Here below is the main call to the Discourse_Relation:

```
disc_relation(
NoFr                 = current number of utterance
View                 = current view
ClauseType           = current clause type
Relevance            = current type of relevance
Intensionality       = current type of intensionality
Aspect               = current type of aspect
[PreCh, Ch]          = preceding and current Change in the World
[PreSt, St]          = preceding and current State of the FSDA
Verb                 = current main verb predicate
Support              = current existing support verbs
[PreCS, CS]          = preceding and current semantic propositional category
Focalizers           = current existing focalizers
PrecDiscRel          = preceding discourse relation
NewDiscourseRelation.
```

Contents of the call are tabulated in the Tables 1 and 1cont. above, and are discussed here below in detail. Whenever an achievement is met, the algorithm tries to hypothesize an egression; consequently it looks for the beginning of the process or its inception. It crawls back in the stack of discourse structures trying to identify an inception, objective or a narration preceded by an inception. Otherwise, it takes the first narration it meets and tries an inference by means of cause_result predicate which encodes logical sequences in the external knowledge of the world – again see chapter V.

```
disc_relation:
        NoFr, View=external, Relevance=foreground, Factuality=factual,
        Aspect=achiev_tr, Change=culminated, Semantic_Prop=NRel,
        Output_Discourse_Relation=egression(PNoFr-Node))
    :-
        one disc_struc(At, PrecNoFr1-NoCl, Topics, MainRel, _, TempRel, inception,
            Strc, objective, Point),
        analyze_relation(NoFr, PrecNoFr1, MainRel, NRel, Topics),
        PNoFr=PrecNoFr1,
        Node=NoCl, !.
```

The call to analyze_relation checks whether the current Topic of Discourse is of type main or expected; then it recovers the topics of the discourse structure from the stack and tries to establish some semantic relation between the two sets of entities, the current and the previous one. The call to infer_relation looks for the inception verb or for a social_engagement verb (illocutionary speech acts). Semantic categories with some examples are listed here below:

Semantic Categories

```
stative_cat([state, existence]).
```

```
social_engagement([decide, promise]).
result_verb([result, manage]).
inception_verb([set, start, begin]).
narration_verb([say, tell]).
evaluation_verb([consider, regard]).
obligation_verb([require, demand]).
definition_verb([be, mean]).
modal_verb([can, must, shall, may, should, would, could, will, ought_to]).
permit_verb([may, allow]).
internal_intens([subjective, mental_activ, emotive]).
internal_extens([perceptive, state, presuppositive]).
result_sequence(activity, result).
result_sequence(activity, accomplishment).
result_sequence(perceptive, result).
relation_role(purpose, _, purpose).
relation_role(advers, _, adverse).
relation_role(cause, _, cause).
relation_role(temp_coinc, _, circumstance).
relation_role(result, culminated, result).
relation_role(cond, _, condition).
relation_role(motiv, _, motivation).
relation_role(conc, _, evidence).
relation_role(hypoth, _, hypothesis).
focalizer_type(sure, evidence).
focalizer_type(certainly, evidence).
```

4. Discourse Structure Representation

We take this level of representation to be composed of relations of various kinds which interact with the domain and the state of discourse in order to check for their semantic consistency. However, differently from other approaches, in our case Discourse Structure is the result of all previous computations: we simply let previous semantic descriptions interact with an algorithm that takes care of structural descriptions in terms of UP and DOWN nodes by means of carefully organized PUSH and POP actions. We have been inspired by L.Polanyi's (1988) and B.Webber's(1988) proposals, who suggest that a structural representation should be composed of Subordination and Coordination relations or by Adjunction and Attachment operations between the clauses that make up the text under analysis. In our case, we see that a stretch of text or a discourse segment characterised by a set of Coordinates - or Same_Level structures, as we call them - corresponds to a Topic Chain in which for instance, some properties of one Participant in the discourse are described. As Webber(1988:6) comments, if one wants to take discourse segmentation as a factor in context change, "then it cannot be done post facto, after a text has been read and understood: it must be doable on-line". Discourse segments are units which may be made object of coreference by appropriate deictic demonstrative pronouns. Furthermore, we assume that there is a one-to-one mapping between Reference-Intervals, as proposed by J.Allen and produced by our algorithm for temporal reasoning, and discourse segments: in other words, a discourse segment must be assigned the same Temporal or Discourse Focus.

In Webber's model, the interpretive constraints for discourse deixis produced by "this" and "that" are the following (ibid., 15):

"1. the interpretation of this and that must come from a sequent(a mental correlate of discourse segment) corresponding to a discourse segment on the right frontier(that is the segments in the discourse tree segmentation whose meaning, purpose, etc. the listener can be taken as actively attending to);
2. their interpretation must be compatible with that of their matrix clause."

The process of discourse segmentation is explained by Webber as follows(ibid., 6):

"Multi-clause segments correspond to non-terminal nodes of the tree, and single-clause segments terminal nodes;

- To start, an initial root node is established. (This will not necessarily be the final root node after segmentation is complete.)
- Clauses are processed in linear order.
- A new single-clause segment (terminal node) is added to the growing tree in one of two ways:
- by attachment or by adjunction:
  - A node is attached to an existing non-terminal node by making it the new rightmost daughter of that node.
  - A node Cj is adjoined to an existing non-terminal node S_i by creating a new non-terminal node S_k and attaching S_i as its left daughter and Cj as its right daughter. If S_i was the root node S_k becomes the new one. If S_i was an internal node, then S_k replaces S_i in the tree.
  - A node Cj is adjoined to an existing terminal node C_i by creating a new non-terminal node S_k, inserting it in the tree in place of C_i, attaching C_i as its left daughter and Cj as its right daughter."

From the description of discourse structuring we may assume that the rightmost node is always and only corresponding to the current latest and lowest clause being processed: in our representation structural relations are not represented in tree like form but take advantage of indentation and the linear sequential order in which clauses in the text are being processed. Since trees are built from left to right, the rightmost daughter corresponds literally to what in our sequential structure might be called the latest daughter.

There is only one example in our texts of a deictic with discourse reference, which we report here below, divided up roughly into clauses:

Text 2.

1.The three friends went all outside. 2.As they were walking in the garden, 3.John said to himself 4."Sara will marry that man", without any resentment. 5.Richard would marry her. 6.He felt strongly about all this.

When we get to the utterance which contains "all this" and is made up of a single clause no.6, the discourse segment available is made up of two clauses: Sara will marry that man / Richard would marry her. The system may compute "this" as a pronoun coreferring with the meaning conveyed by that discourse segment. We implemented one such mechanism that is used to bind discourse deictic anaphora with events of the previous utterances as long as they belong to the same Discourse Segment. We discuss it in Book 1 - Chapt. VII, to be published, and also in Chapter 8 here below.

In Polanyi's model there are four possible parses intervening between two adjacent clauses A and B at any point in the analysis:

1. A is coordinated with B.
2. B is embedded relative to A.
3. B is subordinate relative to A.
4. A is superordinate to B.

Subordinate and Coordinate Nodes are created by the algorithm as the analysis proceeds. In order to embed some clause under a Subordinate node a PUSH action is executed; to exit the stack a POP action should be performed. Coordinate nodes are usually lists of clauses at the same level of attachment. As Polanyi notes, clauses attached under the same mother are accessible and pronominalization should be expected to hold in the Topic Chain by any daughter or rightmost node. On the contrary, whenever a POP to a higher level structure obtains, we should expect pronominalization in a Topic Chain to be barred. However, in case two characters are present in the story, a Subordinate node could indicate the local shift from one to the other of the two characters and this should be marked off by the explicit mention of some property of the entity in focus. A POP from this level could be still performed by some pronoun, provided that the other entity is coreferred by the explicit mention of a property. The same result is achieved by our algorithm of discourse structure which receives as input Discourse States and Topic Structure, as well as Discourse Relations and Temporal Relations. However, a finer-grained description would require more local computation which could be directed at the assessment of the semantic congruence of discourse segments as they are produced independently by our algorithm. As Polanyi comments,

> "How semantic congruence is ascertained is an important issue. This process of semantic analysis is a world-knowledge and inference-driven semantic matching process making use of extra-linguistic knowledge, the meaning of the words and the structures encountered to perform an analytic and possible matching operation on the semantic values encoded in the semantic frames associated with the various nodes." (ibid.617)

Since we assume that extra-linguistic knowledge should be brought to bear independently by the system only when needed, we take semantic congruence to be just a contextually driven process.

Semantic relations in any given text are the main task to be faced when building structural representation. These relations are described by Discourse Relations and Temporal Relations. Consequently we label the nodes of the DSR with this information, as well as with facts or situations containing relations in which Topics are involved. We must point out that we use Discourse Relations as local markers of congruence in adjacency. Hierarchical structures are not further checked nor elaborated even though the mechanism we set up with Discourse Moves, which is the topic of the following section, enacts what can be regarded a de facto hierarchy which however receives no further scrutiny nor labeling at DRs level.

Discourse Relations are computed from aspectual, semantic category, temporal and syntactic information: differently from what both Polanyi and Mann & Thompson(1987) assume we note that there is no intervention of conceptual level reasoning. As to Coordination, Polanyi says that semantic congruence is obtained by a set of Generalised Union Operations on clauses which express propositions conveying the values one function (the unifying property) has for a series of alternative arguments (the coordinated properties). In our case, once Discourse Segments are built, local reasoning could be invoked in order to ascertain whether Generalised Union Operations could be performed. In her example, a coordination obtains between the following sentences:

a. John is a very good athlete.
b. He can run a four-minute mile.
c. He throws a mean hardball, too.

in which the unifying property is the one expressed by the first sentence, and the following sentences are instances of this property: they must be in an ISA Relation with one another proceeding to the right. Other conditions are represented by the fact that they should all refer to the same Participant, and they should express the "most restrictive relevant natural set", in other words, they should form a sequence from the more general to the more specific property. This is the only example she discusses in her paper, and we don't know how her theory would work on more complex cases, such as the ones we present in this book. However, as Polanyi comments, the details of the underlying mechanism are left for further research!

In our system, information on the structure of discourse can be gathered from an extended number of sources. In particular, the Module for the Resolution of Anaphora at Discourse Level, is itself a local finite state machine that parses the text, at the level of utterances. These indications should be consistent with the DSR as proposed in what follows. Also relevant to the issue under discussion is the Rhetorical Structure Representation, where we indicate the list of Topics present in a given utterance as well as the Discourse Domain, be it Objective or Subjective, together with the Subject of Consciousness in case there is one. Finally the Main Spatial Location and the Main Temporal Location are used to assign indices to entities in the world: they should be consistent with other discourse markers.

We could say, that every time text progression is marked by the presence of a number of clauses related to the same Main Topic, these clauses should be regarded as a Segment or an Episode at the level of Semantic Relations affecting a given Entity in the text.

Every time a New Entity is introduced in the text, some interruption is brought to bear on the DRS, and this should be captured by an upward movement from one structural level to another.

It would seem that a POP action should take place every time a new Topic is added in prominent position, and it was not included in the previous list of Topics; in addition, the new attachment level is determined by the congruence of the current Clause as to the participants in the main Semantic_Relation, to the level in which these are present as Topics. One of the prediction that the model enables us to do, is that in case Pronominalization occurs, it will affect all the Topics visible at a certain level. A POP action will cause an UP node to be produced and this in turn will indicate that a nominal head has been used to introduce or reintroduce a given Topic.

On the contrary, a PUSH action takes place every time the previous Topic, be it Expected or Main, is asserted as Secondary and there is a persistence of the same previous Topics.

The existence of a Subjective Domain with a Subject of Consciousness requires the permanence at a certain level of Coordination.

In fact pronominalization processes may be affected by DSs only negatively in that pronouns are not free to select an antecedent from the pool/history of available entities present in the DModel. Pronouns are referentially poor when compared to nominals and in particular proper nouns. These problems are tackled at length in Book I, to appear. In fact, what may happen is that a pronoun cannot be used in case the antecedent is not uniquely identifiable and may induce the addressee/reader into error. Thus it is more a matter of generation than of analysis in picking up the right DS.

4.1. Discouse Segments and Moves

In conclusion, a Discourse Structure is a set of Segments or stretches of Discourse or Text which are marked off by nodes: the following nodes are generated by our algorithm,

1. **ROOT** - to mark the beginning of a story
2. **UP** - to mark a break in the current Segment and a movement upward
3. **SAME_LEVEL** - to mark a subordination or coordination of a clause to the current Segment
4. **DOWN** - to mark an embedding movement in the current Segment

The definition of *Root* is self-explanatory, and we will not comment on it. As to the *UP* node, it occurs whenever there is an interruption in the current Segment: this might be caused either by a return to a previous Topic by means of a nominal expression which denotes some property of the Topic, or by the appearance of a new Topic. In the former case, the algorithm will indicate clause and utterance number of the attachment node; in the latter case, the *UP* node will simply be attached to the root.

The *Same_Level* node is used to set off segments of discourse. They are so regarded by the algorithm on the basis of two main rhetorical strategies:

1. a sequence of clauses can be analysed as a Segment because of its underlying Domain, and it must be a Subjective Domain. In this case, the Discourse Focus does not move forward and is stuck to the clause setting the beginning of the Segment. Discourse Relations may either be Descriptions, Elaborations, or Explanations;
2. a sequence of clauses is analysed as a Segment because it has the same Main Topic. In this case, the Discourse Focus is moved forward and the story progresses by enumerating a number of properties related to the same entity. Discourse Relations may be Narrations or any other previously mentioned Relation.

The second strategy is simply a Default strategy, and is clearly inherent in the first one. The *Down* node is used to mark off the beginning of a possible Segment of discourse, or simply a movement backward of the story where the main topic is however the same as the current one. In the latter case, a past perfect could be used to trigger the appropriate Temporal Relation, a BEFORE relation, and the related Discourse Relation, an Elaboration relation. In more formalized terms:

1. Discourse Segment

It is a stretch of text which has the same Spatial and Temporal Location, the same Main Topic and the same Point of View.

Technically, it may only contain *DOWN* and/or *SAME_LEVEL* movements; it is included in one single temporal Reference Interval;

it may be characterized by one or more Discourse Structures.

2. New Discourse Segment

A New Discourse Segment is created whenever either one or all of the following conditions obtain in the text:

i. Anytime a story/news begins;
ii. A new participant is introduced and is treated as a salient topic, i.e. it persists on the scene;
iii. The narration resumes previously introduced Main Topics and sets them in Foreground.

As a result, any reasoning based on cognitive means should build upon the structural representation as it is independently worked out by our algorithm, by adding further internal structure. We assume that conceptual reasoning implied by Rhetorical Structure Theory as proposed by Mann and Thompson, or by Polanyi could not possibly disrupt our structural representation, which is mainly Topic based and relies on local semantic relations rather than on global relations.

Consider the result of each move onto the discourse structure and the Reference Intervals which constitute the local computations we perform. *Same_level* moves are quite straightforward, in that they simply build up more structure at both levels, temporal and relational. *Down* moves constitute an internal additional level which has access to relations to its left, but usually preludes to an *Up* move. Now consider *Up* moves: there are two possible strategies, we said above, which can motivate such a move: either a new Topic appears in discourse, or some previously mentioned topic is resumed. From the relational point of view things are completely different: in case a new Topic appears it constitutes a break in the local semantic and temporal structure because there will certainly be a new time focus asserted and no semantic relations are entertained locally. This should usually cause the algorithm to go as up as possible to the root node level. In the second case, topicality is overrun by semantic relations, on the basis of which one could decide to establish links with the adjacent or the attachment node.

5. THE ALGORITHM

We shall enter in more detail the actual algorithm that builds Discourse Structures, Temporal Relations and Intervals and Discourse Relations from the current semantic and grammatical information and from that available from previous computation. It is important to highlight the fact that discourse structure is a relevant type of text representation where a certain type of information is being encoded efficiently and that it is dependent on logical form and other semantic representations discussed previously. In addition, Discourse Structure Representation as presented below, is essential for summary or paraphrase generation processes, as shall be commented in the final section of the following chapter.

5.1. Semantic Components of Discourse Structure

For each discourse structure we collect the information shown in the following ten discourse markers from the current and the adjacent utterance:

1. DiscMove:Move(PrecUtterNo-PrecClNo)
2. clause:CurrUtterNo-CurrClNo
3. topics:[Type:Semid:PredHead]
4. main_fact:MainRel([ListArgs, Semid:PredHead], Pol, SpaceLoc)
5. ref_int:tint(MainTimeRef, [ListTimeRefs])
6. temp_rel:TempRelation(TimeRef1, TimeRef2)
7. disc_rel:DiscRelation
8. disc_str:Att_Node(ClNo)-[List-ClNos]
9. disc_dom:DiscDomain
10. p_o_view:subject_of_point_of_view

Each discourse structure starts out by indicating a given Discourse Move from the ones listed above and by the individuation of a given attachment node, represented by an utterance number and a clause number. Then we have the current values for utterance and clause - notice that an utterance may be made up by more than one clause. Marker 3 lists the current topics, their semantic identifier in the DM, their type and predicate. In 4 we have the main relation where we have the semantic predicate appearing in the DM and its semantic arguments represented by a semantic identifier and a predicate head, then we have the polarity and the spatial index for that relation. In 5 we have the time interval representing the reference interval for the current discourse segment made up by a main time reference and a list of subordinate time reference indices. In 6 we have a temporal relation which is the logical relation intervening between two adjacent time references in the current time interval. In 7 we have a discourse relation again elaborated by evaluating the relation intervening between two adjacent discourse structures in the current segment.

- Topics, their types, and their semantic identifiers
- Temporal Relations
- Discourse Relations

- Main propositional relation or predicate and its semantic role
- Preceding Discourse Move
- Preceding Discourse Level
- Preceding Discourse Relation
- Preceding Discourse State

Thus we proceed as follows:

1. we recover all current Topics, with their type, their predicate, their semantic Id;
2. from previous computation we recover the main propositional Relation, the Temporal Relation and the Discourse Relation;
3. we recover from preceding discourse structure computation the Preceding Relation, Preceding State, Preceding Move and Discourse Level;
4. we pass all the information gathered to the main call, disc_move, which has the following arguments:
   PreNoCl = number of preceding clause;
   NoCl = number of current clause;
   PreTops = list of preceding topics built as a triplet, Type:Ind:Pred;
   Tops = list of current topics;
   TRel = Temporal Relation
   TInt = Time Interval for the current Discourse Segment
   PreDisRel = preceding Discourse Relation
   DisRel = current Discourse Relation
   PreState = preceding State of the FSDA
   State = current State of the FSDA
   PreDiscLev = preceding Discourse Level
   DisLev = Discourse Level
   PreDisMove = preceding Discourse Move
   DisMove = Discourse Move
   Att_Cl = attachment node in terms of Discourse Level and Clause number

And here below is the corresponding Prolog code:

```
clause_d_structure( NoFr, Node, NoCl, Tops, DisRel, TRel, Tint, Rel, State, DisMove,
DisLev, Att_Cl) :-
    findall(Type:Ind:Pred, (trova_topics(NoFr, Type, Pred, Ind)), Tops),
    info( NoFr, Node, Prop, _, _,_, _,_, Rel, TRel, DisRel, _, _),
    stato(NoFr, State), PreNoCl is NoCl - 1,
    d_struct( _, _, PreNoCl, PreTops, PreDisRel, _, _, PreState, PreDisMove,PreDisLev),
    disc_move(PreNoCl, NoCl, PreTops, Tops, TRel, PreDisRel, DisRel, PreState, State,
    PreDisLev, DisLev, PreDisMove, DisMove, Att_Cl),
    build_temp_int(Move, NoFr-NoCl, FrCl, TRel, Tint, Strc),
    asserta(disc_struc(At,NoFr-NoCl, Tops, MainRel, Tint, TRel, DisRel, Strc, DisDom,
    Point)).
```

The basic goal of the algorithm is that of deciding the Discourse Move and Level of attachment. This is done at first by matching Discourse Relations of the current and the previous utterance, then by considering special cases of current Discourse Relation like "result, purpose", and then by considering special Temporal Relations as shown by the following list of calls:

```
disc_move(PreNoCl, NoCl, PreTops, Tops, TRel,PrDMove, DRel, PDRel, PreState,
State, PreLev, Lev, Move, Att_Cl) :-
    check_disc_rel(DRel, PDRel, TRel, PrDMove, Move),
    disc_level(PreNoCl, Move, PrDMove, PreLev, PreTops, Tops, NoCl, Lev, Att_Cl).

    check_disc_rel(DRel, DRel, TempRel, PrDMove, level):-
        on(DRel, [explanation, setting, description, evaluation, definition]).

    check_disc_rel(setting, _, TempRel, PrDMove, up):- PrDMove\=nil.
    check_disc_rel(result, hypothesis, TempRel, PrDMove, down).
    check_disc_rel(DRel, PDRel, before(_,_), PrDMove, bottom).
    check_disc_rel(purpose, PDRel, TempRel, PrDMove, down).
    check_disc_rel(DRel, PDRel, overlap(_,_), PrDMove, level):- PrDMove\=nil.
    check_disc_rel(DRel, PDRel, finished_by(_,_), PrDMove, bottom).
    check_disc_rel(DRel, PDRel, TempRel, PrDMove, down):-
        on(DRel, [evaluation, explanation, definition]).
        check_disc_rel(narration, inception, TempRel, PrDMove, level).
        check_disc_rel(DRel, result, TempRel, PrDMove, down).
        check_disc_rel(inception, PDRel, TempRel, PrDMove, up).
        check_disc_rel(obligation, PDRel, TempRel, PrDMove, up).
        check_disc_rel(hypothesis, PDRel, TempRel, PrDMove, up).
```

In case these procedures fail, a number of remaining cases are considered which however only rely on the state of the FSDA, by matching the previous state with the current one, as in the following list:

```
disc_move(PreNoCl, NoCl, PreTops, Tops, _,PreDisMov,_,_,PreSt, St, PreLev, Lev,
DisMov, Att_Cl) :-
    d_move(PreSt, St, DiscMove),
    disc_level(PreNoCl, DisMove, PreDisMove, PreLev, PreTops, Tops, NoCl, Lev,
        Att_Cl).

d_move([shifting], [shifting], up) .
d_move([shifting], [retaining], down) .
d_move([resume], [continue, continue_analyze], up) .
d_move([retaining], [continue, continue_analyze], level) .
d_move([retaining], [change], up) .
d_move([continue], [continue], level) .
d_move([continue_analyze], [continue_analyze], down) .
d_move([continue, retaining], [resume, retaining], up) .
```

```
d_move([continue], [resume], up) .
d_move([change], [resume], down) .
d_move([nil], _, down) .
d_move(_, _, level) .
```

When the Discourse move has been decided it is passed on to the following call, which has to decide where in the preceding discourse structure the current segment can sensibly be attached. The default information will be: attach to the adjacent discourse segment. However, default information can be contradicted by an *UP* move which requires some resetting of discourse structure and a new node to be created.

```
disc_level(_, down, _, PreLev, PreTops, Tops, 1, 1, new(1-1)).
disc_level(PreNoCl, level, bottom, PreLev, _, _, _, Lev, down(NoFr-PreNoCl)) :-
    Lev is PreLev + 1.
disc_level(PreNoCl, down, _, PrecLev, _, _, _, Lev, down(NoFr-PreNoCl)) :-
    info(PreNoFr, Node, _/temp_seq, _, _, _, _, _, _, _, _, _, _),
    Lev is PreLev + 1.
disc_level(PreNoCl, level, _, PreLev, PreTops, Tops, NoCl, Lev, Att_Cl) :-
    move_to_topic(PreTops, Tops, NoCl, PreLev, Lev, Att_Cl),!.
disc_level(PreNoCl, up, _, PreLev, PreTops, Tops, NoCl, Lev, Att_Cl) :-
    (PreNoCl > 0,
    move_to_latest_topic(PreTops, Tops, PreNoCl, PreLev, Lev, Att_Cl) ;
    infer_topics(PreNoCl, Tops, Lev, Att_Cl),! ;
    Att_Cl=to(1-1), Lev=1 ).
disc_level(PreNoCl, down, level, PreLev, Tops, NoCl, Lev, Att_Cl) :-
    move_to_topic(Tops, NoCl, PreLev, Lev, Att_Cl),!.
disc_level(_, _, _, PreLev, _, _, Lev, down(NoFr-PreNoCl)) :- Lev is PreLev + 1.
```

As can be easily noticed from the code listed above, whenever a DOWN move is performed, the current Level is updated by 1; on the contrary, whenever the attachment is to some previous higher node, the level is inherited from there. However the most difficult decision is assuming the current Main, Expected or Secondary Topic as a continuation of some previously asserted Topic, and deciding what relevance it has for the current state of discourse. In fact, we might take as relevant, current Topics limited only to those independently assigned by the FSDA as Main or as Expected. Then, when searching up in the list of previous discourse structures we still have to decide whether the match has be made with a Main, a Secondary or an Expected Topic, disregarding by default Potential Topics.

```
move_to_latest_topic(Topics, NoCl, _, NewLev, At) :-
    (d_struct(NoFr, _, PreNoCl, PreTopics, _, _, _, _, _, Lev),
    match_topics(Topics, PreTopics, _, Func),
    move_up(Topics, NoCl, _, NewLev, At),!.

move_up(Topics, NoCl, _, Lev, to(A-B)) :-
    NoCl > 0, PreNoCl is NoCl - 1,
    move_to_latest_topic(Topics, PreNoCl, _, Lev, to(A-B)).
```

```
move_to_topic(Topics, NoCl, PreLev, Lev, Func(NoFr-PreNoCl)) :-
    (PreNoCl is NoCl - 1,
    d_struct( NoFr, _, PreNoCl, PreTopics, _, _, _, _, _, Lev),
    match_main_topics(Topics, PreTopics), Func=level,!
    ;
    NewNoCl is NoCl - 1,
    move_to_latest_topic(Topics, NewNoCl, PrecLev, Lev, Fun(NoFr-PreNoCl)),!
    ;
    PrecNoCl is NoCl - 1,
    d_struct(NoFr, _, PreNoCl, PreTopics, _, _, _, _, _, Lev),
    match_secondary_topic(Topics, PreTopics, NoFr), Fun=level).
```

The main call is to Match Topics, which takes into consideration only Main and Expected Topics, and a first match is attempted. In case of failure, Main adjacent topics and Main and Secondary topics are tried. Finally, the algorithm looks for a match in one of the previously asserted topic structures, as recorded in Discourse Structure.

Discourse Structure includes also information about Time Focus, Time Reference, Time Interval or Reference Interval which contains all time references related to a given discourse segment. The actual construction of temporal interval can thus take place only at discourse structure level, in particular when a discourse move has been decided:

```
build_temp_int(_, 1-1, _, TempRel, tint(T1, []), Strc):-
    TempRel=Rel(T1, T2),
    Strc = 1-[1],
    retractall(current_temp_int(_, _, _)),
    assert(current_temp_int(1-1, tint(T1, []), Strc)).

build_temp_int(Move, NoFr-NoCl, At, TRel, Tint, CurrStr):-
    time_focus(_, TFoc),
    TRel= TR(Tes1, Tes2),
    PreNoCl is NoCl - 1,
    current_temp_int(_-PreNoCl, tint(OldTFoc, OldInts), OldNoCl-Strc),
    build_interval(NoCl, PreNoCl, OldNoCl, OldTFoc, TFoc, Move, Tes1, TR, OldInts,
    Strc, NewTFoc, NewInts, CurrStr),
    Tint=tint(NewTF, NewInts),
    assert(current_temp_int(NoFr-NoCl, Tint, CurrStr)).

build_interval(2, PrecNoCl, OldNoCl, TF, TF, Move, Tes1, TR, OldInts, Strc, TF,
NewInts, CurrStr):-
    NewInts=[Tes1],
    append(Strc, [2], NewStr),
        CurrStr = OldNoCl-NewStr.
```

We include below the structures related to the English texts listed under 3.2 in the Introduction and discussed in Book I, to appear, which are devoted to Domain of Point of

View, and the whole discourse structure for Story 1. We shall discuss in more detail the UP moves in each text analysed.

Text 1

In this text there are two UP moves: the first one is in utterance no.6 and is determined by topicality; the second one is in the last utterance and is determined both by topicality and semantic relations. In the first case, the move does not create a discontinuity in Reference Interval and in Discourse Structure: in fact, we can see that the Domain has always the same Point of View, Mary. In the second case, the move constitutes a break in the discourse structure and all semantic relations are set to the new attachment point.

```
root:new(1-1)
clause:1-1
topics:[expected:id2:john]
main_fact:give([id2:john, id4:rose, id3:mary], 1, univ)
ref_int:tint(tes(f5_sa01), [])
disc_rel:narration
disc_str:1-[1]
disc_dom:objective
p_o_view:narrator

    down:down(1-1)
    clause:2-2
    topics:[secondary:id4:rose, expected:id3:mary]
    main_fact:take([id3:mary, id4:rose], 1, univ)
    ref_int:tint(tes(f6_sa02), [])
    disc_rel:result
    disc_str:1-[2]
    disc_dom:objective
    p_o_view:narrator

    same_level:from(2-2)
    clause:2-3
    topics:[secondary:id4:rose, expected:id3:mary]
    main_fact:put([id3:mary, id4:rose, id10:hair], 1, univ)
    ref_int:tint(tes(f6_sa02), [f6_sa02])
    disc_rel:result
    disc_str:1-[2, 3]
    disc_dom:objective
    p_o_view:narrator

      down:down(2-3)
      clause:3-4
      topics:[main:id3:mary, secondary:id13:present]
      main_fact:know([id3:mary, id15:give], 1, univ)
      ref_int:tint(tes(f6_sa02), [f8_sa03])
```

disc_rel:evaluation
disc_str:3-[4]
disc_dom:objective
p_o_view:narrator

down:down(3-4)
clause:3-5
topics:[main:id3:mary, secondary:id13:present]
main_fact:give([id3:mary, id13:present, id14:exist], 1, univ)
ref_int:tint(tes(f6_sa02), [f7_sa03])
disc_rel:narration
disc_str:4-[5]
disc_dom:subjective
p_o_view:mary

down:down(3-5)
clause:4-6
topics:[main:id3:mary, secondary:id20:[mary, john], expected:id19:steve]
main_fact:say([id19:steve, id23:enjoy], 1, univ)
ref_int:tint(tes(f6_sa04), [])
disc_rel:narration
disc_str:5-[6]
disc_dom:objective
p_o_view:narrator

same_level:level(4-6)
clause:4-7
topics:[main:id3:mary, secondary:id20:[mary, john], expected:id19:steve]
main_fact:enjoy([id20:[mary, john], id20:[mary, john]], 1, univ)
ref_int:tint(tes(f6_sa04), [f7_sa04])
disc_rel:narration
disc_str:5-[6, 7]
disc_dom:subjective
p_o_view:mary

same_level:level(4-7)
clause:5-8
topics:[secondary:id3:mary, expected:id21:indefinite]
main_fact:shocking([id21:ev], 1, univ)
ref_int:tint(tes(f6_sa04), [f7_sa04, f4_sa05])
disc_rel:evaluation
disc_str:5-[6, 7, 8]
disc_dom:subjective
p_o_view:mary

same_level:from(5-8)

clause:5-9
topics:[secondary:id3:mary, expected:id21:indefinite]
main_fact:shocking([id21:ev], 1, univ)
ref_int:tint(tes(f6_sa04), [f7_sa04, f4_sa05, f2_sa05])
disc_rel:evaluation
disc_str:5-[6, 7, 8, 9]
disc_dom:subjective
p_o_view:mary

up:to(4-7)
clause:6-10
topics:[expected:id3:mary]
main_fact:herself([id32:form], 0, univ)
ref_int:tint(tes(f6_sa04), [f7_sa04, f4_sa05, f2_sa05, f2_sa06])
disc_rel:explanation
disc_str:5-[6, 7, 8, 9, 10]
disc_dom:subjective
p_o_view:mary

same_level:level(6-10)
clause:7-11
topics:[main:id3:mary, secondary:id19:steve]
main_fact:feel([id3:mary, infon166:[determination, hostility]], 1, univ)
ref_int:tint(tes(f6_sa04), [f7_sa04, f4_sa05, f2_sa05, f2_sa06, f5_sa07])
disc_rel:explanation
disc_str:5-[6, 7, 8, 9, 10, 11]
disc_dom:subjective
p_o_view:mary

up:to(1-1)
clause:8-12
topics:[secondary:id3:mary, expected:id2:john]
main_fact:smile([id2:john], 1, id39)
ref_int:tint(tes(f6_sa08), [f5_sa01])
disc_rel:narration
disc_str:1-[12]
disc_dom:objective
p_o_view:narrator

same_level:from(8-12)
clause:8-13
topics:[secondary:id3:mary, expected:id2:john]
main_fact:go([id2:john, id39:away], 1, id39)
ref_int:tint(tes(f6_sa08), [f5_sa01, f6_sa08])
disc_rel:result
disc_str:1-[12, 13]

disc_dom:objective
p_o_view:narrator

Text 2

This text contains two UP moves: the first one is in utterance no.8, where the woman Sara reappears as main character in subject position of a main clause, which however is a consequent of a conditional clause. We assume here that both the temporal and the semantic relations are to be connected with the adjacent text span rather with the topicality determined one. The second UP move which is performed at the end of the text, is to utterance no. 2 and is a return to reality from a long stretch of text which constitutes a subjective domain from John's point of view. In this case, both temporal and semantic relations are entertained with the attachment point, i.e. clause(2-3).

root:new(1-1)
clause:1-1
topics:[expected:id3:friend]
main_fact:go([id3:friend, id2:outside], 1, id2)
ref_int:tint(tes(f5_sa09), [])
disc_rel:narration
disc_str:1-[1]
disc_dom:objective
p_o_view:narrator

same_level:level(1-1)
clause:2-2
topics:[main:id3:friend, secondary:id7:john]
main_fact:say([id7:john, id7:john, id10:marry], 1, id2)
ref_int:tint(tes(f5_sa09), [f7_sa10])
disc_rel:result
disc_str:1-[1, 2]
disc_dom:subjective
p_o_view:john

same_level:level(2-2)
clause:2-3
topics:[main:id3:friend, secondary:id7:john]
main_fact:walk([id3:friend, id15:garden], 1, id2)
ref_int:tint(tes(f5_sa09), [f7_sa10, f4_sa10])
disc_rel:circumstance
disc_str:1-[1, 2, 3]
disc_dom:objective
p_o_view:narrator

down:down(2-3)
clause:2-4
topics:[main:id3:friend, secondary:id7:john]

```
main_fact:marry([id8:sara, id9:friend], 1, id2)
ref_int:tint(tes(f7_sa10), [])
disc_rel:evaluation
disc_str:3-[4]
disc_dom:subjective
p_o_view:john

same_level:level(2-4)
clause:3-5
topics:[secondary:id3:friend, expected:id8:sara]
main_fact:marry([id3:friend, id8:sara], 1, id2)
ref_int:tint(tes(f7_sa10), [f5_sa11])
disc_rel:evaluation
disc_str:3-[4, 5]
disc_dom:subjective
p_o_view:john

same_level:level(3-5)
clause:4-6
topics:[main:id7:john, secondary:id8:sara]
main_fact:feel([id7:john, id10:this], 1, id2)
ref_int:tint(tes(f7_sa10), [f5_sa11, f5_sa12])
disc_rel:explanation
disc_str:3-[4, 5, 6]
disc_dom:subjective
p_o_view:john

same_level:level(4-6)
clause:5-7
topics:[main:id7:john, expected:id8:sara]
main_fact:person([id8:sara], 1, id2)
ref_int:tint(tes(f7_sa10), [f5_sa11, f5_sa12, f5_sa13])
disc_rel:explanation
disc_str:3-[4, 5, 6, 7]
disc_dom:subjective
p_o_view:john

same_level:level(5-7)
clause:6-8
topics:[main:id7:john, secondary:id8:sara]
main_fact:absurd([id7:john], 1, id2)
ref_int:tint(tes(f7_sa10), [f5_sa11, f5_sa12, f5_sa13, f9_sa14])
disc_rel:explanation
disc_str:3-[4, 5, 6, 7, 8]
disc_dom:subjective
p_o_view:john
```

same_level:level(6-8)
clause:7-9
topics:[main:id7:john]
main_fact:absurd([id30:demand], 1, id2)
ref_int:tint(tes(f7_sa10), [f5_sa11, f5_sa12, f5_sa13, f9_sa14, f5_sa15])
disc_rel:explanation
disc_str:3-[4, 5, 6, 7, 8, 9]
disc_dom:subjective
p_o_view:john

up:to(5-7)
clause:8-10
topics:[main:id8:sara, secondary:id7:john]
main_fact:accept([id8:sara, id7:john], 1, id2)
ref_int:tint(tes(f7_sa10), [f5_sa11, f5_sa12, f5_sa13, f9_sa14, f5_sa15, f5_sa16])
disc_rel:evaluation
disc_str:3-[4, 5, 6, 7, 8, 9, 10]
disc_dom:subjective
p_o_view:john

down:down(8-10)
clause:8-11
topics:[main:id8:sara, secondary:id7:john]
main_fact:absurd([id7:john], 1, id2)
ref_int:tint(tes(f7_sa10), [f7_sa16])
disc_rel:narration
disc_str:10-[11]
disc_dom:subjective
p_o_view:john

up:to(2-3)
clause:9-12
topics:[secondary:id8:sara, expected:id18:richard]
main_fact:begin([id18:richard, id38:sing], 1, id2)
ref_int:tint(tes(f5_sa09), [f7_sa10, f4_sa10, f5_sa17])
disc_rel:inception
disc_str:1-[1, 2, 3, 12]
disc_dom:objective
p_o_view:narrator

Text 3

In this text, there is only one UP move, and it is performed at the end. The utterance connects naturally with the first utterance of the text and both from a temporal and a semantic point of view the relation is entertained with the one contained in the first utterance.

root:new(1-1)

```
clause:1-1
topics:[expected:id2:mary]
main_fact:pick_up([id2:mary, id4:phone], 1, univ)
ref_int:tint(tes(f5_sa18), [])
disc_rel:narration
disc_str:1-[1]
disc_dom:objective
p_o_view:narrator

 same_level:from(1-1)
 clause:1-2
 topics:[expected:id2:mary]
 main_fact:call([id2:mary, id3:jason], 1, univ)
 ref_int:tint(tes(f5_sa18), [f6_sa18])
 disc_rel:narration
 disc_str:1-[1, 2]
 disc_dom:objective
 p_o_view:narrator

 same_level:level(1-2)
 clause:2-3
 topics:[main:id2:mary, secondary:id9:husband]
 main_fact:think([id2:mary, id11:consider], 1, univ)
 ref_int:tint(tes(f5_sa18), [f6_sa18, f5_sa19])
 disc_rel:elaboration
 disc_str:1-[1, 2, 3]
 disc_dom:objective
 p_o_view:narrator

 same_level:level(2-3)
 clause:2-4
 topics:[main:id2:mary, secondary:id9:husband]
 main_fact:consider([id9:husband, infon43:[base, untruthful]], 1, univ)
 ref_int:tint(tes(f5_sa18), [f6_sa18, f5_sa19, f7_sa19])
 disc_rel:evaluation
 disc_str:1-[1, 2, 3, 4]
 disc_dom:subjective
 p_o_view:mary

   down:down(2-4)
   clause:3-5
   topics:[main:id2:mary, secondary:id16:thing]
   main_fact:there_be([id15:something], 1, univ)
   ref_int:tint(tes(f6_sa18), [])
   disc_rel:explanation
   disc_str:4-[5]
```

disc_dom:subjective
p_o_view:mary

up:to(1-1)
clause:4-6
topics:[secondary:id2:mary, expected:id3:jason]
main_fact:answer([id3:jason], 1, univ)
ref_int:tint(tes(f10_sa21), [f5_sa18])
disc_rel:narration
disc_str:1-[6]
disc_dom:objective
p_o_view:narrator

Story 1

In the story of three little pigs there is a first UP move in utterance no.2 which however is not a discontinuity in the relational structure. The second UP move is in utterance no. 9 and is only determined by a change in topicality. The third UP move is in the following utterance, which requires the stack of relations to be reset to the new attachment point: the main relation is one of RESULT and this has no connection with the local environment but only connects to the attachment point. Consequently, also the stack of Reference Intervals is set to the new reference point. Then we find another UP move in utterance 15 with no change in topicality but a change in event structure. On the contrary in the next UP move, in utterance 18 there is a change in topicality: the wolf reappears. Then, when we get to the end of the text, we have a sequence of UP moves the first of which is the result of the wolf's blowing, seen from the point of view of the house, by means of inchoativization, in utterance 21. Then in utterance 22, the next UP move indicates the result of blowing from the wolf's point of view - he falls to the ground! Finally, in utterance 23, we see the result of the wolf's attempt to destroy Jimmy's house, from the little pigs' point of view, another UP move. Comments on the criteria to build coherent reference-intervals for temporal relations in case of UP moves are added locally.

C1/C'erano una volta tre fratelli porcellini che C2/vivevano felici nella campagna.
root:new(1-1)
clause:1-1
topics:[main:id3:porcellino]
main_fact:esserci([id3:porcellino], 1, id2)
ref_int:tint(tes(f5_po1), [])
temp_rel:contains(tes(f5_po01), td(f5_po01))
disc_rel:setting
disc_str:1-[1]
disc_dom:objective
p_o_view:narrator

same_level:from(1-1)
clause:1-2
topics:[main:id3:porcellino]

main_fact:vivere([id3:porcellino, id2:campagna], 1, id2)
ref_int:tint(tes(f5_po1), [f4_po1])
temp_rel:during(tes(f4_po01), tes(f5_po01))
disc_rel:setting
disc_str:1-[1, 2]
disc_dom:objective
p_o_view:narrator

C3/Nello stesso luogo però viveva anche un terribile lupo che C4/si nutriva proprio di porcellini grassi e teneri.

up:to(1-1)
clause:2-3
topics:[main:id9:lupo, secondary:id3:porcellino]
main_fact:vivere([id9:lupo, id13:luogo], 1, id2)
ref_int:tint(tes(f5_po1), [f4_po1, f4_po2])
temp_rel:finished_by(tes(f4_po02), tes(f5_po01))
disc_rel:setting
disc_str:1-[1, 2, 3]
disc_dom:objective
p_o_view:narrator

same_level:from(2-3)
clause:2-4
topics:[main:id9:lupo, secondary:id3:porcellino]
main_fact:nutrire([id9:lupo, id9:lupo, id10:porcellino], 1, id2)
ref_int:tint(tes(f5_po1), [f4_po1, f4_po2, f3_po2])
temp_rel:during(tes(f3_po02), tes(f5_po01))
disc_rel:setting
disc_str:1-[1, 2, 3, 4]
disc_dom:objective
p_o_view:narrator

C5/Questi allora, C6/per proteggersi dal lupo, decisero di costruirsi ciascuno una casetta.

up:to(1-2)
clause:3-5
topics:[secondary:id9:lupo, expected:id3:porcellino]
main_fact:decidere([id3:porcellino, id17:costruire_si], 1, id2)
ref_int:tint(tes(f3_po3), [])
temp_rel:after(tes(f3_po03), tes(f5_po01))
disc_rel:inception
disc_str:4-[5]
disc_dom:objective
p_o_view:narrator

down:down(3-5)
clause:3-6

topics:[secondary:id9:lupo, expected:id3:porcellino]
main_fact:proteggere([id3:porcellino, id3:porcellino, id9:lupo], 1, id2)
ref_int:tint(tes(f3_po3), [finf1_po3])
temp_rel:overlap(tes(finf1_po03), tes(f3_po03))
disc_rel:purpose
disc_str:5-[6]
disc_dom:objective
p_o_view:narrator

C7/Il maggiore, Jimmi, che era saggio, lavorava di buona lena e C8/costruì la sua casetta con solidi mattoni e cemento.

down:down(3-6)
clause:4-7
topics:[main:id24:porcellino, secondary:id25:casa]
main_fact:lavorare([id24:jimmi], 1, id2)
ref_int:tint(tes(f6_po4), [])
temp_rel:finished_by(tes(f4_po04), tes(f3_po03))
disc_rel:elaboration
disc_str:6-[7]
disc_dom:objective
p_o_view:narrator

same_level:level(4-7)
clause:4-8
topics:[main:id24:porcellino, secondary:id25:casa]
main_fact:costruire([id24:jimmi, id25:casa], 1, id2)
ref_int:tint(tes(f6_po4), [f6_po4])
temp_rel:after(tes(f6_po04), tes(f3_po03))
disc_rel:result
disc_str:6-[7, 8]
disc_dom:objective
p_o_view:narrator

C9/Gli altri, Timmy e Tommy, pigri e oziosi, se la sbrigarono in fretta C10/costruendo le loro casette con la paglia e con pezzetti di legno.

down:down(4-8)
clause:5-9
topics:[main:id32:porcellino, id35:casa]
main_fact:sbrigarsi([id32:porcellino, id36:fretta], 1, id2)
ref_int:tint(tes(f3_po5), [])
temp_rel:after(tes(f3_po05), tes(f6_po04))
disc_rel:evidence
disc_str:8-[9]
disc_dom:objective
p_o_view:narrator

same_level:level(5-9)
clause:5-10
topics:[main:id32:porcellino]
main_fact:costruire([id32:porcellino, id35:casa], 1, id2)
ref_int:tint(tes(f3_po5), [fger36_po5])
temp_rel:after(tes(fgerund36_po05), tes(f3_po05))
disc_rel:result
disc_str:8-[9, 10]
disc_dom:objective
p_o_view:narrator

C11/I due porcellini pigri passavano le loro giornate C12/suonando e C13/cantando una canzone C15/che diceva C14/chi ha paura del lupo cattivo?

same_level:level(5-10)
clause:6-11
topics:[main:id32:porcellino, secondary:id9:lupo]
main_fact:passare([id32:porcellino, id44:giornata, id45:st], 1, id2)
ref_int:tint(tes(f3_po5), [fger36_po5, f6_po6])
temp_rel:finished_by(tes(f6_po06), tes(f3_po05))
disc_rel:elaboration
disc_str:8-[9, 10, 11]
disc_dom:objective
p_o_view:narrator

same_level:level(6-11)
clause:6-12
topics:[main:id32:porcellino, secondary:id9:lupo]
main_fact:suonare([id32:porcellino], 1, id2)
ref_int:tint(tes(f3_po5), [fger36_po5, f6_po6, fger40_po6])
temp_rel:during(tes(fgerund40_po06), tes(f3_po05))
disc_rel:narration
disc_str:8-[9, 10, 11, 12]
disc_dom:objective
p_o_view:narrator

same_level:level(6-12)
clause:6-13
topics:[main:id32:porcellino, secondary:id9:lupo]
main_fact:cantare([id32:porcellino, id43:canzone], 1, id2)
ref_int:tint(tes(f3_po5), [fger36_po5, f6_po6, fger40_po6, fger41_po6])
temp_rel:during(tes(fgerund41_po06), tes(f3_po05))
disc_rel:narration
disc_str:8-[9, 10, 11, 12, 13]
disc_dom:objective
p_o_view:narrator

down:down(6-13)
clause:6-14
topics:[main:id32:porcellino, secondary:id9:lupo]
main_fact:avere([id49:chi, infon242:paura], 1, id2)
ref_int:tint(tes(f3_po5), [f4_po6])
temp_rel:before(tes(f4_po06), tes(f3_po05))
disc_rel:evaluation
disc_str:13-[14]
disc_dom:subjective
p_o_view:pro

down:down(6-14)
clause:6-15
topics:[main:id32:porcellino, secondary:id9:lupo]
main_fact:dire([id43:canzone, id50:avere], 1, id2)
ref_int:tint(tes(f3_po5), [f7_po6])
temp_rel:during(tes(f7_po06), tes(f3_po05))
disc_rel:narration
disc_str:14-[15]
disc_dom:objective
p_o_view:narrator

As said at the beginning of this section, whenever an UP move takes place there might be a disruption of a locally built reference-interval for temporal reasoning, as a direct consequence of the fact that discourse structure might show the need to resume a previously discussed topic or introduce directly a new one. In the former case it would seem that reference intervals should reflect a local connection with the previous interval; however, in the latter case, it seems clear that the appearance of a new topic when presented in the world by means of a presentational syntactic structure, it is locally bound. Now consider the case at hand: the wolf is being locally evoked by the three little pigs, but is not physically present: in other word it is treated as an intensional entity and not as an extensional one. However, the wolf actually appears and we pass suddenly from fantasy to reality. The reference interval includes the last bit of temporal structure and starts up a new stretch.

C16/Ma ecco che improvvisamente il lupo apparve alle loro spalle.
up:to(6-15)
clause:7-16
topics:[main:id32:porcellino, expected:id9:lupo]
main_fact:apparire([id9:lupo], 1, id2)
ref_int:tint(tes(f1_po7), [f7_po6])
temp_rel:after(tes(f1_po07), tes(f3_po05))
disc_rel:contrast
disc_str:14-[]
disc_dom:objective
p_o_view:narrator

C17/Aiuto, aiuto gridarono i due porcellini e C18/cominciarono a correre più veloci che potevano verso la loro casetta, per sfuggire al terribile lupo.

same_level:from(7-16)
clause:8-17
topics:[main:id32:porcellino, secondary:id9:lupo]
main_fact:gridare([id32:porcellino, id59:aiuto], 1, id2)
ref_int:tint(tes(f3_po5), [f7_po6, f1_po7, f4_po8])
temp_rel:after(tes(f4_po08), tes(f1_po07))
disc_rel:result
disc_str:14-[15, 16, 17]
disc_dom:objective
p_o_view:narrator

down:down(8-17)
clause:8-18
topics:[main:id32:porcellino, secondary:id9:lupo]
main_fact:cominciare([id32:porcellino, infon314:correre], 1, id2)
ref_int:tint(tes(f4_po8), [])
temp_rel:after(tes(f7_po08), tes(f4_po08))
disc_rel:inception
disc_str:17-[18]
disc_dom:objective
p_o_view:narrator

same_level:from(8-18)
clause:8-19
topics:[main:id32:porcellino, secondary:id9:lupo]
main_fact:correre([id32:porcellino, infon324:sfuggire], 1, id2)
ref_int:tint(tes(f5_po8), [])
temp_rel:after(tes(f9_po08), tes(f4_po08))
disc_rel:rationale
disc_str:17-[18, 19]
disc_dom:objective
p_o_view:narrator

In this case, the UP move simply registers the gap intervening in narration whenever more than one participant in one event is present: the narrator must necessarily alternate his descriptions by focussing each time on one or a set of participants at a time, in case their personal stories are not concurrent. Clearly this is also representable in a plan, as said at the beginning of this chapter: but it is also clearly determined by discourse and text structure or by the plot texture. Since the wolf and the little pigs have different and conflicting aims in mind, their individual story should be narrated separately. In this case, the UP move simply establishes a connection between what the wolf was doing a while ago, when he first appeared physically on the scene: however, the way in which it is linguistically expressed, imposes a local temporal connection, limiting the meaning of the UP move to a topic alternation.

Consider RESULT relations: sometimes they have a CAUSE and some other times they don't. In particular, C17 does not have a corresponding CAUSE and the same applies below to C21. Literally, only the infinitival SFUGGIRE contains a discourse marker PER that indicates RATIONALE. However, from a Discourse level point of view, we may note that also GRIDARE is a RESULT of the wolf APPEARing in the previous utterance. This should also be marked, but only by means of knowledge of the world, which would not be available. The infinitival SFUGGIRE is then computable as the REASON or RATIONALE of the RUNning event. The meaning conveyed by the RUNning event in itself is that of INCEPTION. Notice that the clause is coordinated locally to the SHOUTing clause and is simply in a SEQUENCE relation with it. However, again, one might recognize a CAUSE/RESULT relation to the APPEARance of the wolf which would then affect not just one clause but two. Perhaps the solution to this problem lies in the assumption that clauses may entertain multiple Discourse Relations within their Discourse Segment with other clauses - more on this topic in the following chapter.

C19/Questo intanto si leccava già i baffi C20/pensando al suo prossimo pasto così invitante e saporito.
up:to(7-16)
clause:9-19
topics:[secondary:id32:porcellino, expected:id9:lupo]
main_fact:leccarsi([id9:lupo], 1, id2)
ref_int:tint(tes(f4_po8), [f3_po9])
temp_rel:started_by(tes(f3_po09), tes(f4_po08))
disc_rel:elaboration
disc_str:17-[18, 19]
disc_dom:subjective
p_o_view:lupo

same_level:from(9-19)
clause:9-20
topics:[secondary:id32:porcellino, expected:id9:lupo]
main_fact:pensare([id9:lupo, id32:porcellino], 1, id2)
ref_int:tint(tes(f4_po8), [f3_po9, fger4_po9])
temp_rel:after(tes(fger4_po09), tes(f4_po08))
disc_rel:elaboration
disc_str:17-[18, 19, 20]
disc_dom:objective
p_o_view:lupo

The same argument applies to the next UP move, which is again a topic alternation but it has no consequences on the temporal sequence of events. Now 10-21 is a RESULT of what happened in 8-18, however we don't need/want to relabel 8-18 as a CAUSE. To sum up, it would seem that CAUSE-EFFECT/RESULT pairs of DRs may present themselves in texts as chains of RESULT/EFFECT DRs which need a reformulation whenever a subsequent event turns them into CAUSES. The simplest way out of this rather unmanageable recursive trap is to admit to the existence of RESULT/EFFECT clauses which are attached to some previous event that might or might not be classified as CAUSE, and is obviously related to some adjacent previous clause. By allowing clauses to entertain multiple DRs, we also automatically allow some redundance. And CAUSES need not always be specified nor can they be attached to one single only event: they may have – and usually do have – multiple effects; the same applies to RESULT/EFFECTS which may have – and usually do have – multiple CAUSES. This is also what is being discussed at lenght in the following chapter.

C21/Finalmente i porcellini riuscirono a raggiungere la loro casetta C22/e vi si chiusero dentro C23/sbarrando la porta.

up:to(8-18)
clause:10-21
topics:[main:id32:porcellino, secondary:id9:lupo]
main_fact:riuscire([id32:porcellino, id77:raggiungere], 1, id35)
ref_int:tint(tes(f5_po10), [f4_po8])
temp_rel:after(tes(f3_po10), tes(f4_po08))
disc_rel:result
disc_str:18-[21]
disc_dom:objective
p_o_view:narrator

down:down(10-21)
clause:10-22
topics:[main:id32:porcellino, secondary:id9:lupo]
main_fact:chiudere([id32:porcellino, id32:porcellino], 1, id35)
ref_int:tint(tes(f5_po10), [f4_po8, f5_po10])
temp_rel:after(tes(f5_po10), tes(f3_po10))
disc_rel:evidence
disc_str:21-[22]
disc_dom:objective
p_o_view:narrator

same_level:from(10-22)
clause:10-23
topics:[main:id32:porcellino, secondary:id9:lupo]
main_fact:sbarrare([id32:porcellino, id76:porta], 1, id35)
ref_int:tint(tes(f5_po10), [f4_po8, f5_po10, fger61_po10])
temp_rel:after(tes(fger61_po10), tes(f5_po10))
disc_rel:result
disc_str:18-[21, 22, 23]
disc_dom:objective
p_o_view:narrator

C24/Dalla finestra cominciarono a deridere il lupo C25/cantando la solita canzoncina: chi ha paura del lupo cattivo.

down:down(10-23)
clause:11-24
topics:[main:id32:porcellino, secondary:id9:lupo]

main_fact:cominciare([id32:porcellino, id87:deridere], 1, id35)
ref_int:tint(tes(f3_po11), [])
temp_rel:after(tes(f3_po11), tes(f5_po10))
disc_rel:inception
disc_str:23-[24]
disc_dom:objective
p_o_view:narrator

same_level:level(11-24)
clause:11-25
topics:[main:id32:porcellino, secondary:id9:lupo]
main_fact:cantare([id32:porcellino, id43:canzone], 1, id35)
ref_int:tint(tes(f3_po11), [fger65_po11])
temp_rel:after(tes(fger65_po11), tes(f3_po11))
disc_rel:elaboration
disc_str:23-[24, 25]
disc_dom:objective
p_o_view:narrator

The same argument applies to the next UP move, which is again a topic alternation but it has no consequences on the temporal sequence of events: notice that the discourse relation is PARALLEL meaning just the fact that what is happening to the wolf parallels what the previous stretch of discourse was narrating.

C26/Il lupo stava intanto pensando al modo di penetrare nella casa.

up:from(11-25)
clause:12-26
topics:[main:id32:porcellino, expected:id9:lupo]
main_fact:pensare([id9:lupo, id97:penetrare], 1, id2)
ref_int:tint(tes(f3_po11), [fger65_po11, f5_po12])
temp_rel:finished_by(tes(f3_po12), tes(f3_po11))
disc_rel:parallel
disc_str:26-[25]
disc_dom:objective
p_o_view:narrator

C27/Esso si mise ad osservare attentamente la casetta C28/e notò che C29/non era davvero molto solida.

down:down(12-26)
clause:13-27
topics:[main:id9:lupo, secondary:id35:casa]
main_fact:mettersi([id9:lupo, id102:osservare], 1, id2)
ref_int:tint(tes(f6_po13), [])
temp_rel:after(tes(f3_po13), tes(f3_po11))
disc_rel:inception
disc_str:26-[27]

disc_dom:objective
p_o_view:narrator

same_level:level(13-27)
clause:13-28
topics:[main:id9:lupo, secondary:id35:casa]
main_fact:notare([id9:lupo, id106:essere], 1, id2)
ref_int:tint(tes(f6_po13), [f6_po13])
temp_rel:after(tes(f6_po13), tes(f3_po13))
disc_rel:evidence
disc_str:26-[27, 28]
disc_dom:objective
p_o_view:narrator

same_level:level(13-28)
clause:13-29
topics:[main:id9:lupo, secondary:id35:casa]
main_fact:solido([id35:paglia], 0, id2)
ref_int:tint(tes(f6_po13), [f6_po13, f5_po13])
temp_rel:after(tes(f5_po13), tes(f6_po13))
disc_rel:contrast
disc_str:26-[27, 28, 29]
disc_dom:objective
p_o_view:narrator

Here below we have another case of a RESULT DR preceded by a clause computed as NARRATION, as far as the relation intervening with the previous stretch of discourse is concerned. It is a fact that CAUSE/RESULT relations are often built as a sequence in which the Result follows the Cause, so that in order to tell a Cause once the Result is achieved one has to search backward. In logical terms, CS relations are transitive and asymmetric as will be discussed in detail in the following section.

C30/Soffiò con forza un paio di volte C31/e la casetta si sfasciò completamente.

same_level:level(13-29)
clause:14-30
topics:[main:id9:lupo, secondary:id35:casa]
main_fact:soffiare([id9:lupo], 1, id2)
ref_int:tint(tes(f6_po13), [f6_po13, f5_po13, f5_po14])
temp_rel:after(tes(f3_po14), tes(f6_po13))
disc_rel:narration
disc_str:26-[27, 28, 29, 30]
disc_dom:objective
p_o_view:narrator

same_level:level(14-30)
clause:14-31

topics:[main:id9:lupo, secondary:id35:casa]
main_fact:sfasciare([id35:casa], 1, id2)
ref_int:tint(tes(f6_po13), [f6_po13, f5_po13, f5_po14])
temp_rel:after(tes(f5_po14), tes(f3_po14))
disc_rel:result
disc_str:26-[27, 28, 29, 30, 31]
disc_dom:objective
p_o_view:narrator

Here again we see that the UP move is a consequence of a topic alternation; but there is no local temporal connection with the previous stretch of discourse. The reason is simply that so far the text described what the wolf was doing to the little house where the little pigs were hidden. When we look back at utterance 12, clause 26, which is the new attachment point established independently by the algorithm, we discover that this is where we left the little pigs.

C32/Spaventatissimi i due porcellini corsero a perdifiato verso la casetta del fratello.
up:to(11-25)
clause:15-32
topics:[secondary:id9:lupo, expected:id32:porcellino]
main_fact:correre([id32:porcellino, id25:casa], 1, id2)
ref_int:tint(tes(f3_po15), [f3_po11])
temp_rel:after(tes(f3_po15), tes(f5_po14))
disc_rel:narration
disc_str:25-[32]
disc_dom:objective
p_o_view:narrator

C34/"Presto, fratellino, aprici! C33/Abbiamo il lupo alle calcagna".
down:down(15-32)
clause:16-33
topics:[main:id32:porcellino, secondary:id9:lupo]
main_fact:avere_calcagna([id32:porcellino, id9:lupo], 1, id2)
ref_int:tint(tes(f3_po15), [f4_po16])
temp_rel:during(tes(f4_po16), tes(f3_po15))
disc_rel:evaluation
disc_str:32-[33]
disc_dom:subjective
p_o_view:porcellino

same_level:level(16-33)
clause:16-34
topics:[main:id32:porcellino, secondary:id9:lupo]
main_fact:aprire([id24:jimmi, id32:porcellino], 1, id2)
ref_int:tint(tes(f3_po15), [f4_po16, f2_po16])
temp_rel:during(tes(f2_po16), tes(f3_po15))

disc_rel:narration
disc_str:32-[33, 34]
disc_dom:subjective
p_o_view:porcellino

C35/Fecero appena in tempo ad entrare e tirare il chiavistello.
same_level:level(16-34)
clause:17-35
topics:[main:id32:porcellino, secondary:id125:chiavistello]
main_fact:fare_tempo([id32:porcellino, id126:entrare], 1, id25)
ref_int:tint(tes(f3_po15), [f4_po16, f2_po16, f9_po17])
temp_rel:after(tes(f7_po17), tes(f3_po15))
disc_rel:narration
disc_str:32-[33, 34, 35]
disc_dom:objective
p_o_view:narrator

The next UP move is again a topic alternation and has no consequences on the temporal sequence of events: in fact, we can see that the discourse relation is again a PARALLEL relation.

C36/Il lupo stava già arrivando deciso a non rinunciare al suo pranzetto.
down:down(17-35)
clause:18-36
topics:[secondary:id70:pranzo, expected:id9:lupo]
main_fact:arrivare([id9:lupo], 1, id2)
ref_int:tint(tes(f3_po15), [tes(f3_po18)])
temp_rel:finished_by(tes(f3_po18), tes(f3_po15))
disc_rel:parallel
disc_str:35-[36]
disc_dom:objective
p_o_view:narrator

C37/Sicuro di abbattere anche la casetta di mattoni il lupo si riempì i polmoni di aria C38/e cominciò a soffiare con forza alcune volte.
down:down(18-36)
clause:19-37
topics:[main:id9:lupo, secondary:id25:casa]
main_fact:riempire([id9:lupo], 1, id2)
ref_int:tint(tes(f4_po19), [])
temp_rel:after(tes(f3_po19), tes(f3_po15))
disc_rel:narration
disc_str:36-[37]
disc_dom:objective
p_o_view:narrator

up:to(18-36)
clause:19-38
topics:[main:id9:lupo, secondary:id25:casa]
main_fact:cominciare([id9:lupo, id146:soffiare], 1, id2)
ref_int:tint(tes(f4_po19), [tes(f4_po19)])
temp_rel:after(tes(f4_po19), tes(f3_po19))
disc_rel:inception
disc_str:36-[37, 38]
disc_dom:objective
p_o_view:narrator

C39/Non ci fu niente da fare.
same_level:level(19-38)
clause:20-39
topics:[main:id9:lupo, secondary:id152:niente]
main_fact:esserci([id152:cosa], 0, id2)
ref_int:tint(tes(f4_po19), [tes(f4_po19), tes(f4_po20)])
temp_rel:after(tes(f4_po20), tes(f4_po19))
disc_rel:contrast
disc_str:36-[37, 38, 39]
disc_dom:objective
p_o_view:narrator

The next UP move is again a topic alternation, but it has some consequences on the discourse and temporal structure of events. In particular, we can see that the previous clause was structurally dependent on a previous segment, being a down move. The previous clause is an INCEPTION and has as one of its topics, the "casa"/house the next utterance is addressing. In addition, we know that there is a CONTRAST relation between what was uttered in clause 38, which constitutes the new attachment point, and the semantic contents of the next utterance.

C40/La casa non si mosse di un solo palmo.
up:to(19-38)
clause:21-40
topics:[secondary:id9:lupo, expected:id25:casa]
main_fact:muovere([id25:casa], 0, id2)
ref_int:tint(tes(f3_po21), [f4_po19])
temp_rel:after(tes(f3_po21), tes(f4_po19))
disc_rel:contrast
disc_str:39-[40]
disc_dom:objective
p_o_view:narrator

The next UP move is a topic alternation but has no consequences on the temporal sequence of events. The interesting thing to notice is the separation of INTENTIONALITY and temporal sequencing. In particular, the meaning conveyed by the next clause is strictly connected to what the wolf did in clause 39, utterance 19, even though it is temporally in a sequence with the adjacent stretch of discourse. Thus, we use EGRESSION with the indices of the previous utterance-clause pair to indicate that discourse relation. Again, EGRESSION might also be computed as RESULT/EFFECT of some previous action/s and the CAUSE would in that case be the INGRESSION computed in 18-36.

C41/Alla fine esausto il lupo si accasciò a terra.
up:to(18-36)
clause:22-41
topics:[main:id9:lupo, secondary:id25:casa]
main_fact:accasciarsi([id9:lupo, infon818:terra], 1, id2)
ref_int:tint(tes(f4_po22), [f3_po21])
temp_rel:after(tes(f4_po22), tes(f3_po21))
disc_rel:egression(19-38)
disc_str:40-[41]
disc_dom:objective
p_o_view:narrator

The next UP move is a topic alternation but has no consequences on the temporal sequence of events. In fact it is more or less contemporary to what is happening to the wolf. The question to be addressed here, is how should we regard the reference to the set of three little pigs, which constitutes the Expected Topic and is the entity id3, to be found in utterance 1, clause 1 of the text. This is clearly not what the system should do: the closest reference to little pigs as Main Topics is recovered instead in utterance 17, clause 35, which is where in the story the two lazy little pigs manage to enter their brother's sturdy house. The reference interval is the result of a local computation and assumes that parallel to the discourse structure it takes the latest UP move as its attachment point.

C42/I tre porcellini si sentivano al sicuro nella solida casetta di mattoni.
down:down(22-41)
clause:23-42
topics:[secondary:id9:lupo, expected:id3:porcellino]
main_fact:sentirsi([id3:porcellino, infon837:sicuro], 1, id25)
ref_int:tint(tes(f4_po22), [tes(f4_po23)])
temp_rel:finished_by(tes(f4_po23), tes(f4_po22))
disc_rel:narration
disc_str:41-[42]
disc_dom:objective
p_o_view:narrator

C43/Riconoscenti i due porcellini oziosi promisero al fratello C44/che da quel giorno anche essi avrebbero lavorato sodo.
up:to(15-32)
clause:24-43
topics:[main:id32:porcellino, secondary:id9:lupo]
main_fact:promettere([id32:porcellino, id3:porcellino, id169:lavorare], 1, id25)

ref_int:tint(tes(f4_po22), [tes(f4_po23), tes(f245_po24)])
temp_rel:after(tes(f245_po24), tes(f4_po22))
disc_rel:inception
disc_str:41-[42, 43]
disc_dom:objective
p_o_view:narrator

down:down(24-43)
clause:24-44
topics:[main:id32:porcellino, secondary:id9:lupo]
main_fact:lavorare([id32:porcellino], 1, id25)
ref_int:tint(tes(f4_po22), [tes(f244_po24)])
temp_rel:before(tes(f244_po24), tes(f4_po22))
disc_rel:narration
disc_str:43-[44]
disc_dom:objective
p_o_view:narrator

Chapter 5

DISCOURSE RELATIONS AND CAUSALITY

1. INTRODUCTION

In this chapter we intend to propose a Model of Causal Relations (hence CRs) which encompasses different levels of linguistic representations and features and will be applied to free unlimited texts in order to evaluate its robustness.

In order to characterize CRs in texts we will proceed by re/formulating properties of Discourse Relations as they can be derived from the annotated examples reported in two available databases, DiscourseGraph Bank and Penn Discourse TreeBank. We will also characterize CRs from a theoretical point of view by drawing from current linguistic and computational literature. Finally, we will present an evaluation based on the two annotated databases and showing what can be achieved by the use of linguistic information and what knowledge of the world may contribute to improve the performance of the system. For this task we will use the Hybrid robust version of GETARUNS, which is further commented and described in Chapter IX below.

CRs have always constituted a very thorny issue in the linguistic and philosophical literature and to cover all related issues we need to address the whole gamut of linguistic information, i.e.,

- pragmatic information, where inferences and reasoning is carried out using knowledge of the world;
- semantic information, where features like negation, opacity, aspectual features, event structure, modality and mood, temporal properties of propositions and quantification may be individuated, both intra and intersententially;
- syntactic information, which encompasses also the lexical level and has access to features from constituency and functional structural representation, as well as syntactic properties of governing predicates in terms of subcategorization and selectional restrictions. Important lexical properties of predicates to be taken into account are Semantic Roles.

Our goal is to find if and in what measure CRs are dependent on Knowledge of the World, and what kind of constraints surface syntactic structure plays on the nature of CRs, eventually what kind of information needs to be stored in the lexicon in order to spot CRs.

2. General Principles and Properties of CRs

As a general starting point we may note that natural CRs – i.e. causality relations related to natural facts of the physical world in which we live - are usually left unexpressed unless the text is dealing with explanatory descriptions and experimental work in scientific literature and educational academic and school related literature.

Whenever CRs are reported of exceptional physical events we will have to take it into consideration, also in its possibly abnormal dimension, which is usually so when compared to usual commonplace similar facts – e.g. the tsunami is an abnormal ocean wave which is caused by landslide or earthquake.

In order to express CRs in text, two clauses must be used: one expressing Motivation or Cause, and another expressing Result or Effect. It is not always the case that Causes are expressed fully: in many cases they may be left implicit as if they can be understood by the addressee. What is usually reported in texts is the effect of some previous event which might – or might not be reported in the previous text, and may be adjacent or non adjacent to the current sentence. CRs may be expressed at a propositional level, thus intersententially by means of a connective,

- John built a house because his wife is a person difficult to please

or without the presence of a connective,

- John built a house. His wife is a person difficult to please.

but also intrasententially,

- John built a house to please his wife.

CRs may also be expressed as a sequence of nominal expressions in a nominal compound as in,

- The tsunami disastrous effects

where the "Tsunami" is the CAUSER-Subj of the effects.

As will be shown below, we will also have to consider situations in which Causes are not expressed by clauses but simply by Prepositional Phrases as for instance in the example below that we take from DiscourseGraph Bank:

15250 Relation: ce
[A] for his outspoken opposition to the Vietnam War

[B] The late Prime Minister Olof Palme was blacklisted from the White House

Eventually, Cause may be simply part of the lexical meaning of the verb/noun, and may be extracted by some system of semantic decomposition in lexical primitives or templates, as for instance suggested by Jackendoff or Talmy, which will be discussed in detail below.

2.1. Different Structural Ways of Expressing CRs

The list below taken from Meier (2002), shows all possible different syntactic realizations of Causality Relations:

2.1. Because of the rain, the leaves of the tree are wet.
2.2. Because it has been raining, the leaves of the tree are wet.
2.3. It has been raining. Therefore the leaves of the tree are wet.
2.4. It has been raining, and the leaves of the tree are wet.
2.5. It has been raining. The leaves of the tree are wet.
2.6. The leaves of the tree are wet because it has been raining.
2.7. It has been raining. Consequently the leaves of the tree are wet.
2.8. It has been raining heavily for the last few days, with the result that the garden is now completely swamped.
2.9. The leaves of the tree are wet because of the rain.
2.10. So airlines have only themselves to blame if air does not secure a bigger part of the apparently static common carrier market due in turn to the growth of private carriers.
2.11. As it has been raining, the leaves of the tree are wet.
2.12. His English parents -- which was how he thought of his mother and her husband -- had little money, being unambitious academics.
2.13. And to my own dismay I began to feel so claustrophobic in the cathedral that I had to leave.
2.14. Next, for her own good, Marie-Louise demanded that her daughter jump to the floor from a table, several times. The only result was exhaustion and despair in the victim.
2.15. “Very well, I will,” said he, agreeing as much to what had not been said as to what had: his difficulty in keeping up with his wife's unspoken languages was the main reason he had been pleased to leave her.
2.16. She caused his death. (verb cause)
2.17. She killed him. (causative verb)

We need then to add those cases in which the Cause relation is semantically constituted by Purpose, Comment, Rationale, Telicity or Outcome, and Means, and is expressed by nonfinite clauses, as shown in the following examples taken from Balkanski (1992):

2.18. Mary bought a suit to wear at the meeting,
2.19. John is not sure what to do, to put it briefly.
2.20. Bush warned his press secretary to prevent a leak.

2.21. Mary awoke one morning to find the house in an uproar.
2.22. Mary pays her rent by building furniture.

As shall be discussed in detail in section 6, the meaning conveyed by nonfinite expressions is totally different from the one obtained in the finite clausal examples and is related to the (NON)-FACTIVITY of event or action indicated in the clause. Generally speaking CAUSES need to be separated from REASONS/Motivations: whereas the former express contingent relations entertained in the world under certain circumstances, the latter involve rational, i.e. human intervention. For instance Quirk et al. make the following four-way distinction:

a) Cause and effect: “the construction expresses the perception of an inherent objective connection in the real world” (Quirk et al. 1985: 1103) – see 2.1 above.
b) Reason and consequence: “the construction expresses the speaker’s inference of a connection” (Quirk et al. 1985: 1104) and may not have any correspondance in the actual world:
   2.23. The Pope himself probably survived only because he isolated himself from everybody else in his huge palace.
c) The reason clause can also express the motivation of a rational agent, “the intention of an animate being that has a subsequent result” (Quirk et al. 1985: 1104),
   2.24. I sometimes think that was the real reason you married me, not for security but because you needed somebody else’s emotion to stimulate your creativity.
d) Finally, the reason clause can express a relationship between a circumstance and following result: the circumstantial clause combines reason with a condition that is assumed to be fulfilled or about to be fulfilled, the construction expressing a relationship between a premise in the subordinate clause and the conclusion in the matrix clause (Quirk et al. 1985: 1104).
   2.25. Since the weather has improved, the game will be held as planned (Quirk et al. 1985: 1104)
e) In contrast, reason clauses may also express an indirect reason relationship, where “the reason is not related to the situation in the matrix clause but is a motivation for the implicit speech act of the utterance” (Quirk et al. 1985: 1104). As an example of this consider:
   2.26. My bank account is empty, because I checked it this morning.

Other topics we will be dealing with in this chapter regard the use of discourse markers or connectives which is motivated by the need to make explicit the relation intervening between two adjacent clauses. As will be discussed in detail in the sections below, whenever a discourse connective is used, CRs are more readily expressed. The presence of an explicit connective in most cases is self-explanatory and may be related to the need to keep the discourse open. However, it is likewise important to verify under which discourse structural conditions such discourse markers are added, and when they may be omitted. Generally speaking, CRs need causative verbs to be expressed or else discourse markers.

We may safely assume that lexical connectives can be redundant in some cases, seen that CRs may also be expressed without their use: in these cases the discovery of discourse relations is left to the reader. From a stylistic point of view, there will be two separate sentences, connected by what is usually referred to as *parataxis*. On the contrary, when the connector are lexically expressed the two clauses specifying MOTIVATION/CAUSE and RESULT/EFFECT are connected in a *hypotactic* way.

2.2. Lexicalized Causal Meaning: LCS and FrameNet

As noted above, causes need causative verbs to be expressed or else discourse markers. From a conceptual point of view, all predicates belonging to the following aspectual classes may contain an abstract CAUSE operator:

- accomplishments
- non reversible accomplishments
- gradual accomplishments
- achievements
- punctual achievements

Predicates belonging to these classes may also be regarded as containing two additional features:

- intentionality
- animacy

However, it may be proven that CRs may be non-intentional and have a non-animate causer as it would happen with all natural events.

In this perspective, we follow Ray Jackendoff by postulating the existence of a certain number of primitive operators among which is the CAUSE operator. For instance, the sentence,

- John built a house

may be conceptually decomposed and represented into the following representation,

CAUSE(John-SUBJ,
BE-IN-THE-WORLD/EXISTENCE(house-OBJ),
$Evs_{i,j}$ (Ev_i ...Ev_j))

Which can be paraphrased as follows,

John caused the house to be in existence/world in the time span intervening between Ev_i and Ev_j, where the final event represent the Accomplished Result State. More on these topics in section 6.

Predicates belonging to STATE or ACTIVITY cannot be used to express Causes and consequently cannot be decomposed into the lexicalized conceptual causal operator. On the contrary they may be regarded the preferred target of RESULT clauses.

In the LCS lexicon freely downloadable from http://www.umiacs.umd.edu/~bonnie/verbs-English.lcs on the total number of lexical items present, which amount to 9000 entries, over 5000 have a CAUSE operator incorporated in their lexical meaning representation. LCS entries contain cross reference to Levin verb classes, to WordNet sense, to PropBank argument list which have been mapped to a more explicit label set of Semantic Roles which can be regarded more linguistically motivated than the ones contained in FrameNet which are more pragmatically motivated. However, for our purposes, LCS notation is more perspicuous because of the presence of the CAUSE operator, and is more general: on a total number of 9000 lexical entries, 5000 contain the CAUSE operator. On the contrary, in FrameNet on a total number of 10000 lexical entries, only 333 are related to a CAUSE Frame; if we search for the word "cause" in the definitions contained in all the Frames the number increases to 789 but is still too small compared to LCS. Here below is one example of LCS entries:

```
(:DEF_WORD "prevent"
 :CLASS "059"
 :WN_SENSE (("1.5" 01387332)
          ("1.6" 01669882))
 :PROPBANK ("arg0 arg1 arg2(from)")
 :THETA_ROLES ((1 "_ag_th_prop(from)"))
 :LCS (cause (* thing 1)
     (go circ (* thing 2)
    ((from 3) circ (thing 2) (at circ (thing 2) (* nil 27))))
     (prevent+ingly 26))
 :VAR_SPEC ((27 (aspect prog))) )
```

To recover the same information from FrameNet, either the definition or the Frame Elements had to be inspected. In particular, Prevent is part of the Frame PREVENT which has Preventing_Cause as Frame Element. "Purge" is part of the Frame Removing and in order to know that it is a causative verb one needs to read the definition which paraphrases the content of the Frame Elements by saying that The Agent is a person (or other force) that causes the Theme to move.

FrameNet – FrameNet 1.3 - uses the following FRAMEs related to Causation to classify predicates:

Causation
- Cause
- Cause_begin_motion
- Cause_change
- Cause_change_of_consistency
- Cause_change_of_phase
- Cause_change_of_position_on_a_scale
- Cause_confinement
- Cause_expansion
- Cause_fluidic_motion
- Cause_harm

Cause_impact
Cause_motion
Cause_of_shine
Cause_temperature_change
Cause_to_amalgamate
Cause_to_be_dry
Cause_to_be_sharp
Cause_to_be_wet
Cause_to_continue
Cause_to_end
Cause_to_experience
Cause_to_fragment
Cause_to_make_noise
Cause_to_make_progress
Cause_to_move_in_place
Cause_to_resume
Cause_to_start
Cause_to_wake

The following template is used as a super frame for causality relations,

Causation_scenario

and encompasses all the following Frame Elements and Frame targets,

```
{ident = 217, name = Causation_scenario, }
  fe -> ALL OF
   {ident = 3693, name = Cause, }
    target_ref ->
     made
      frame_target ->
       {ident = 5, name = Causation, }
       {ident = 54, name = Arriving, }
       {ident = 64, name = Self_motion, }
       {ident = 259, name = Building, }
       {ident = 268, name = Cooking_creation, }
       {ident = 280, name = Intentionally_create, }
       {ident = 400, name = Reparation, }
       {ident = 408, name = Manufacturing, }
       {ident = 683, name = Cause_change, }
       {ident = 1085, name = Make_acquaintance, }
      ,
    target_ref ->
     caused
      frame_target ->
       {ident = 5, name = Causation, }
```

```
,
{ident = 3694, name = Effect, }
 target_ref ->
  led
   frame_target ->
    {ident = 5, name = Causation, }
    {ident = 56, name = Cotheme, }
    {ident = 73, name = Leadership, }
    {ident = 90, name = Talking_into, }
```

All predicates thus described will have a Causer or an Agent as Subject. The number of predicates thus classified in FrameNet is however very small, less than 548 over 10195 examples, 349 of which are constituted by verb predicates. FrameNet also elaborates a limited number of inference relations of type Causative_of to identify Cause-Effect relations which are based on Frame Elements or Semantic Roles:

ident = 3139, name = Causative_of: Cure --> Recovery
ident = 2647, name = Causative_of: Change_of_leadership --> Leadership
ident = 2663, name = Causative_of: Eventive_cognizer_affecting --> Purpose
ident = 3015, name = Causative_of: Giving --> Getting
ident = 1209, name = Causative_of: Apply_heat --> Absorb_heat
ident = 1208, name = Causative_of: Cause_to_move_in_place --> Moving_in_place
ident = 2728, name = Causative_of: Grinding --> Ground_up
ident = 1998, name = Causative_of: Killing --> Death
ident = 2594, name = Causative_of: Endangering --> Run_risk
ident = 2774, name = Causative_of: Cause_to_end --> Process_end
ident = 2130, name = Causative_of: Imposing_obligation --> Being_obligated
ident = 2542, name = Causative_of: Hiding_objects --> Eclipse

To these 12 inferential rules there are two other similar cases based on the relation Inchoative_of:

ident = 2844, name = Inchoative_of: Coming_to_believe --> Awareness
ident = 1238, name = Inchoative_of: Change_position_on_a_scale --> Position_on_a_scale

2.3. WordNet, VerbOcean and Cause-Effect Relations

Cause Effect relations are dependent on facts of the world and constitute knowledge of the world. In other words, they cannot be derived from linguistic properties of the text. In WordNet the following 220 or so relations are reported, we list some of them here below in the format: cs(Cause index, Effect index):

cs(200013442, 200009805).
cs(200014590, 200009805).
cs(200017738, 200018458).
cs(200018031, 200018644).
cs(200037906, 200038045).
cs(200039309, 200039057).
cs(200045186, 201452083).
cs(200051406, 200051279).
cs(200052062, 200052840).
cs(200053789, 200002143).
cs(200066451, 200016821).
cs(200068375, 200067743).
cs(200083947, 200074063).
cs(200097065, 200094964).
cs(200138658, 200138909).
cs(200140937, 200140363).
cs(200149082, 200149731).
cs(200150780, 200150444).
cs(200153724, 200152756).
cs(200155596, 200155084).
cs(200164725, 200164388).
cs(200167804, 200158819).
cs(200170328, 200169382).
cs(200170582, 200170483).
cs(200173224, [200158081, 200172114]).
cs(200173827, 200173705).
cs(200174378, 200173956).
cs(200175268, 200179555).
cs(200175935, 200175388).
cs(200176545, 200176104).
cs(200181884, 200181629).
cs(200184403, 201249365).
cs(200185374, 200185374).
cs(200193498, 200192676).
cs(200207661, 201815328).
cs(200209671, 200209493).
cs(200211930, 200211486).
cs(200215332, 200216063).
cs(200216484, 200216222).
cs(200216677, 200215001).
cs(200217890, 200218146).
cs(200218465, 200218299).
cs(200218668, 200219109).
cs(200219644, 200219370).
cs(200220373, 200220272).
cs(200220504, 200219507).
cs(200221402, 200164533).
cs(200242403, 201778989).
cs(200246253, 201779664).
cs(200252877, 200252740).
cs(200255269, 200255423).
cs(200258652, 200258213).
cs(200259088, 200259859).
cs(200259713, 200258521).
cs(200261276, 200261606).
cs(200262285, 200260887).
cs(200268049, 200267598).
cs(200269963, 200269813).
cs(200272277, 200272165).
cs(200289432, 200289607).
cs(200290032, 200290685).
cs(200291365, 200291205).
cs(200293010, 200293275).
cs(200299862, 200300201).
cs(200300448, 200300319).
cs(200309646, 200309461).
cs(200310972, 200310783).
cs(200311317, 200309849).
cs(200311784, 200311612).
cs(200312214, 200311485).
cs(200313984, 200313029).
cs(200315864, 200315280).
cs(200317807, 201414286).
cs(200320487, 200320369).
cs(200320830, 200320978).
cs(200322518, 200322396).
cs(200327278, 200327120).
cs(200330720, 200330961).
cs(200349043, 200348938).
cs(200349285, 200349174).
cs(200376671, 200376518).
cs(200377600, 200377769).
cs(200395938, 200395807).
cs(200399493, 200397666).
cs(200399709, 200397666).
cs(200406271, 200406072).
cs(200407541, 200407401).
cs(200411656, 200411760).
cs(200412961, 200410666).
cs(200472835, 200471542).
cs(200562446, 200403772).
cs(200563274, 200404146).

cs(200577163, 201612822).
cs(200582994, 200582840).
cs(200583375, 200022398).
cs(200632077, 200633716).
cs(200634658, 200633716).
cs(200655894, 200656764).
cs(200658752, 200659045).
cs(200755028, 200753559).
cs(200769883, 200770206).
cs(200784705, 201261992).
cs(200788109, 201826205).
cs(200795500, 200795711).
cs(200801099, 200794578).
cs(200807505, 200807650).
cs(200816880, 200817136).
cs(200857882, 201341375).
cs(200883915, 200883766).
cs(200884615, 200881999).
cs(200885494, 200881672).
cs(200903723, 200250254).
cs(200915832, 200919067).
cs(200919360, 200919225).
cs(200919962, 200921313).
cs(200920424, 200921157).

The corresponding lexical values are reported in Appendix I. The problem with these relations is that in many cases they are reporting orthographic variants (see agonize, agonise) or else they only include the same linguistic description (see air, air), being thus deprived of any usefulness.

We also looked at another lexical list called VERBOCEAN, available at http://semantics.isi.edu/ocean/

The list contains a number of semantic relations one of which, HAPPENS-BEFORE constitutes one of the properties that Cause-Effect relations must have. However, only a small percentage of the 6500 verbs entertaining that relation can be also computed as Cause-Effect relations. For instance, we report here below a select short list where we marked with an asterisk cases which could be treated as such:

bomb [happens-before] invade :: 15.258472
bomb [happens-before] loot :: 15.893175
bomb [happens-before] loot :: 15.893175
bomb [happens-before] occupy :: 13.791149
bomb [happens-before] occupy :: 13.791149
bombard [happens-before] destroy :: 12.407347
*boycott [happens-before] contest :: 11.831781
*boycott [happens-before] contest :: 11.831781
brutalize [happens-before] murder :: 16.543608
build [happens-before] assemble :: 10.646834
build [happens-before] assemble :: 10.646834
build [happens-before] convert :: 8.527320
build [happens-before] demolish :: 16.549256
build [happens-before] dismantle :: 13.004022
build [happens-before] equip :: 8.727628
build [happens-before] expand :: 9.125721
build [happens-before] expand :: 9.125721
build [happens-before] inspect :: 10.877988
*build [happens-before] install :: 9.389751
*build [happens-before] install :: 9.389751
*build [happens-before] lease :: 10.811572

*build [happens-before] run :: 9.454894
*build [happens-before] sell :: 10.350507
*build [happens-before] sell :: 10.350507
build [happens-before] transform :: 8.902804
*build [happens-before] use :: 9.588662
burn [happens-before] bury :: 13.562610
burn [happens-before] char :: 12.395452
burn [happens-before] char :: 12.395452
burn [happens-before] extinguish :: 12.771544
burn [happens-before] plant :: 10.348880
burn [happens-before] plant :: 10.348880
buy [happens-before] assemble :: 8.914474
*buy [happens-before] distribute :: 8.867975
*buy [happens-before] distribute :: 8.867975
*buy [happens-before] donate :: 9.503991
*buy [happens-before] donate :: 9.503991
*buy [happens-before] have :: 9.276482
buy [happens-before] put :: 8.583570
buy [happens-before] put :: 8.583570
*buy [happens-before] resell :: 12.505550
*buy [happens-before] resell :: 12.505550
*buy [happens-before] swap :: 8.803371
*buy [happens-before] use :: 9.428121
*buy [happens-before] use :: 9.428121
call [happens-before] announce :: 10.258568
call [happens-before] dismiss :: 9.712657
call [happens-before] label :: 10.114944
call [happens-before] like :: 8.902841
call [happens-before] like :: 8.902841
call [happens-before] name :: 9.703518
call [happens-before] say :: 9.141204
call [happens-before] say :: 9.141204
cause [happens-before] aggravate :: 11.918791
cause [happens-before] aggravate :: 11.918791
cause [happens-before] ease :: 9.014679
cause [happens-before] ease :: 9.014679
cause [happens-before] exacerbate :: 13.402510
cause [happens-before] exacerbate :: 13.402510
*challenge [happens-before] attack :: 9.124541
*challenge [happens-before] confront :: 13.463043
challenge [happens-before] dismiss :: 10.062619
*challenge [happens-before] overturn :: 13.342745
*challenge [happens-before] overturn :: 13.342745
challenge [happens-before] reject :: 10.159693
*chase [happens-before] arrest :: 12.971321
*chase [happens-before] capture :: 10.388343

*chase [happens-before] catch :: 11.891366
*chase [happens-before] catch :: 11.891366
chase [happens-before] disperse :: 12.594124
chase [happens-before] hunt :: 9.996422
chase [happens-before] hunt :: 9.996422
*chase [happens-before] kill :: 11.208660
chase [happens-before] pull :: 11.264111
chase [happens-before] pull :: 11.264111
choke [happens-before] strangle :: 14.555605
choke [happens-before] strangle :: 14.555605
*claim [happens-before] renounce :: 10.939372
*combat [happens-before] eliminate :: 10.259578
*combat [happens-before] eliminate :: 10.259578
*combat [happens-before] eradicate :: 11.870437
*combat [happens-before] eradicate :: 11.870437

What the majority of cases really encode is the need of a temporal sequence between the two events if they happen in the world. This is interpretable as a sufficient condition in most cases and in some other cases as a necessary condition. But no Causal relations are really implied in most cases.

2.4. Talmy's Theory

The force dynamic model of causation (Talmy, 2000; Wolff, 2003) represents a particular approach to causation that specifies the basic dimensions of meaning associated with various causal concepts such as CAUSE, ENABLE and PREVENT. Interesting prediction derive from this model. In particular, causal conjunctions, including adverbs, and causal prepositions can be used to express generative but not preventive causation (Dancygier & Sweetser, 2000). Three types of subordinating conjunctions can be used to talk about causal relations: causal (because, since), temporal (after, when), and conditional (if). In all cases, the main clause expresses the *result* and the subordinate clause expresses the *cause*. Causal subordinating conjunctions explicitly assert a causal relation. Causal subordinators typically introduce a clause that might be best characterized as expressing a reason. Although the precise connection between causes and reasons has not yet been fully articulated, we assume, along with Lakoff and Johnson (1999), that reasons can be conceptualized, in an extended sense, as causes.

Temporal conjunctions are exemplified here below,

2.27a. Liberman left the Republican Party after George W. Bush was nominated.
b. Fiona stopped the car when she saw the elephant.
c. George W. Bush was nominated before Liberman left the Republican Party.

Clark and Clark (1977) make the interesting observation that the subordination relation is critical in implying a causal reading. If the *result* is subordinate to the *cause*, as in (c), the sentence loses its causal interpretation, even though it describes the same sequence of events as in (a). According to Talmy (1976), in English and other languages, *results* are generally construed in terms of *causes*, not vice versa, and it is for this reason that sentences with *before* do not receive a causal interpretation.

Causation can also be expressed by counterfactuals and conditional expression using the *conditional if*, examples of which are shown below,

2.28a. If you are found guilty, you will go to prison.
b. If I win the lottery, I will buy a Ferrari.

In these sentences, a particular *result* is understood to be contingent upon a particular *cause*. *If-then* statements can also be used in *counterfactual* statements. *Conditionals* and *counterfactuals* are closely related, as exemplified by the sentences in (c-d) which are very similar to those in (a-b).

c. If John had been found guilty, he would have gone to prison.
d. If John had won the lottery, he would have bought a Ferrari.

Coordinating conjunctions most often associated with causation are *and* and *so*. *So* explicitly *asserts* a causal relation of some sort, while *and* can *imply* causation in certain contexts .

Conjunctive adverbs (e.g., consequently, thus, therefore, as a result) and lexical cues phrases (e.g., that's why) may also be used to expresses causes, as in:

2.29a. Ralph totaled the car. As a result, his auto insurance rates increased.
b. John drank a lot of coffee. That's why he stayed awake.

Causal prepositions also include from, by and with.

We can then distinguish two types of causative verbs: *Periphrastic* and *Lexical*. *Periphrastic* causative verbs fall into the three basic categories of causation posited by the force dynamic model: CAUSE-type verbs (a), PREVENT-type verbs (b), and ENABLE-type verbs (c) (Wolff et al., 2002; Wolff & Song, 2003):

2.30a. bribe, cause, compel, convince, drive, have, impel, incite, induce, influence, inspire, lead, move, persuade, prompt, push, force, get, make, rouse, send, set, spur, start, stimulate
b. bar, block, constrain, deter, discourage, dissuade, hamper, hinder, hold, impede, keep, prevent, protect, restrain, restrict, save, stop
c. aid, allow, enable, help, leave, let, permit

Lexical causatives can be divided into three main subclasses according to the type of result they encode: change of state (a), change of location in a particular manner (b) and certain kinds of light or sound emission (c) (Levin & Rappaport Hovav, 1994; Pinker, 1989; Smith, 1970).

2.31a. awake, balance, bend, break, burn, capsize, change, chill, clog, close, collapse, crack, crumble, decompose, decrease, deflate, defrost, degrade, dissolve, divide, drain, enlarge, expand, explode, flood, fold, freeze, hush, ignite, increase, melt, open, pop, rip, reproduce, rupture, scorch, shatter, shrink, sink, snap, split, tear, thaw, topple

b. bounce, coil, drift, drop, float, glide, move, revolve, roll, rotate, slide, spin, swing, turn, twirl, twist, whirl, wind

c. shine, beam, buzz, jingle, ring, rustle

3. The Hypothesis

Whenever a situation has to be expressed or described in linguistic terms it will take a certain number of sentences to unfold in a text or discourse. Argumentations and descriptions are usually made up by spans of text that express sequences of events related to one main event or the FOCUS (a title or the headlines of a newspaper article) and a number of accompanying sentences reporting additional information related to the main Topic in the form of EXPLANATION-EVIDENCE, EVALUATION, PARALLEL, GENERALIZATION, ATTRIBUTION and ELABORATIONS. In addition, in narratives, it would be quite normal to have sequences of sentences introducing new participants and new events, which would be unrelated at first with the previous stretch of discourse which can be labeled NARRATION or just (TEMPORAL)SEQUENCE.

As a general starting point we can posit the existence of a subdivision into two major typologies of discourse relations: unmarked, default discourse relations like SEQUENCE or NARRATION, ELABORATION, PARALLEL, EVALUATION and perhaps EXPLANATION and EVIDENCE, which will be called UDRs for short.

Whenever the author, narrator, speaker needs to introduce *special* or *specific* argumentations and descriptions he/she will do so by using specialized Discourse Relations like, CONTRAST, CONDITION, CAUSE-RESULT, VIOLATED-EXPECTATION, ANTITHESIS, COUNTERFACTUALS etc. . These relations are specialized in the sense that they require some additional linguistic means to be used in order to apply. The pragmatics of these DRs would be related to the needs hinted at by the defining label (to contrast, to express conditional statements, etc.) which is different from the one assumed to apply with UDRs, namely that of adding new information. These specialized DRs will be called SDRs for short.

Traditionally, coherence relations have been binarily classified into two major classes: either semantic vs. pragmatic relations (van Dijk, 1979; Schiffrin, 1987); or internal vs. external relations (Halliday and Hasan, 1976); or, finally, in RST, into presentational vs. subject matter relations. Presentational relations (Antithesis, Background, Concession, Enablement, Evidence, Justify, Motivation, Preparation, Restatement, Summary) are those whose intended effect is to increase some inclination in the reader, such as a desire to act, or to heighten the degree of positive regard for, belief in, or acceptance of, the nucleus. Subject matter relations (Cause, Circumstance, Condition, Elaboration, Evaluation, Interpretation, Means, Purpose, Result, Solutionhood) are those whose intended effect is that the reader recognize the relation in question (Mann, 2005).

We can assume as our starting hypothesis that CAUSES must be expressed whenever the EFFECTS are unexpected, unwanted, unattested, in other words whenever the FACT constituting the effect clause is new, surprising, negates or contradicts the evidence. To achieve such a pragmatic result, EFFECT clauses must contain at least one of the major or more than one of the following linguistic components:

A. Minor components

- NEGATION
- MODALITY OPERATOR (adverb, modal verb, adjective, etc.)
- QUANTITY OPERATOR (quantifiers, intensifiers, adjectives, etc.)
- DISCOURSE MARKER indicating ADVERSE or CONTRARY meaning (but)

B. Major Lexical Components

- DISCOURSE MARKERs indicating cause (because, because_of, the_reason, caused_by, cause_of, due_to, as, etc.)
- DISCOURSE MARKERs indicating result (why, result_from, as_a_result, that_means_that, with_the_aim_of, so_that, so, etc.)
- LEXICALIZED NEGATION (refuse, reject, etc.)
- ATTITUDINAL VERBS (think, believe, expect, criticize, attack, etc.)
- EMOTIONAL VERBS (concern, worry, doubt, fear, etc.)
- QUANTITY GRADING VERBS (rise, soar, slump, cut_down, etc)
- EVALUATIVE PREDICATES (wrong, right, improve, worse, etc.)
- NECESSITY PREDICATES (must, ought_to, need, have_to, etc.)
- (EVENTIVE DEVERBAL) NOUNS and ADJECTIVES indicating (natural) catastrophe, illegal dangerous events (attack, crash, weapon, bribe, etc.)
- PREDICATES (adjectives, adverbials, verbs, nouns) indicating novelty, discovery (scientific and not)
- PREDICATES (adjectives, adverbials, verbs, nouns) indicating problematic and troublesome situations and events

C. Structural Components

- Resultative Infinitivals
- Adjunct Gerundives headed with FOR, BY
- Adjunct PP or NPs

D. Referential Components

- SUBJect pronominals corefer
- Possessive pronominal corefers to a previous argument
- The second sentence in the discourse pair starts with a deictic pronoun THIS/THAT

Two typical examples of these properties are contained in the following two sentence pairs from PDTB:

(578)
Relation: Cause
Connectives: because
[Arg1] This is not the case

[Arg2] Some diaries simply aren't worth snooping in

(1301)
Relation: Cause
Connectives: because
[Arg1] That isn't surprising
[Arg2] Regular TV series ratings have slumped in the past five years , and premiering new shows is `` a crap shoot

4. Data Analysis: The CRs Examples Annotated in DGBank and PDTBank

The data analysis will be concerned with the individuation of linguistic criteria to subdivide CRs as they have been selected and annotated in the two databanks available at HLT. DGBank is the corpus of annotated Discourse Relations built at ISI by Carlson et al. (2001) which contains 8910 relations and clause pairs, 466 (thus constituting approximately the 5% of all relations) of which have been labeled as CE, i.e. Cause-Effect. The PDTB contains only 1515 discourse relations, 204 of which have been labeled as CAUSE (approximately 13%).

The two corpora are markedly different however: the PDTB only contains "implicit" or lexically unexpressed discourse markers. In other words, sentence pairs related by a given Discourse Relation are not connected by an explicit lexical connector. They are also usually made of two separate sentences; however the structures selected may also respond to phonological criteria as reported in the Technical Manual(Wolf et al.)

As a basic rule, discourse segments (DSs) here will be assumed to be

- clauses delimited by commas or full-stops, since commas and full-stops are assumed to be equivalents of phrase boundaries in speech (cf. Hirschberg & Grosz (1992))
- elements of text (especially modifiers) that are separated by commas. The idea here is that commas that are equivalent to intonational phrase boundaries in speech should denote DSs.
- attributions, as in "John said that…". This is empirically motivated. The texts used here are taken from news corpora, and there, attributions can be important carriers of coherence structures. For instance, consider a case where some Source A and some Source B both comment on some Event X. It should be possible to distinguish between a situation where Source A and Source B make basically the same statement about Event X, and a situation where Source A and Source B make contrasting comments about Event X.

Here are some refinements of these basic rules:

- Clauses delimited by commas or full-stops are DSs. Commas are not DS-boundaries if they separate elements of a complex NP, or in cases like the following:

- *[It wasn't known to what extent, if any, the facility was damaged.]* (Marcu (2000))

- Elaborations (cf. Section 3.1.1 on MUC-7 annotation tags) are separate DSs:
  - *[Mr. Jones,][spokesman for IBM,] [said...]*
- Infinitival clauses are separate DSs (to has to be substitutable by in order to):
  - *[The arm can be fitted to allow it to grasp, lift and turn objects of differing sizes][to suit a variety of tasks.]*

  Discourse Graphbank documentation Wolf, Gibson, Fisher & Knight
  Page 9 of 23 December 2003 contact: fwolf@mit.edu
- Infinitival complements of verbs are not treated as separate DSs:
  - *[The machinery is of the type used to make small parts in metal cutting shops.]* (Marcu (2000))
- Participial complements of verbs are not treated as separate DSs:
  - *[The company misled many customers into purchasing more credit-data services.]* (Marcu (2000))
- Gerund forms that are clausal modifiers are treated as DSs:
  - [*the prices benefited from price reductions*][*arising from introduction of the consumption tax*]
- Prepositional phrases are treated as DSs if they are clausal modifiers:
  - *[With the ground stone being laid,] [they were able to move on.]*
- Whenever a source for a statement is mentioned, the statement and the source are treated as separate DSs.
  - *["Gorbachev deserves more credit than Reagan does,"] [Thomas Cronin said.]*
- DSs can contain ellipses (elided part in bold):
  - *[Human workers remain responsible for keeping inventory][and coordinating different aspects of the production line.]*
- Time-, space-, personal- or detail-elaborations are treated as DSs:
  - *[This past year,][the original robot was replaced with one able to perform more tasks.]*
  - *[Andy Russell,][a spokesman for IBM]*
- Strong discourse markers (e.g. *because*, *although*, *after*, *while*) are assumed to delimit DSs:
  - *[IBM will benefit][because we will be helping to train the (computer-integrated manufacturing) workers and decision makers of today and tomorrow.]*" (pagg.8-9, Wolf et al.)

On the contrary the DGB contains all types of discourse relations, with both expressed and unexpressed connectors, both inter and intrasententially organized. In particular, as far as CRs are concerned, we have the following distribution of data:

- 190 sentence pairs: 1) lexically unexpressed discourse marker;
- 136 clause pairs: 1) result/effect expressed as infinitival preceded by to/in_order_to; 2) intrasententially
- sentence pairs: 1) lexically expressed discourse markers (68 because + 21 because_of + 4 cause, caused_by); 2) intersententially

- 38 clause pairs: 1) result/effect expressed as gerundive preceded by by/for; 2) intrasententially
- 35 sentence pairs: 1) lexically expressed discourse markers (as, as_a_result, so. so_that, as_a_means_of, part_of, since, since_then, when, due_to); 2) intersententially
- 8 are non classified because not in agreement with the annotators
- 70 contain negation markers (not, no, none, nothing, never, neither, nor)
- 39 sentences in a pair are Relative Clauses
- 82 NPs intervene in the discourse relations either directly as one segment or indirectly
- 13 PPs and APs treated as segments
- 23 cases of pronominal coreference

Overall, we end up with 2/5 of all CRs with no lexical connector and 2/3 having one discourse marker; 2/5 of all CRs constituted by intrasentential structures and 3/4 having an intersential structure. Thus, by far the majority of discourse segments annotated are not between two clauses with finite verb.

What we really question is the criterion of using phonological methods to spot discourse segments of a non-clausal size. In particular those cases in which a phrase is selected which plays the role of an adjunct, generically. We report here below the critical cases, with line number reported in order to individuate them in the database, and then discuss them in more detail:

26590 Relation: ce
[A] No dummies ,
[B] the drivers pointed out they still had space on their machines for another sponsor 's name or two .

15250 Relation: ce
[A] for his outspoken opposition to the Vietnam War
[B] The late Prime Minister Olof Palme was blacklisted from the White House

24651 Relation: ce
[A] as a result of lower per capita consumption of beef , eggs , whole milk , butter , lard and edible tallow .
[B] the decline in animal products occurred

8405 Relation: ce
[A] given Vouet 's fame and his value on today 's market .
[B] the price was `` more than reasonable , and assuredly advantageous ,

16985 Relation: ce
[A] With Japan 's cash - flush banks aligned against it , though ,
[B] raising money may be difficult .

17020 Relation: ce
[A] but as the largest underwriters in the Eurobond market ,
[B] they might be able to scuttle borrowings there , too .

25911 Relation: ce
[A] Obstruction of Congress in Sept. and Oct. 1985 ,
[B] five - year imprisonment and $ 250,000 fine .

25936 Relation: ce
[A] False statements to Congress on Sept. 5 , 1985 ,
[B] five - year imprisonment and $ 250,000 fine .

25951 Relation: ce
[A] False statements to Congress by North on Sept. 12 , 1985 ,
[B] five - year imprisonment and $ 250,000 fine .

25966 Relation: ce
[A] False statements by North to Congress on Oct. 7 , 1985 ,
[B] five - year imprisonment and $ 250,000 fine .

25986 Relation: ce
[A] Obstruction of Congress in Aug. 1986 ,
[B] five - year imprisonment and $ 250,000 fine .

26001 Relation: ce
[A] Obstruction of Congress in Nov. 1986 ,
[B] five - year imprisonment and $ 250,000 fine .

26016 Relation: ce
[A] Obstruction of a presidential inquiry in Nov. 1986 ,
[B] five - year imprisonment and $ 250,000 fine .

26031 Relation: ce
[A] False statements on Nov. 23 , 1986 ,
[B] five - year imprisonment , $ 250,000 fine .

26046 Relation: ce
[A] Destroying or falsifying government documents ,
[B] three - year imprisonment and $ 250,000 fine .

26066 Relation: ce
[A] Receipt of an illegal gratuity ,
[B] two - year imprisonment and $ 250,000 fine .

26091 Relation: ce
[A] Conversion of traveler 's checks to personal use ,

[B] 10 - year imprisonment , $ 250,000 fine .

26106 Relation: ce
[A] Conspiracy to defraud the Treasury and the Internal Revenue Service ,
[B] five - year imprisonment , $ 250,000 fine .

26370 Relation: ce
[A] to set up a meeting ,
[B] `` It means no one will go out of their way

In most of the examples above, the discourse relations may be recovered by adding a dummy BE/GET predicate – or other similar light predicates. In some cases, the decision to treat the INFINITIVAL as a RESULTATIVE adjunct is disputable to say the least, as in 26370. Also consider 24651 where the predicate OCCUR cannot possible occur without a modifier, be it an adverbial, a gerundive or a PP. Eventually 26590 does not easily lend itself to a classification as CE, the relation being very far-fetched to be acknowledgeable by most readers.

Anyhow, the most critical question is the fact that non-clausal discourse segments, not possessing themselves any internal propositional structure but inheriting it from the main governing predicate, cannot be computed as being in a discourse relation with the rest of the clause to which they belong. Here we are not denying the fact that a semantic relation EXIST, but simply that it cannot be computed as a DISCOURSE relation. What has been annotated is simply the existence of an ADJUNCT which entertains a CAUSE/EFFECT relationship with the EVENT described by the governing predicate which it modifies. For instance, in the cases reported again here below,

15250 Relation: ce
[A] for *his* outspoken opposition to the Vietnam War
[B] *The late Prime Minister Olof Palme* was blacklisted from the White House

24651 Relation: ce
[A] as a result of lower per capita consumption of *beef , eggs , whole milk , butter , lard and edible tallow* .
[B] the decline in *animal products* occurred

8405 Relation: ce
[A] given *Vouet's* fame and *his* value on today 's market .
[B] ' '*the price* was `` more than reasonable , and assuredly advantageous ,

16985 Relation: ce
[A] With Japan's *cash-flush banks* aligned against **it** , though ,
[B] *raising money* may be difficult .

17020 Relation: ce
[A] but as the largest underwriters *in the Eurobond market* ,
[B] they might be able to scuttle borrowings *there* , too .

we marked in bold all cases of pronominal coreference, bridging and other cases of nominal anaphora which indicate strong cohesion between arguments and adjuncts of the same predicate. Then the use of such prepositions as GIVEN, AS, FOR, WITH, is a strong indication that they can easily be interpreted as adjuncts with the semantic relation of CAUSE of the event described by the predicate.

So we consider that from a computational point of view, we want to distinguish CAUSAL relations at propositional level from those intervening at non-propositional level. In particular, adjuncts are interpreted when computing the structure of the whole proposition and no separate discourse segment may be assigned to them because they lack an independent propositional meaning.

As to PDTB, we analysed all of the 204 CRs pairs and we came out with similar results. On a first perusal of the structures we discovered that these examples are highly paraphrastic, using copulative or light verbs together with extended nominalization to convey the meaning of events. Overall, we counted 218 cases of copulative as main verbs (be, there_be, become, have), which makes at least one for each sentence pair. On the contrary, the same verbs in the DGB only amount to 126 cases, about 27% of sentence pairs only. We also counted the number of clauses overall and the mean length per discourse relation is much higher in PDTB – 3,1, when compared to DGB - 2,3.

In PDTB Cause annotated sentence pairs, there is a consistent use of negation: there are 83 sentences containing negation, i.e. 40.7%: if we compare this with DGB, where we had 70 negation items – i.e. 15% of the all examples – we can see that it is much higher.

5. A Semantics of Causality Relations

Generally speaking, most of the CRs annotated in the two corpora must in fact be interpreted as some other type of relation, notably, CIRCUMSTANCE, RATIONALE, PURPOSE, MEANS. Also cases in which the DR is marked by the presence of a discourse marker such as BECAUSE which is regarded almost as unambiguous as to its meaning, the relation is not expressible as CAUSE. In this section we will use examples taken from the two corpora to illustrate the necessity to distinguish semantically CRs as they have been encoded according to their meaning and their import in a framework like QA which requires fine-grained distinctions to be made. In particular, whenever WHY questions need to be answered and a MULTI-question scenario be instantiated, the meaning associated implicitely or explicitely with each question needs to be clearly specified in order to look for the appropriate answer. For instance, in many cases when somebody asks "why does X happen" the question is open to two interpretations: it could truly be asking for the cause of X, or it could be asking how we KNOW X will happen.

Consider one example which may be paraphrased as

5.1. the CAUSE why B HAPPENED was A.

7160 Relation: ce
[A] apparently because of television cameras nearby .

[B] four other young boys who showed up at one of the campuses left

As may be noticed, the presence of an adverb of opacity or doubt like APPARENTLY, influences the veridicity of the reported event by introducing a modality/intensionality operator. On the contrary the majority of cases of CEs must be paraphrased differently as,

5.2. the REASON why B HAPPENED was A.

5074 Relation: ce
[A] because of executive privilege .
[B] as president , Nixon was immune from judicial subpoena

In nonfinite structures like infinitivals and gerundives, the most recurrent semantic paraphrase would be something like,

5.3. the INTENDED REASON why B HAPPENED was A

where we are left with the possibility that A might or might not have happened, as shown by the following examples,

6114 Relation: ce
[A] to create pieces
[B] Lewczenko worked as an maintenance man while building a glass - cutting machine at home

6119 Relation: ce
[A] to prove himself as a cutter.
[B] to create pieces

from the context available it would be impossible to deduct that the RESULT indicated in the A fragment actually happened. We may consider the latter example, 6119, as a case of PURPOSE clause, where the speaker conveys the aim, the goal of the action expressed in the governing clause, B.

Now consider the following pair,

5724 Relation: ce
[A] by using the profits from arms sales to Iran
[B] to purchase supplies for the Contras .

which is derived from the following complete sentence,

[A] North 's activities in these countries were central to Walsh 's legal strategy to show that the former National Security Council aide conspired to defraud the United States and steal government property by using the profits from arms sales to Iran to purchase supplies for the Contras, where we derive that the gerundive is used in a Factive context, so that the final reading will correspond to the semantic paraphrase contained in 5.1. Besides, the A clause contained in 5724 expresses MEANS, that is the instrument by means of which the action expressed in A is carried out.

As in previous cases – see Chapt. 1 on Logical Form - I will be using a Davidsonian event semantic representation (see Davidson 1967) and further developed by Higginbotham (1985, 1989), in which events are individuals of an abstract kind and contribute to the overall semantic representation of a proposition by introducing a variable 'e'. Again following Higginbotham (1983) we assume that finite tense introduces quantification over the event. Thus, in a. below

a. John left.

We have the following representation,

b. Exist leave(John, e)

which can be paraphrased,

'There was an event, e: e is a leaving by John.'

Using this representaiton for rationale clauses, the argument structure of rationale is given in 5.3 (see Whelpton, 1):

5.3. RATIONALE (x, e, ^p) <-> x brings about e with the intention that p

RATIONALE has three argument positions, one ranging over individuals, one ranging over events and one ranging over propositions. The conditions on reference state that the individual must bring about the event (i.e. be the 'agent' of the event) with the intention that the proposition come to be true. Other conditions require the governing predicate denote an event, and that the SUBJect of the RATIONALE be related to the SUBJect of the main event.

In English RESULTATIVES, the main verb names an action or process while a dependent predicate phrase names either the result state or the extent of the action. Simpson (1983) points out that if the main verb is transitive or unaccusative, the dependent predicate names the result state which the patient achieves, as in (a) examples. If the main verb is unergative, or a transitive verb with unexpressed patient, the dependent predicate names the extent of the action as in (b) examples.

5.4a. I painted the car yellow.
I cooked the meat to a cinder.
I shot John dead.
The milk froze solid.
The vase broke into little pieces.
b. I laughed myself sick.
I shouted myself hoarse.

I cried myself to sleep.
I worked my fingers to the bone.
She drank him under the table.

As can be easily gathered from these examples, RESULTATIVES constitute cases of felicitous performance of the action named by the main verb. This is however also due to the use of PAST TENSE, which by itself, at least in English and in other languages, is PERFECTIVE or TELIC, i.e. describes actions which actually happened in the past. From this point of view, all actions narrated in the past may be computed as FACTIVE. However, there may be cases in which the action described in the event is negated or contradicted by a following utterance. We will comment on the importance of Aspectual information and its relation with Tense here below.

Resultatives, Means Clauses and Rationale Clauses all share properties also belonging to canonical Causality Relations expressed by discourse markers: they are irreflexive, asymmetric, and transitive. However, transitivity affects utterances with Rationale clauses in a different manner from other cases, as also commented by Balkanski and shown in the following examples:

4.5.a. Mary reset the printer by pressing the button
b. Mary pressed the button to reset the printer

The two sentences express the same content but the meaning in example (b) is not transmitted appropriately. The Rationale clause leaves open the possibility that something might happen after the action of PRESSing the button and the RESULT might not be achieved. Example (a) might be felicitous continued by specifying details of the action with more granularity, structurally by embedding recursively; on the contrary, example (b) does not allow this possibility as shown by,

4.6.a. Mary fixed her problems by resetting the printer by pressing the button
b. Mary pressed the button to reset the printer to fix her problems
c. ??Mary pressed the button to fix her problems to reset the printer

In both (b-c) examples the two Rational infinitivals are linked to the main verb and cannot create a Causality chain as happens in (a). Using LF as shown above we may end up with the following representation for sentence 5.5a.,

LF: *Exist xl,x2, press(x1) & past(xl) & agt(xl,Mary)*
& obj(x1, Button) & in_order_to(x1, x2)
& reset(x1) & obj(x2, Printer)

where Balkanski introduces the operator IN_ORDER_TO to indicate the meaning of the Rationale Clause. As suggested by Webber, representations in a Discourse Model may have to refer to events and entities which may not (yet) exist in the real world, but nonetheless they may become object of coreference by means of pronominal and nominal expressions.

Meaning as expressed by Semantic Roles, also needs to be taken into account and requires deep scrutiny. In particular, we want to be sure that such influencing factors as

INTENTIONALITY, VOLITIONALITY and OCCASIONALITY all receive an appropriate representation in the final Logical Form, so that the appropriate inferential and reasoning processes can be fired. We will now look into Talmy's latest publication and also in the comments and additional interesting points made by some of his colleagues a more recent paper.

Talmy (2000) in his chapter on causality, makes a very fine-grained subdivision of circumstances in which agency and events may entertain different relations, which need to be expressed by appropriate semantic roles. For instance he presents a long list of distinct types, from which we extrapolate the ones that we assume interesting to our framework (ibid., 472-474):

5.1. Talmy's Taxonomy of Causal Semantic Relations

- Autonomous event
- The vase broke.
- Resulting-event causative or basic causative
- The vase broke from a ball rolling into it.
- Causing event causative
- A ball rolling into it broke a vase.
- Instrument causative
- A ball broke the vase by rolling into it.
- Author causative – i.e. with unintended outcome
- I broke a vase with my rolling a ball into it.
- Agent causative – i.e. with intended outcome
- I broke the vase by rolling a ball into it.
- Undergoer situation (not causative)
- I lost the pen somewhere in the kitchen.
- Purpose situation
- I hit the snail to kill it.

As said above, the force dynamic model of causation (Talmy, 2000; Wolff, 2003) represents a particular approach to causation that specifies the basic dimensions of meaning associated with various causal concepts such as CAUSE, ENABLE and PREVENT. From a force dynamic perspective, the concept of CAUSE belongs to a family of concepts that includes ENABLE and PREVENT, among others. Differences among the concepts are captured in terms of various patterns of tendency, relative strength, rest, and motion between an affector and patient. These basic dimensions, or components, of meaning are referred to as the "structural" aspects of causal meaning, by means of which various causal expressions can be classified. In this theory, an *affector* is the entity that ACTS ON another entity and the *patient* is an entity that is ACTED ON by another entity. Consider the following examples:

5.8a. Strong winds caused the bridge to collapse.
b. Vitamin B enables the body to digest food.
c. Corn oil prevents butter from burning.

Wolff and Song (2003; Wolff, Song & Driscoll, 2002), introduced a version of Talmy's theory, the force dynamic model, in which the model defines the concepts of CAUSE, ENABLE and PREVENT with respect to three binary dimensions: 1) the *patient's* intrinsic tendency for the *result*, 2) whether the *affector* and *patient* act in concordance, and 3) occurrence of the *result*. In a CAUSE situation (a), for example, the tendency of the *patient* (the bridge) is not for the *result* (i.e., not to collapse), but the *affector* (strong winds) does not act in concordance with this tendency and the *result* occurs. In an ENABLE situation (b), the tendency of the *patient* (the body) is for the *result* (to digest food); the *affector* (Vitamin B) acts in concordance with this tendency, even assisting in its realization, and the *result* occurs. In a PREVENT situation (c), the tendency of the *patient* (butter) is for the *result* (burning), the *affector* (corn oil) is not in concordance, and the *result* does not occur.

5.2. Reclassifying CRs

Eventually one may posit the existence of a bipartition in the semantic classification of CRs:

CLASS I: one the one side we have CRs which represent the propotypical situation in which an AGENT or CAUSER does X which is linked to another EVENT Y which is interpretable as the OUTCOME or the EFFECT/RESULT of X. Constraints applying on this kind of CRs are the asymmetric condition, the transitive condition and the temporal sequence;

CLASS II: on the other side we have subjective relations where the goal of the text is that of explaining the RATIONALE, the MOTIVATION, the PURPOSE, the MEANS, the CIRCUMSTANCE of the Causal Event X.

In order to verify our theoretical stand, we engaged ourselves in a reclassification of the DRs annotation of DGB. At first we wanted to limit our experiment to CRs and to a select but significant sample. We thus chose 115 sentence pairs which were representative of both classes we individuated.

At the bottom of each sentence pair to better specify processing and interpretive aspects I added three more items, FACT, COREF, POLAR.

FACT: - has a binary value, EXTENSIONAL vs INTENSIONAL, where the first expresses the factivity of the events contributing to the annotation of a Discourse Relation as Cause-Rationale-Means-Purpose-Circumstance/Effect, the second one indicates the presence of opaque operators which may express different types of modality;

COREF: may assume three values, YES, indicating the presence of pronominal expressions linked by coreferentiality in the two separate sentences; NO, no coreferentiality taking place; HYP, there is at least one nominal expression coreferring or cospecifying another nominal expression by means of inferential processes (hyponymic or hypernymic, etc.), or simply by repetition of the same linguistic description.

POLAR: may assume two values, where YES means that the proposition have positive polarity; NO has a number of different values: it may point to the presence of negation, but also lexicalized negation. We also marked with NO cases of events carrying negative judgement, affect describers, depending on our knowledge of the world.

The 5 DRs may be paraphrased as follows, where A indicates the Effect/Consequent clause and B the other:

CAUSE
There is an inherent objective connection in the real world between A and B
RATIONALE
The intended reason why A happened is B
A happened in order to do/carry out B
A happened following/according to the contents of B
MEANS
A happened by means of B
CIRCUMSTANCE
A happened independently of(no intentionally, no volitionality) B, which
(will) take place consequently
PURPOSE
A happened with the aim to do/carry out B

Notice that all relations apart from Purpose have a transitive property and are asymmetric (B causes/motivates A happening and happens before A). Purpose relations have the opposite property: they are typically non realized in the world and constitute the consequent of the A event/action.

Eventually we got the following results:

PURPOSE: 22
RATIONALE: 41
MEANS: 7
CIRCUMSTANCE: 2
CAUSE: 44

84 – FACT: EXTENS
32 – FACT: INTENS
(6 are PURPOSE, 1 CIRCUMSTANCE, 11 RATIONALE, 14 CAUSE)

80 - COREF: YES
20 – COREF: HYP
16 – COREF: NO

75 - POLAR: YES
15 – POLAR: YES/NO
23 – POLAR: NO/NO
4 – POLAR: NO/YES

5.3. Explicit and Implicit CRs: Are they Interchangeable?

Marcu and Echihabi (2002) carried out a study with the aim of detecting relations automatically. They reported that Contrast relations were signalled by a discourse marker in 26% of the cases where they appeared. Relations labelled as Explanation-Evidence were found to be signalled also around 26% of the time. This level or signalling is, obviously, a problem for an automatic system that purports to identify relations based on discourse markers, such as the one proposed by Marcu (Marcu, 2000a, 2000b).

However, they trained an automatic classifier to recognize the relations that were not signalled by a discourse marker. The classifier was trained on examples of actual relations, versus examples of non-relations (random pairs of units, sometimes each taken from different documents), using lexical patterns. It learnt to distinguish relations that were not signalled by a discourse marker, increasing accuracy over a discourse-marker-based method by as much as 77%. This however has been carried out on automatically classified DRs. When tested on manually annotated date, the same algorithm has been reported to achieve an accuracy of 57%, which is a very poor result.

We want to assume that use of discourse markers is not optional. The strong hypothesis would be that in order to be able to omit/insert a causality discourse marker some structural and semantic conditions have to obtain. In addition, it seems that inserting BECAUSE corresponds to testing the causality reading of the DR. For instance, one of the relations marked in DGB, is not a DR but just a complement:

95 instance:2475 file:42
DU1: to release a 408-page FDIC report ,
DU2: Seidman told reporters at a luncheon

Which can be paraphrased as,

- Seidman told reporters at a luncheon that they had to release a 408-page FDIC report

But not,

** Seidman told reporters at a luncheon BECAUSE they had to release a 408-page...

On the contrary, in all other cases, whenever a Causality relation is implied, the sentence can be reformulated using BECAUSE. Consider the following examples taken from the DGB:

96 instance:1884 file:31 - PURPOSE
DU1: to produce chemical weapons .
DU2: the plant was built
- the plant was built BECAUSE they/one (wanted, intended) to produce chemical weapons

73 instance:939 file:15 - RATIONALE
DU1: He died in Dec. 21 Pan Am plane crash in Scotland while on his way to New York
DU2: to observe the signing of an agreement for Namibian independence from South African rule .
- He died in Dec. 21 Pan Am plane crash in Scotland while on his way to New York BECAUSE he (wanted, intended) to observe the signing of an agreement for Namibian independence from South African rule .

However, no such reformulation is allowed when there is CAUSE DR, there are two separate clause with finite tense, and there is no discourse marker. Consider,

79 instance:435 file:7
DU1: these early PCs triggered explosive product development in desktop models for the home and office .
DU2: PC shipments annually total some $ 38.3 billion world - wide.
- These early PCs triggered explosive product development in desktop models for the home and office *BECAUSE PC shipments annually total some $38.3 billion world-wide.

59 instance:4689 file:76
DU1: Tenor Enrico Caruso was a guest as the temblor struck .
DU2: He was tossed from his bed
- He was tossed from his bed *BECAUSE tenor Enrico Caruso was a guest as the temblor struck.

5.4. Implicit Discourse Markers and Reclassification

We then applied the same scheme of reclassification to the whole of CAUSE relations - 205 discourse unit pairs - contained in the PDTB. The overall picture we got was totally reversed. Here below are the final counts:

51 - COREF: NO
31 - COREF: (HYP) HARD COREF
66 - COREF: HYP
52 - COREF: YES

We have decided to introduce a new category (HYP) for hard to get coreferentiality cases which not only calls for the right resource to be available but difficult to implement inferential mechanisms. As can be gathered, now the majority of cases are no longer made of Pronominal coreference but Nominal coreference and in particular, there is 40% of cases which are either hard to compute or contain no coreferential link at all.

In order to better evaluate this situation we examined the content of this 40% of cases in order to discover the nature of the semantic interpretation needed to fire the Causality relation. We found the following:

34 - Idiomatic or Rhetorical Statements
11 - Generic Statements

In other words, half of the cases of lack or hard coreference are constituted by Idiomatic or Rhetorical and Generic Statements, which are inherently nonfactual.

6. Towards a General Model of CRs

Attempts at producing Automatic Discourse Relations Classification are very few in the literature: Ken Barter in 1995 produced an interactive algorithm and an evaluation limited though to a small number of examples. As reported above, Marcu and Echihabi (2002) carried out a study with the aim of detecting discourse relations automatically. They trained an automatic classifier to recognize the relations that were not signalled by a discourse marker. The classifier was trained on examples of actual relations, versus examples of non-relations (random pairs of units, sometimes each taken from different documents), using lexical patterns. It learnt to distinguish relations that were not signalled by a discourse marker, increasing accuracy over a discourse-marker-based method by as much as 77%. This result refers to an experiment carried out on automatically classified DRs. When tested on manually annotated data, the same algorithm has been reported to achieve an accuracy of 57%, which is a very poor result.

Another experiment has been reported lately, see Verbene 2006 and Verbene et al. 2006 where the authors make use of DGB data to answer Why questions. They also attempt a reclassification task as we did with the following results:

> "...During the manual classification, we assigned the answer type *cause* to 23.3 percent of the questions and *motivation* to 40.3 percent. We were not able to assign an answer sub-type to the remaining pairs (36.4 percent). These questions are in the broader class *reason* and not in one of the specific sub-classes. None of the question-answer pairs was classified as *circumstance* or *purpose*. Descriptions of *purpose* are very rare in news texts because of their generic character (e.g. People have eyebrows to prevent sweat running into their eyes). The answer type *circumstance*, defined by Quirk (cf. section 15.45) as a combination of reason with conditionality, is also rare as well as difficult to recognize. For evaluation of the question analysis module, we mainly considered the questions that did get assigned a sub-type (motivation or cause) in the manual classification. Our question analysis module succeeded in assigning the correct answer sub-type to 62.2 percent of these questions, the wrong sub-type to 2.4 percent, and no sub-type to the other 35.4 percent." (ibid. 44).

Besides noting the difficulty of the manual classification task for some subtypes of Causal Relations, the authors general remark is that using Discourse Relations on top of syntactic representation is by far more advantageous than not using it, in the task of answering Why questions.

We will now present in detail the contents of the algorithm from a technical and linguistic point of view. The algorithm performs these actions:

1. collects linguistic information from parser output
2. translates linguistic information into Semantic and Pragmatic Classes
3. assigns Discourse Relation on a clause-by-clause level: some will be specific, some generic or default
4. detects the presence of Causality Relations according to the algorithm traced above
5. determines coreference relations between Discourse Units thus classified

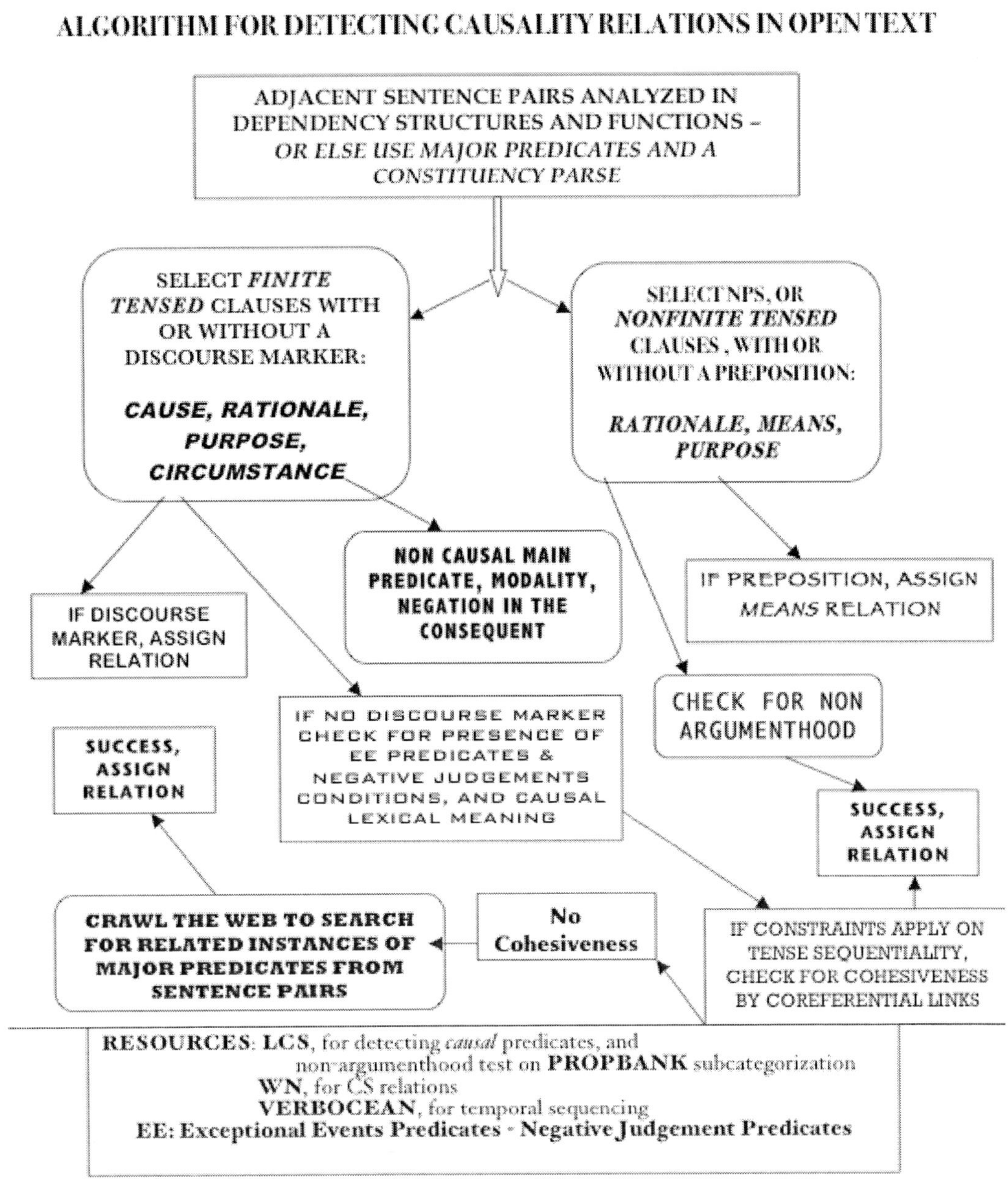

Figure 3. The Algorithm for Causality Relations Detection in open domain unrestricted text.

Input to the algorithm is reported in Table 2.: the list of linguistic items represents clause level information as derived from dependency structure – related to the example “he was not frozen in place by rigid ideology”:

Table 2a. Linguistic Information from Dependency Structure

Speech	Predicate	Tense	Voice	Modal	Neg
direct	freeze	past	passive	nil	not

Table 2b. Linguistic Information from Dependency Structure continued

Aux	Foc	Aspect	Mood
nil	nil	Accomplishment	Indic

Lexical aspect is derived from LCS following the approach presented in Dorr & Olsen(1997). The remaining linguistic items are quite straightforward to describe from the output of a dependency parser. Table 2c contains the semantic interpretation of the initial features, which is wrought by means of combining features together and the use of external knowledge to tell different classes of verbs apart, which we take from WordNet, LCS, FrameNet and PropBank. For instance, Auxiliary and Tense contribute to produce COMPTENSE, etc.; Point of view depends on Speech and semantic class of verb; Factuality depends on Mood, Modality; Relevance depends on negation and Viepoint. A full set of rules is reported in the previous chapter.

Table 2c. Informational Structure derived from Linguistic Information

ClauseType/SemRole	View-point	Comp-Tense	Factuality	Relevance
main/prop	external	past	no	Back-ground

Table 2d. Discourse Structure derived from Informational Structure

DISCREL	DISCDOMAIN	DISCSTRUCTURE
narration	objective	down(1-2)

The second step takes as input the forms shown here above in Table 2c, and the list of arguments and adjuncts and produces the output of Table 2d. The second step is represented here below by three sets of rules:

1. the first rule looks for clause governed by BE/HAVE, i.e. copulative constructions in which the verb has no semantic relevance
2. the second rule looks for all cases of clauses be it finite or nonfinite
3. the third rules takes into account adjunct PPs, governed by a preposition, which have already received their interpretation by the parser

Finally, as explained above and indicated in Figure 3 below, the rules elaborated for the detection of Causal Relations are fired after the other DRs have already been decided. The rules have the task of recovering the Cause/Circumstance whenever a Result/Effect has already been decided by the previous algorithm. To this aim, we try to take advantage of the information encoded in two resources: WordNet and FrameNet. In order to spot Negative Judgement predicates we use Laswell Value Dictionary and the Harvard IV dictionary available at http://www.webuse.umd.edu:9090/tags/.

As discussed above, DISCOURSEREL is recomputed after the first pass.

In case a RESULT or a RATIONAL clause has been previous computed, the system looks for the most adequate adjacent clause to become a CAUSE or an OUTCOME. This is done by checking Temporal and Coreferentiality constraints. The outcome of this pass is to relabel some previously labeled Discourse Relations which constitute default relations, into the one required by the context.

7. Results and Evaluation

In order to carry out the evaluation we assumed that the gap existing between Discourse Units (hence DUs) and Syntactic Units (hence SUs) should be minimal. To that end, we compared the three corpora at hand with the task to be realized. As it turned out, PDTB resulted unsuitable for either tasks, the DRR and DSR. The reason for that is simply due to the arbitrariness of correspondences existing between Syntactic Units and Discourse Units. The annotators had syntactic structures available from PTB and did not impose themselves a strict criterion for the definition of what a DU might correspond to. The result is an average proportion of 3.2 clauses per DU, a fact that makes the corpus unsuitable for either tasks. In their ppt presentation of annotation guidelines, downloadable from PDTB website, Eleni Miltsakaki et al. summarize in one slide what counts as a legal Discourse Unit, which they refer to as Argument:

A single clause (tensed/untensed); A single sentence; Multiple sentences; NPs that refer to clauses; Some nominal forms expressing events or states.

So basically any syntactic unit may actually become a discourse Argument, and the correspondence Clause-DU is completely lost. The problem is that in order to take automatic decisions, criteria to be used become hard to define, and refer to pragmatic and semantic domain rather than simply and more safely to syntax. This situation should also affect machine learning methods which would use general linguistic features to build their models and then would be at a loss when trying to scale them to different syntactic structures.

So finally we are left with two corpora, DGB and RST. The latter in particular is very strictly compliant with a syntax based unit correspondence. DGB, even though not intended to respond to such a criterion, has an average ratio of clauses per DU of 2.2. We decided to cope with this inconsistency by assigning a Discourse Relation to a corresponding larger Unit in case the smaller one was missing when computing the same sentence, on the basis of the presence of the same main predicate.

General data for the two corpora are tabulated here below:

Table 3a. General Data and EDU/Sentence Ratio

	No. sentences	No. words	No. EDUs	Ratio EDU/Ss
RST-test	799	19300	2346	2.9
DGB	3110	72520	8910	2.8

Table 3b. Quantitative Evaluation of DU Segmentation

	No. EDUS	My No. EDUS	Recall	Precis.
RST-test	2346	2281	97.2	87.9
DGB	8910	8910	100	89.8

Results reported in S&M report an F-measure of 84.7% when using the PennTreebank structure and 83.1% when using Charniak's parser.

Table 3c. F-measure values for DGB experiment

	Causality Relations	Condition	Contrast	Other Relations
DGB	38.13%	48.25%	44.34	59.13

The overall F-measure for DGB is 54.57%.

8. Lexical Appendix

A. Predicates derived from PDTB

Negative Judgement and Exceptional Events
disagree, limit, criticize, defend, lose, lack, hurt, take_a_beating, object, refuse, eliminate, be_under_pressure, have_policy_against, soar, ignore, differ_from, rise, loss, excessive, challenge, step_up, increase, defeat, force, cut_down, slump, acquire, sell, buy, be_bigger, be_biggest, be_slimmer, stick_with, grow

Periphrastic Causality
convince, opinion, strive, be_another_story, be_uncertain, be_chance, be_likely, feel_like, be_difficult, puzzle, expect, believe, decide, take_step, know, consider

B. Predicates derived from DGB

Negative Judgement and Lexicalized Negation
avoid, refuse, reject, deny, delay, divert, affect, play_down, dismiss, disheartening, disappear, disrupt, disease, distrust, limit, hamper, prevent

Positive Judgement
encourage, foster, help, favor, recommend, support, aid, agree, accept, accuse, criticize, attack, deter, sue, discuss, dispute, consider

Exceptional Event and Gradual Unexpected Change
rise, raise, grow, exaggerate, underestimate, reduce, shrink, expand, drop, loss, gain, spend, pay, decline

Lexicalized Causality
decide, force, arrest, discover, solve, start, begin, continue, have_to, should, require, need

Periphrastic Causality
create, provide, kill, injure, build, close, open, destroy, buy, sell, resign, leave, lose, win, resume, return, get_back, borrow, hire

Chapter 6

TEXT GENERATION

1. INTRODUCTION

In order to generate a text, a computer program needs some computational theory of human language ability for language generation. Starting from the 70s' there has been a long tradition of TUS – Text Understanding System – which have tried to represent the internal psychological operations human beings actually perform when planning and actually uttering a discourse or writing a text. However, computer programs are only intended to simulate processes which can only be surmised to take place in the human mind in a certain order. We consequently assume that the following basic components are required:

a. a knowledge base containing events, entities and their properties
b. communicative intentions and goals - for a given audience/domain
c. rhetorical structure building rules
d. a lexicon and criteria for lexical choice
e. a grammar and criteria for structural choice

Points b. and c. together realize what is usually called the planning component, whereas points d. and e. the realization component of a text generation system. As to point a., it is necessary to have an inferential basis onto which build a sensible content for any text: in case such a component is lacking there must be some set of axioms telling us which lexical items to choose in order to build up a sequence of sensible actions and participants in the actions for a given topic/domain we may choose.

In short, we must know *what to say* and *how to say it.*

Some of the most important issues to be tackled in building such a system are:

1. how to build a coherent and cohesive sequence of sentences
2. how to choose from among a number of possible candidates the most adequate description for a given entity
3. at each step of the generation process, expressing only relevant information

As to point 1. there is a tight link between component b. and c. above which determines the most adequate sequence of rhetorical segments: directive text is different from narrative text as we saw in previous chapters. It is clear, for instance, that a sequence of directives must follow some sequential order which in turn must have some logical coherence. Take a simple recipe: you stir only after you pour some ingredient in a bowl and not viceversa. The same would apply to a narration: some actions can be performed only after some other action takes place. In other words, we need knowledge of the world to order facts and to select entities and their properties.

Here again however, we are confronted with a different task according to whether we are either answering some queries in a question-answering system, or we are generating descriptions of some object whose features are elaborated in a knowledge base from some analogic input. None of these two tasks actually interests us, since our only concern is narrative text, which is what the book is about. So we shall limit ourselves to generation of narrative text, and this could be done at least in three ways:

a. by summarizing the contents of some previously analysed text
b. by generating the text itself from a pool of topics and preorganized text structures
c. by answering some question on the basis of a Discourse Model

Whereas b. will be dealt with in this chapter, a. and c. will be developed in the following Chapter VII. What linguistic information constitutes an adequate input to the tactical component ? In order to answer this first question we need to decide how much work has to be assigned to the planner. From the subdivision of labour between the two components, we shall be able to ascertain what is left to the grammar itself and the lexicon.

1.1. Generating Modes

We can surmise that generation can be realized at least in three different modes:

A. from a random choice of predicates in the lexicon preceded by a planning phase that determines the goals the text has to achieve, the message and rhetorical structure which is more appropriate, the realization of the information as a grammatical sequence of utterances where coherence and cohesion is achieved;
B. by paraphrasing the contents of Discourse Model on the basis of Discourse Structures;
C. by summarizing the contents of the Discourse Model on the basis of the most relevant facts related to the most relevant entity.

In what follows, we shall try to account for the internal processing of two types of application for text generation: the first one is a random chooser from a pool of predicates and the second one is a summarizer from a discourse model as produced by the output of Getarun. In both cases, we do not resort to canned text nor to templates: rather, we aim at building text plans at discourse level and then to specify semantic structure sufficient for sentence level generation. Semantic specifications are very much in terms of feature-structure, where on the basis of a set of fixed slots we try to fill a value which is then turned into some lexical item independently realized by the surface generator.

But before going into the details of the applications we shall discuss some general problems related to Italian.

1.2. Text Generation in Italian

Generating text in Italian is intrinsically bound to the peculiarities of its surface grammar. Summarizing is a task that requires full discourse structure information which in our case is made available from Getarun and feeds directly the planning component. In turn, grammar and lexicon needed for the tactical component is readily available from the DCG parser.

As we know and as has been extensively discussed in the linguistic literature, Italian is a language that allows and in some cases requires the Subject to be generated in postverbal position. Subject inversion is a free process, i.e. it does not obey such constraints as the D(efinitiness) E(effect), and requires no expletive, as is the case with other languages like English, German or French. In fact, Italian is regarded as a language with empty expletives. Choice for auxiliaries is determined on the basis of syntactic category: unaccusatives require "be", while the other categories require "have". However, passive and impersonal constructions also require "be" as auxiliary. In addition, Object NP can be expressed as clitic and be thus obligatorily positioned in front of tensed verb.

Here are some examples, where we include verbal features in brackets, a literal translation and finally an approximate English rendering:

1. Arriva [Arriva_3/pers/sing_pres/ind]
   lit. Arrives |He is arriving|
2. Arriva Gino [Arriva_3/pers/sing_pres/ind Gino]
   lit. Arrives John |John is arriving|
3. E' arrivata Maria
   [E'_3/pers/sing_pres/ind arrivata_3/pers/sing/fem_past/partic Maria]
   lit. Is arrived Mary |Mary has arrived|
4. Gino l'ha conosciuta ieri
   [Gino l'_acc ha_3/pers/sing_pres/ind conosciuta_3/pers/sing/fem_past/partic ieri]
   lit. John her has known yesterday |John met her yesterday|
5. Cosa hanno detto i tuoi amici?
   [Cosa hanno_3/pers/plur_pres/ind detto_3/pers/sing/mas_past/partic i_mas/plur tuoi_2/pers/plur/mas amici_plur/mas]
   lit. What have said the your friends |What did your friends say|
6. Gino ha visto ieri Maria sull'autobus
   [Gino ha_3/pers/sing_pres/ind visto_3/pers/sing/mas_past/partic ieri Maria sull' autobus_mas]
   lit. John has seen yesterday Mary on the bus |Yesterday John saw Mary on the bus |

As can be noticed from the features associated to the verbal morphemes, agreement on the past participle should include Gender as well as Number which in case of unaccusatives should agree with the Subject. However, as example 4 shows, agreement goes with the Object with transitive verbs. Also notice the apostrophe which deletes the final vowel of clitic pronouns: in this case no information is available on the gender, only case can be inferred.

Example 5 is a case of obligatory postverbal Subject: "Cosa i tuoi amici hanno detto" is ungrammatical. Notice the use of the article in front of a possessive pronoun which is again obligatory and can be dispensed with in case of names denoting family relations like brother, sister, mother etc.

Finally, example 6 shows two important features of Italian and other Romance languages: first, adjuncts can be freely interspersed between Subject and verb or verb and Object, in other words there is no adjacency constraint applicable. Second, Italian has amalgamated prepositions, i.e. a preposition with article which in turn can undergo epenthesis by the use of the apostrophe. In the latter case, generation of the compound preposition requires gender and number information to be made available beforehand, or else it should be generated afterwards.

1.3. Lexical Choice

As a first approximation, we do not want to modify the lexicon in order to introduce a higher quantity of information if required. Since Italian is a language that requires Gender and Number features in its Agreement to be determined before Lexical Form Selection can adequately take place we would like the Grammar to be able to propagate and solve all problems related to Agreement. As we saw in previous Chapters, the semantics can at times be responsible for the information related to Gender, in particular when the current entity is a person and not a thing. Problems related to Number on the contrary are basically semantic in nature. The entity asserted in the Discourse Model should be individuated either as set, or as individual or else as a generic class entity. In the ontology we may also find locations which again may be assigned the same semantics as entities.

2. Mode A: Random Generation

Criteria for generating short stories may vary according to genre and to contents. Story generation should be minimally constrained in the sense that the generation process should be endowed with the minimal world knowledge necessary to bring it into life. This would be represented by a startup frame containing the minimum information required to establish a sensible framework. Goal specification could be instantiated by defining genre linked frames which are differentiated by their Topic.

Let's assume we intend to generate a story which has one main character and a number of secondary characters which are in the relation of "friend" to the main character. We may also assume that they all share a common social role, the one of "student"; they live in the same spatiotemporal location but in different houses and attend the same "school". This will conform to the following startup frame:

Frame 1
Topic = student_story

Main_Character = proper_name
Main_Social_Properties = [student, hockey_player]
Main_Relational_Properties = [friend, daughter, sad, happy]
Spatial _Locations = [school, home, [town, [south_italy]]]
Temporal _Locations = [last_week, yesterday, today]
Means_of _Transport = [bicycle, bus, car]
Main_relations = [go, get_back, arrive, study, play, win, lose]
Main_interests = [hockey, watching_tv, reading]

The aim of the planning process is to build up a sequence of predicate argument structures from the predicates included in the frame. The frame is made up of a certain number of attributes and their values are templates which can be used to trigger a corresponding lexical entry. This frame could give rise to a number of short descriptions of a main character and the events associated with him.

Consider again the frame or schema above and its attributes: we need only specify main properties and relations; secondary relations derive from searching into the lexicon for selectional restrictions associated with main properties and other properties may be recovered in the same way. For instance, by using semantic relations and aspectual classes available in our lexicon, we only need to specify verbal predicates that involve change of the world, while all verbs indicating perceptual activities, states and other processes that can be applied to humans are freely available to build comments, elaborations and other background events. No adjectives are included: these again can be picked up from the lexicon on the basis of their semantic restrictions. The ontology includes only extensional referring expressions and relational linguistics expressions.

However, in order to build a coherent text, we need to build a plan based on a sequence of *narration units* (hence NU) each one will be expanded in one *episode*. Narratives – as Propp and other structuralists like Greimas and Brémond taught us – are structurally organized around a climax which in turn is started out by an initial state of equilibrium where the characters of the story exhibit their usual connotative features. After story setup has taken place – regarding spatiotemporal locations – an uncouth and unexpected event happens in which the protagonist does some exemplar deed or is the victim of some fatal doom. As a reaction to that initial event, he flees from home/homeland and travels in search of some help/fortune. Adventures follow up to a climax. Then the return home constitutes the second part of the narrative structure. This would be the plot of typical myths. If we look at fairy tales again there is a structural organization with an opening setup, a shocking event that breaks out unexpected, a climax and a final part of the plot where the original equilibrium is reestablished or some transformation takes place.

Each NU can be made up by an utterance which in turn may be realized as a simple or a complex sentence. The internal structure of each sentence is determined by rhetorical structure and rhetorical strategy. In particular, once it is clear that we want to generate a narrative text which is a description, we may choose a narration type and then associate a strategy to the plan creation phase. This could be paraphrased as follows:

Create a sequence of episodes each one based on the strategy of Narratives, alternated with Elaborations; the beginning of the story is constituted by a setting which is built on the basis of Topic-Dominant-Chaining strategy.

Once the Plan has been built, Main Relation predicates are chosen and are passed on to the Semantic Structure creator that assigns suitable arguments and adjuncts to each Main Relation. The following text has been built accordingly:

Text 1.

Sheila is a student and lives in a small town in the south of Italy. She has a lot of friends: they go to the same school. Last week she went to play hockey with her team but she lost. When she got back home she was very sad. Her father cheered her up.

In plan-based text generation, the sequence of possible events is preorganized and constrained; however, this approach fits well into a strongly domain-limited model of generation. We want to assume that in narrative text generation, the overall plan is not prescriptive in the sense that there is no fixed order of discourse units the generator has to follow in order to achieve coherence and cohesion.

In our system, we created a general planning model which could be adapted to specific domain simply by adding domain-dependent plans, which in turn are strictly related to domain-dependent concepts. Knowledge of the world may be easily added, but knowledge required to execute plans is highly articulated and points to three separate modules: discourse structure, conceptual representation, external knowledge of the world or a list of hierarchically organized conceptual relations, the Tbox. Discourse structure has been discussed in detail above, and external knowledge is of no interest to us seen that it simply encodes superset, subset and part_of relations between objects of the lexicon. As to conceptual representation and their relevance we shall discuss them below.

2.1. Plan Creation from Rhetorical Relations and Conceptual Representations

There are two main problems we are faced with when thinking of a random narration/description generator: choice of actual words, and order in which they should occur. In order to select the appropriate lexical predicate, a number of crossing abstract representation should conspire to produce the most adequate result. In particular, we assume that in a plan there are different levels of abstractions involved: the higher level is represented by relations very similar to RST rhetorical relations. These in turn specialize into tuples of semantic relations which are subsequently used to recover predicates from the lexicon. These tuples may be represented by a semantic class and an associated aspectual class, as for instance in:

narrative(movement, activity).
background(existence, state).

In addition, we need some criteria to establish the order with which events may take place in the world: this is not to be intended in the sense of domain discourse plans for task oriented dialogues above. Of course, we use "happens-before" relations listed in VerbOcean and Causality Relations from WordNet discussed in previous chapter. However, we also want to characterize these notions from a theoretical general point of view. The idea we have in mind is based on conceptual classes onto which linking rules may be established so as to disallow unwanted sequences, as for instance in,

LR1: *(GO(TOx ==>GO(TOx)
LR2: *(STAY(ATx ==> STAY(ATx)
LR3: *(BE(ATx ==> BE(ATx)
LR4: *(BE(ATx ==> GO(TOx)

These rules are axioms made up of two sides: the left is a part of a conceptual representation and is the consequent and the right side is the premise; they can be applied at sequences of relations one of which must be the unrealized or yet to be realized relation, represented by the left template. The right side template can be linked to any of the relations already present in the plan. The variable "x" is linked to the object, location or other semantic type for an argument.

Conceptual Representations (hence CptR) have been introduced by Jackendoff and others, however we refer to Dorr(1993) who introduced a number of augmentation to the original set which we also endorse. In our case (Delmonte, 1990), we already considered CptR the link from the semantics to the knowledge of the world needed to represent meaning in a general and uniform manner, as also Pereira and Grosz suggest,

> "...Dorr's analysis, while here applied to a machine translation problem, could also be used in the kinds of interpretation systems discussed in the next section: in fact some of the techniques used in those systems, particularly the one described by Palmer et al., might be profitably seen as rule-based specializations of Dorr's principle-based analysis."(ibid, 8)

Table 2a. Dorr's Semantic Classes And Conceptual Representations

• Class1 - Position
STAYtemp, CAUSE(STAYtemp, STAYloc, CAUSE(STAYloc, BEtemp, BEloc,
• Class 2 - Change of Position and Load/Spray
GOloc, CAUSE(GOloc, LET(GOloc, Gotemp, CAUSE(Gotemp, LET(Gotemp,
• Class 3/4 - Directed Motion and Manner with Motion and Contact/Effect
(Change of Position) + GOposs, CAUSE(GOposs, LET(GOposs,
• Class 5 - Exchange
CAUSE-EXCHANGE,
• Class 6 Physical State and Psychological State
BEident, STAYident, CAUSE(STAYident, LET(STAYident,
• Class 7 - Change of Physical State
GOident, CAUSE(GOident, LET(GOident,
• Class 8 - Orientation
ORIENTloc, CAUSE(ORIENTloc, LET(ORIENTloc,
• Class 9 - Existence
BEexist, CAUSE(BEexist, LET(BEexist, GOexist, CAUSE(GOexist, LET(GOexist, STAYexist, CAUSE(STAYexist, LET(STAYexist,
• Class 10 - Circumstance

Table 2a. Dorr's Semantic Classes And Conceptual Representations (Continued)

BEcirc, GOcirc, CAUSE(GOcirc, LET(GOcirc, STAYcirc, CAUSE(STAYcirc, LET(STAYcirc,
• Class 11 - Range
GO-EXTident, CAUSE(GO-EXTident, LET(GO-EXTident, GO-EXTtemp, CAUSE(GO-EXTtemp, LET(GO-EXTtemp, GO-EXTloc, CAUSE(GO-EXTloc,
• Class 12 Intention
ORIENTcirc, ORIENTtemp
• Class 13 - Ownership
BEposs, STAYposs, CAUSE(STAYposs
• Class 14 - Ingestion
EAT
• Class 16 - Perception and Communication
HEARperc, CAUSE(HEARperc, LET(HEARperc, SEEperc, CAUSE(SEEperc, LET(SEEperc
• Class 17 - Mental Process
BEperc, GOperc
• Class 18 - Cost
ORIENTident, CAUSE(ORIENTident

On the contrary, Dorr following Jackendoff assumes that the primitives building up each CptR should have a direct correspondence to the syntactic structure in order to achieve a mapping from each field of CptR to maximal projections in syntactic surface structures. In Dorr(1993) we find the following classes of primitives(see Appendix C, 363-368):

Since we endorse LFG as our theoretical framework, and our lexical forms encompass semantic information related to semantic roles, we assume that the correct mapping from lexical forms and CptR is achieved by means of semantic roles and aspectual class. In this way, CptRs map onto and outwards Lexical Forms. C-structure and f-structure representation would be completely lost in our framework once the Discourse Model is being built. On the contrary, the Discourse Model only contains reference to semantic roles and other semantic relations like Poss, which have a correspondence in the CptR.

In accordance with the principle of meaning decomposition, we assume that concepts denoted by lexical items are made up of primitive concepts which can be expressed by the use of a very limited number of templates. The granularity of the description depends strictly on the (sub)domain and the aim of the task at hand. For instance, abstract concepts like "responsible" or "responsibility" when dealt with in a legal subdomain require a specification of preconditions which is different from what is expected in a generic domain (see Delmonte, Dibattista).

A method for the decomposition of lexical information should represent a principled way to organize a taxonomy of the concepts in a language, categorized by sets of features, which however are tightly interleaved with argument structure and the syntactic nature of each argument.

Basic constituents for our CptRs are spatial primitives on the basis of analogical relations existing in the spatiotemporal realm which is at the heart of the meaning of all verbs and deverbal nouns and adjectives. According to Jackendoff and Gruber, human beings seem to base their descriptions of any kind of experience on some crucial concepts drawn directly from what might be called the spatial semantic field. Similarly, temporal sequence is both perceived and expressed on the model of spatial sequence. Events and states are located in time - on a timeline - just as things and entities are located in space. The same prepositions are used both for spatial and temporal expressions.

As Dorr's LCS has shown, it is possible to describe the basic conceptual components of meaning of any verb given a finite number of spatial primitives. Our representation varies slightly from hers in that we introduce additional pieces of meaning of two types: lexicalized negation, and modality. Both negation and modalities are treated as operators in CptR and are attached to them. Modalities describe a bit/portion of meaning of a lexical item when decomposed into conceptual primitive functions, and adds to them a certain modality. This is not to be confused with negation, which is itself an operator preceding and having scope over conceptual functions, as implied by the meaning of lexical items.

The content of CptR is as follows (but see Book I to appear):

A. a set of primary functions which are, GO, BE, STAY, CAUSE, LET, ORIENT, IDENT and might all be preceded by negation NOT;
B. a fixed finite number of semantic fields distinguishing common areas of meaning in real knowledge of the world, like INFORM, POSSESS, EVAL, SUBJ, HYPER, PERCPT, MANIP, FACTV, MENT_ACT, PROPR, MEASU, POSIT, COERC, ASK, REACT, TOUCH, HOLD, HOLE, DIR, DIVID, UNIT, LET, etc.
C. a small number of directions indicators, FROM, TO, INTO, AGAINST, AT, TOWARD
D. a small number of secondary functions which are REP, TR
E. a finite set of modality operators with scope on the verb meaning and its complements, which include the following:
   [exist, nonexist, major, minor, violnt, difclt, perf]

Finally, there is a generic evaluative polarity which simply accompanies the concept and encodes the way in which its meaning is perceived in a default manner as having a positive or a negative import: kill, die, destroy are computed as GO(TO[nonexist] X) negative); on the contrary create, be born, heal are computed as GO(TO[esist] X) positive) - they don't appear in this paper. The following is the complete list of the CptRs contained in our lexicon:

As to Aspectual Classes we use them to define lexical classes rather than sentence level aspectual class, which as said above, is the result of the interaction of an extended number of linguistic elements. Lexical aspect is used to individuate the appropriate internal constituency of the event (see Delmonte, 1997 and above), and also to drive the semantics, which together with the information coming from arguments and adjuncts will be able to trigger the adequate knowledge representation. In particular, as shown in Delmonte 1990, but see also Passonneau 1988, we need to process reference to entities and events in the discourse model, in order to know what predicates are asserted to hold over what entities and when.

As discussed at length in Chapter 3, we use the following lexical aspectual classes:

a. achievement
b. achievement irreversible

c. achievement iterable
d. accomplishment
e. accomplishment ingressive
f. activity
g. state
h. state_result

Meaning associated to each semantic class are expanded into conceptual classes by means of aspectual information. For instance, the following class

11 = exten (GO(TO[end] - (GO(TO[exist] finire/end, creare/create is split into the following two meanings:

Funct(exten, achievement irreversible) CAUSE(GO(TO[end] finire "to end"

Funct(exten, accomplishment) CAUSE(GO(TO[exist] creare "to create"

where Funct may assume only those rhetorical or discourse relation labels that constitute a conceptually admissible link. Elaboration or Description are not allowed by Linking Rules. Narration and Egression would be allowed.

Here below are conceptual representations for Main_relations contained in the Frame for student_story:

Table 2b. Semantic classes and conceptual representations

0 = exten	(STAY/GO/IDENTexten(AT/TO	lavorare/work
1 = subj	(STAY!GO/IDENTin_subj_mind(REP	credere/believe
2 = hyper	(ORIENThyper(TOWARD	fingere/pretend
3 = manip	(STAY/GO/IDENTcirc(AT/TO -	minacciare/threaten
4 = factv	(IDENTfactv(REP(TR	sapere/know
5 = eval	(ORIENTeval(TOWARD	piacere/like
6 = propr	(STAY/GO/IDENTpropr(AT/TOWARD	divenire, assomigliare/ become, seem
7 = ment_act	(STAY/GO/IDENTcirc(AT/TO	dimenticare,comprendere/ forget,understand
8 = process	(STAY/GO/IDENTcirc(REP(AT/FROM	continuare/continue
	(GOcirc(TO[exist]/[end] -	finire, interrompere/finish,interrupt
9 = measu_maj	(STAY/GO/IDENTmeas(AT/TO- [major]	crescere/grow
10 = percpt	(STAY/GO/IDENT(REP(AT/TO -	mostrare,esibire/show,exhibit
11 = exten	(GO(TO[end] - (GO(TO[exist]	finire, creare/end,create
12 = perf	(GOcirc[perf]	battezzare/baptize
13 = percpt	(REP(STAY/GO/IDENT(AT/TO -	ascoltare, udire/listen,hear
14 = inform	(STAY/GO/IDENT(REP(AT/TO -	capire,comunicare/understand, communicate
15 = possess	(STAY/GOposs(AT/TO -	dare, vendere, possedere/give,sell,possess
16 = possess	(GOposs(FROM -	comprare, ricevere/buy,receive
17 = inform	(STAY/GO/IDENT(REP(AT/FROM-	domandare,rispondere,sapere/ask,a nswer, know

Table 2b. Semantic classes and conceptual representations (Continued)

18 = measu_min	(STAY/GO/IDENTmeas(AT/TO-	[minor]diminuire/diminuish
19 = posit	(STAY/GOposit(AT/TO	andare, stare/go,stay
20 = react	(STAY/GOreact(AT/TO	resistere, contraddire/resist,contradict
21 = posit	(GOposit(FROM	venire, arrivare/come,arrive
22 = exten	(GO(TO[nonexist]	distruggere, uccidere/destroy,kill
23 = let	(LET(GOcirc	permettere, aiutare/allow,help
24 = coerc	(GOcoerc(TO[exist]	costringere/oblige
25 = ask_poss	(REP(GOinf(FROM	chiedere/ask
26 = at_posit	(STAY(AT	essere – locativo/be-locative
27 = not_exten	(NOT(GOexten(TO[exist]	mancare, escludere/lack,exclude
28 = not_let	(NOT(LET(GOcirc	ostacolare, vietare/hinder,prohibit
29 = dir	(GO(AFTER	seguire, corteggiare/follow, court
30 = touch	(STAY/GOtouch(AT/TO	toccare,accarezzare/touch,caress
31 = divd	(GOsegmnt(TO	separare/separate
32 = hold	(STAY/GOhold(AT/TO	tenere,acchiappare/keep,catch
33 = hole	(GOhole(INTO	perforare, bucare/pierce,hole
34 = dir_d	(GO(AFTER[difclt]	inseguire/chase
35 = unit	(STAY/GOunite(AT/TO	unire/unite
36 = against	(GO(AGAINST	attaccare, assalire/attack,assail
37 = ingest	(GOingest(INTO	ingerire, ingoiare/ingest,swallow
38 = perf	(GOperf(TO	incaricare/charge
39 = contr	(REP(STAY/GO/IDENTcontr(AT/TO	controllare/control
40 = not_react	(NOT(GO/STAYreact(TO -	cedere,subire/give up, undergo
41 = dir_tow	(GO(TOWARD	dirigere, deviare/direct,deviate
42 = over	(GO(OVER	sorpassare, vincere/overrun,win
43 = through	(GOexten(FROM(TO	andare, tradurre/go,translate

andare[CAUSE(<agent>(GOexten(FROM<source_da>(TO<goal_a><theme_in>))){(en,tn),(e1,t1)}]/go
andare[CAUSE(<agent>(GOposit(FROM[x](TO<prop/v_pred_a>))){(en,tn),(e1,t1)}]/go
andare[CAUSE(<causer>(GOposit(FROM[x](TO<locat_[loc_p_set]>))){(en,tn),(e1,t1)}]/go
arrivare[BE(<th_unaff>(STAYposit(AT<locat_a>))){(en,tn),(e1,t1)}]/arrive
giocare[CAUSE(<actor>(STAYexten(AT(WITH<instr_con>))){(e1(t1,t2,t3))}]/play
giocare[CAUSE(<actor>(STAYexten(AT(WITH<comit_con>))){(e1(t1,t2,t3))}]/play
perdere[NOT(LET(<causer>(GO(OVER<th_aff>)))){(e1,t1),(en,tn)}]/lose
studiare[LET(<address>(STAY(REP(AT<informtn>(FROM<source_info_da>))){(e1(t1,t2,t3))}]/study
vincere[LET(<causer>(GO(OVER<th_aff>))){(e1,t1),(en,tn)}]/win

In the knowledge representation we establish a semantic relation that holds between a sentence and an interval in the spirit of interval semantics. We specify what property of an interval is entailed by the input sentence and then compositionally we construct a representation of the event from the intervals and their associated properties. Here below, we report the relevant part of Delmonte 1990 which contains the mapping from CptR to the theorem prover cast in a version of KL-ONE written in C-Prolog. The inferential engine which has inferential rules associated to CptR has been constructed by conjoined work with D.Bianchi at the University of Parma in a thesis work by Sanson(1990). The inferential procedure has a set of basic rules which decompose CptR on more elementary predicates like BE, as follows:

```
a) [CAUSE (X,E) at t1] => [E] cond = +specific(t1)
b) [STAY ([X],[AT Y]) from t1 to t2] => [BE ([X],[AT Y]) at t3] cond = t1<t3<t2
c) [GO([X],[FROM Y],[TO Z]) at t1] => [BE ([X],[AT Y]) at t2] &
                                      [BE ([X]?[AT Z]) at t3] cond = t2<t1<t3
d) [GO ([X],[(AWAY_)FROM Y],[TO(WARD) Z] from t1, to t2] =>
           NOT [STAY ([X],[AT Y])
           from t1, to t2] & NOT [STAY ([X],[AT Z]) from t1, to t2]
e) [STAY ([X],[AT Y] from t1, to t2] =>
           NOT [GO ([X],[(AWAY_)FROM Y],[TO(WARD)W])
           from t3, to t4] cond = t1<t3<t4<t2
```

The reading of these expressions is quite intuitive: in a) if an agent X causes E than E takes place, under the condition that reference time be specific; b) is the subinterval condition which is cast into J.Allen(1983a, 1983b, 1984) formalism for temporal reasoning; c) shows how a motion predicate is translated into a couple of state predicates and so on. Here below are some excerpts from the implementation into KL-ONE in C-Prolog:

```
i.BE(x,state)
   infer(be(Theme,Location,Time,Mode,_,BEx),true):-
      fact(be(Theme,Location,Time,Mode,_,BEx),
      proof(be(Theme,BEx,Time,circumstantial,_,_),true).
ii.GO(x,y,z,t1) =>BE(y,x,t2) cond = t1<t2
   infer(Theme,Location,Time,Mode,_,GOx),true):-
      proof(go(Theme, _,Source,Location,Tx,Mode,GOx),true),
      immediately_precedes(Tx, Time).
iii.GO(x,y,z,t1) =>BE(y,x,t2) cond = t1>t2
   infer(Theme,Location,Time,Mode,_,GOx),true):-
      proof(go(Theme,Location,_,Dest,Tx,Mode,GOx),true),
      immediately_precedes(Time,Tx).
iv.STAY(x,y,t1,t2) => BE(x,y,t3) cond = t1<t3<t2
   infer(be(Theme,Location,Time,Mode,_,STAYx),Value):-
      proof(stay(Theme,Location,Tb,Te,Mode,STAYx),Value),
      precede_eq(Tb,Time),
      precede_eq(Time,Te).
```

This information is coupled to the CptR associated to each main predicate, with variables added for tense. The output of the theorem prover is a truth value associated to a query about the spatiotemporal location of individuals and events in the world: both predicates and individuals may constitute the query. The same could be applied to the state of the world as regards changes that the world undergoes on certain entities affected by the result of predicates of change. In Delmonte(1990) the listing of the theorem prover is shown. The result of the query for two example sentences are shown here below:

A. "John runs home" with sentence index f03 and the input logical form below, containing the feature -specific for tense interpretation:

```
exA:- assert(run(john,nil,home,t3,f03),-specific)/X,
  run(Theme,Source,Destination,Time,position,Symb,X).
And here is the query and the outputs of the theorem prover:
be_at(john,Source/Destination,Time, f03)?
be_at(john,nil,t2,f03)/true
be_at(john,not nil,t2,f03)/false
```

We have used a predicate like "run" which can assume an activity and an accomplishment meaning depending on tense. In our case, tense being present, we end up with an activity, and activities denote intervals with no boundaries at the end. The output to the query confirms the intuition above, where nil for Source indicates the fact that we do not know the place but there must have been some place when he started running but nothing can be asserted of John in relation to his destination, hence not nil. In case we introduce a specific time reference and an accomplishment motion verb, the computation will change abruptly:

B. "John went home" with sentence index f03bis and the input logical form containing the feature +specific for tense interpretation:

```
exA:- assert(go(john,nil,home,t3,f03),+specific)/X,
  run(Theme,Source,Destination,Time,position,Symb,X).
And here again is the query and the outputs of the theorem prover:
be_at(john,Source/Destination,Time, f03bis)?
be_at(john,home,t4, f03bis)/true
be_at(john,nil,t2,f03bis)/true
be_at(john,not home,t4,f03bis)/false
be_at(john,not nil,t2,f03bis)/false
```

2.2. Comparison with Existing Systems

In our system we have not been using any "frame" nor "scenario". But if we want the description to make sense it should obey some common sense set of rules for sequencing relations and properties. Of course this can only be done in closed domains and for short texts. This is usually done by associating a frame-like description to each relation, with preconditions and postconditions. This is described in Webber & Baldwin, following Dale's system called EPICURE, where context changes by event simulation, i.e. by simulating the effects of the events that the text describes(ibid., 97). In order to do this, each object and state has a unique index, with the set of objects available in a given state constituting its woking set. With respect to objects, an action can change a property of the object, it can add an object to or remove it from the world. The preconditions and postconditions of each action indicate the objects required in the working set for its performance and the changes it makes to objects in the working set as a result. The authors assume that the semantics of any individual event description requires specifying the situations prior to and following the event(ibid., 98). In addition the authors make a default assumption that if an action is not known to affect an object and the text does not indicate that the object has been affected, then one assumes it has not been(ibid., 98).

As an example, the authors quote ADD, in the sense of "add X to Y", which has the precondition that X and Y be in the current working set and as postconditions, that X and Y are absent from the resulting working set and a new object Z is present whose constituents are X and Y. EPICURE generates recipes which start from a list of ingredients, followed by instructions as to what to do with them.

One implementation(ibid.,100) of this is represented below for the sentence,

-Mix the flour, butter and water.
mix(e1, {f,w,b},m) & flour(f) & water(w) & butter(b) & definite({f,w,b})
precond: [manipulable({f,w,b})]
delete: [manipulable({f,w,b})]
postcond: [mixture(m) & manipulable(m) & consituentsOf(m,{f,w,b})]

from the underlying abstract representation:

mix(E,X,Y)
precond: [manipulable(X)]
delete: [manipulable(X)]
postcond: [mixture(Y) & manipulable(Y) & constituentsOf(Y,X)]

As the authors comment, the predicate in the header definite(X), is an instruction that unique antecedents need to be found for each member of the set. If definite is absent, as in the case of interpreting "mix some flour, water and butter" then new entities have to be introduced into the working set.

A more general and comprehensive way to do plan-based generation is represented by task-oriented dialogues as for instance in Carberry(1985), Litman(1985), Litman & Allen(1984). Litman herself presents her approach as follows:

> "...a new model for representing and recognizing implicit relationships between utterances. Underlying linguistic relationships are formulated as discourse plans in a plan-based theory of dialogue understanding. This allows the specification and formalization of the relationships within a computational framework, and enables a plan recognition algorithm to provide the link from the processing of actual input to the recognition of underlying discourse plans. Moreover, once a plan recognition system incorporates knowledge of linguistic relationships, it can then use the correlations between linguistic relationships and surface linguistic phenomena to guide its processing."(ibid., 216)

Plans are actually meta-plans, domain-independent and are rather discourse plans in that they are introduced to represent and reason and generalize about discourse relations. Discourse plans represent plan introduction, plan execution, plan specification, plan debugging, plan abandonment, plan-continuing, and so on, independently of any domain.

Following Hovy(1994, 357) every plan has a *name* and/or a *header*, a parameterized action description that names the plan. Action descriptions are represented as operators on a planner's world model and defined in terms of *prerequisites* or *preconditions*, *decompositions*, and *effects*(Litman,216). Every plan has a set of applicability conditions associated with it, called *constraints*. These are similar to prerequisites, except that the planner never attempts to achieve a constraint if it is false: they are already facts in the knowledge base or discourse model that must hold before the plan may be used. Prerequisites are conditions that need to hold (or to be made to hold) in the world model before the action operator can be applied: the planner might ignore them but the hearer may be confused and some repair action should be executed. Effects are statements that are asserted into the world model after the action has been successfully executed: they are goals of the speaker which should affect the hearer's state of knowledge, opinion and goals and are expressed in the hearer's mental state. Decomposition enables hierarchical planning: it is an ordered list of subgoals to be achieved, where there might be flags for optionality which will allow the planner to ignore them. This is an example of plan reported by Hovy(ibid., 358) where discourse relations are intermingled with modal operators that represented the communicative intent and state of knowledge of both speaker and hearer. In order to do this, Hovy comments on the fact that Rhetorical Relations had to be operationalized and reformulated as relation/plan operators which contained semantic preconditions as well as structurer subgoals with suitable effects. Here below is the frame for Extended-Description:

```
Name:              EXTENDED-DESCRIPTION
Header:            Describe(S, H, entity)
Constraints:       Entity?(entity)
Preconditions
Essential:         KNOW-ABOUT(S, entity) &
                   WANT(S, KNOW-ABOUT(H, entity))
Desirable:         ~KNOW-ABOUT(H, entity)
Effects:           KNOW-ABOUT(H, entity)
Decomposition:Define(S, H, entity)
          optional(Detail(S, H, entity))
          optional(Divide(S, H, entity))
          optional((Illustrate(S, H, entity)) OR
                   Give-Analogy(S, H, entity))
```

Finally, we present Hovy's taxonomy of semantic discourse relations reported in 1994, p. 377, which we split into two tables.

Table 3a. Hovy's Taxonomy of SRs

1.ELABORATION
1.ELABOBJEC 2.ELABPART 3.ELABGENERALITY 4.RESTATEMENT
| | | |
OBJECT ATTRIBUTE SET-MEMBER GENL-SPECIFIC
SUMMARY OBJECTFUNCTION PROCESS-STEP ABSTR-INSTANCE
WHOLE-PART
|
1.5 IDENTIFICATION

2.CIRCUMSTANCE
|
TIME MEANS MANNER INSTRUMENT PARALLELEVENT

3.SEQUENCE
|
SEQTEMPORAL SEQSPATIAL SEQORDINAL

4.CAUSE/RESULT
|
C/RVOL C/RNONVOL PURPOSE
| |
VOLCAUSE NONVOLCAUSE
VOLRESULT NONVOLRESULT

5.GENERALCONDITION
|
CONDITION EXCEPTION EQUATIVE

6.COMPARATIVE
|
CONTRAST OTHERWISE COMPARISON ANALOGY

To this list of semantic discourse relations, Hovy adds Interpersonal and Presentational relations.

Table 3b. Hovy's Taxonomy of SRs

7.EVALUATION 8.BACKGROUND 9.ANTITHESIS

10.EXHORTATION
|
SUPPORT CONCESSION QUALIFICATION
|
SOLUTIONHOOD 11.LOGICALRELATIONS
EVIDENCE
JUSTIFICATION
MOTIVATION

Table 3b. Hovy's Taxonomy of SRs (Continued)

12.PRESENTATIONALSEQ	13.JOIN | CONJUNCTION DISJUNCTION

In Litman, actions may be abstract as opposed to primitive: abstract actions are composed of primitive actions and possibly other abstract action descriptions or plans. Here below are frames for three plans, Introduce-Plan, Continue-Plan, Correct-Plan(Litman, 216-217):

HEADER: INTRODUCE-PLAN(speaker, hearer, action, plan)
DECOMPOSITION: REQUEST(speaker, hearer, action)
EFFECTS: WANT(hearer, plan) & NEXT(action, plan)
CONSTRAINTS: STEP(action, plan) & AGENT(action, hearer)

HEADER: CONTINUE-PLAN(speaker, hearer, step, nextstep, plan)
PREREQUISITES: LAST(step, plan) & WANT(hearer, plan)
DECOMPOSITION: REQUEST (speaker, hearer, nextstep)
EFFECT: NEXT(nextstep, plan)
CONSTRAINTS: STEP(step, plan) & STEP(nextstep, plan) & AFTER(step, nextstep, plan)
AGENT(nextstep, hearer) & CANDO(hearer, nextstep)

HEADER: CORRECT-PLAN(speaker, hearer, laststep, newstep, nextstep, plan)
PREREQUISITES: WANT(hearer, plan) & LAST(laststep, plan)
DECOMPOSITION-1: REQUEST (speaker, hearer, newstep)
DECOMPOSITION-2: REQUEST (speaker, hearer, nextstep)
EFFECTS: STEP(newstep, plan) & AFTER(laststep, newstep, plan)&
AFTER(newstep, nextstep, plan) & NEXT(newstep, plan)
CONSTRAINTS: STEP(laststep, plan) & STEP(nextstep, plan) &
AFTER(laststep, nextstep, plan) &
AGENT(newstep, hearer) &
~CANDO(speaker, nextstep) &
MODIFIES(newstep, laststep)&
ENABLES(newstep, nexstep)

Plans are activated by the parsing module which performs syntactic and semantic analysis; then a speech act recognition might be needed in case imperatives are present in a dialogue system. At the beginning, the system tries to introduce a plan: using the corresponding plan schema, the REQUEST of the user "Show me the generic concept called 'employee'" which is analysed as the speech act REQUEST(user, system, D1:DISPLAY (system, user, E1)) where E1 stands for the generic concept, and the process of forward chaining via plan decomposition, the system postulates that the utterance is the result of the decomposition of INTRODUCE-PLAN(user, system, D1, ?plan) where STEP(D1, ?plan) and AGENT(D1, system). The hypothesis is then evaluated using the set of plan heuristics, e.g. the effects of the plan must not already be true and the constraints of every recognized plan must be satisfiable. To satisfy the STEP constraint a plan containing D1 will be created. The second constraints is already satisfied. Finally, since INTRODUCE-PLAN is not a step in any other plan, further chaining stops. Otherwise, an incremental process of heuristic search would be started. The plan recognizer/builder tries to find the plan for which the input is a step, and then tries to find more abstract plans for which the postulated plan is a step, and so on. After every step of this chaining process, a set of heuristics prune the candidate plan set based on assumptions regarding rational planning behaviour. For example, candidates whose effects are already tried are eliminated, since achieving these plans would produce no change in the state of the world(ibid., 218). Chaining stops also whenever the heuristics cannot uniquely determine an underlying plan.

It is interesting to note that the headers introduced so far recall very closely our discourse states. In fact, plan recognition and generation could be modeled either following a domain or a discourse strategy, where in the first case plan continuation is determined by knowledge of the domain, and in the second by more linguistically coherent relations. CONTINUE-PLAN simply continues a previous topic as in our system; CORRECT-PLAN interrupts a topic for a semantically related topic, resembles very close our RETAINING state; INTRODUCE-PLAN interrupts a topic for a totally unrelated topic, thus resembling our CHANGE. Other plan headers are CONSIDER-ASPECT or EXAMINE which correspond to our CONTINUE-ANALYSE, in which a subpart of a set is looked at more closely, very much like an ELABORATION of some kind. On the contrary, whenever new additional information is required ADD-DATA is called. Other plans are strictly related to the domain: MOVE on the screen, PUT data in a location on the screen, DISPLAY data on the screen, MAKE performs some instruction, etc.

3. Mode B: Paraphrasing and Summarising

Paraphrasing a text requires the generator to have access to the semantic representation present in the Discourse Model. Consider now as a simple example the text we used previously to illustrate temporal interpretation:

Text 1.

a. mario ieri corse a casa
b. maria lo aspettava
c. lei lo insultò

where we would like to have a simplified and shortened or paraphrased version, as in:

a. ieri mario corse a casa
b. maria che lo aspettava lo insultò

where sentence c. has been reformulated as an embedded relative clause. There are two types of semantic information derived from text analysis: the Discourse Model itself is the list of all facts and entities as shown below again.

```
entities_of_the_world
entity(ind,id3,18,facts([
fact(infon6, inst_of, [ind:id3, class:uomo], 1, univ, univ),
fact(infon7, name, [mario, id3], 1, univ, univ),
fact(id5, correre, [agente:id3, locativo:id4], 1, tes(f4_ta), id2),
fact(id9, aspettare, [actor:id8, tema_nonaff:id3], 1, tes(f4_tb), id2),
fact(id11, insultare, [agente:id8, tema_aff:id3], 1, tes(f4_td), id2)])),
entity(ind,id8,12,facts([
fact(infon30, inst_of, [ind:id8, class:donna], 1, univ, univ),
fact(infon31, name, [maria, id8], 1, univ, univ),
fact(id9, aspettare, [actor:id8, tema_nonaff:id3], 1, tes(f4_tb), id2),
fact(id11, insultare, [agente:id8, tema_aff:id3], 1, tes(f4_td), id2)])),
entity(ind,id4,2,facts([
fact(infon8, has_prop, [ind:id4, main_sloc:id2], 1, id1, id2),
fact(infon9, isa, [ind:id4, class:casa], 1, id1, id2),
fact(infon10, inst_of, [ind:id4, class:cosa], 1, univ, univ),
fact(id5, correre, [agente:id3, locativo:id4], 1, tes(f4_ta), id2)])),
loc (ind,id7,0,facts([
fact(infon28, main_tloc, _, 1, tes(f4_ta), _)])),
loc(ind,id2,0,facts([
fact(infon4, main_sloc, [arg:casa], 1, _, _)])),
loc(ind,id1,0,facts([
fact(infon3, main_tloc, [arg:ieri], 1, _, _)]))
```

As can be seen, "Entities of the world" contain a list of the entities making up the Discourse Model; each entity or location has the following information (but see Chapter 1.):

Semantic Type: ind, set, class, ent
Semantic Identifier: constant
Score: numeric value
Facts: list of facts taken from the model in the order in which they occur
Fact: one fact is characterized by an infon index or a semantic identifier, a property which can be a relation of a semantic predicate - a verb or a preposition-like linguistic expression -, a list of arguments, a polarity, two indices for spatiotemporal locations. In turn, the list of arguments may be unary, binary or ternary and is a term made up of a semantic role and a semantic identifier.

Discourse Structures are made up of main relation for each clause with its arguments which are characterized by topic hierarchy and all relevant information to define discourse relations and structure, as follows (but see previous two Chapters):

Utterance-Clause Number: two numeric values
Topic List: list of topics of current clause, which includes a topic type, a semantic identifier, a predicate - the one associated to the topic hierarchy

Shortened Infon: a shortened form of the infon associated to the situation described in the current clause, made up by a relation, the arguments, a polarity and a spatial location

Temporal Relation: a logical relation and its temporal arguments

Discourse Relation: a relation name

Discourse Structure: the structure of discourse at that clause made up of the main node and a structure, a list of nodes attached to it.

discourse_structures

ds(3-3, [main:id8:maria, secondary:id3:mario], insultare([id8:maria, id3:mario], 1, id2), after, narration, 2-[3]),

ds(2-2, [main:id3:mario, secondary:id8:maria], aspettare([id8:maria, id3:mario], 1, id2), finished_by, elaboration, 1-[1, 2]),

ds(1-1, [expected:id3:mario], correre([id3:mario, id4:casa], 1, id2), overlap, narration, 1-[1])]).

We assume that in order to summarize some reductive paraphrase should be computed on the input text. At first we hypothesize that the Summarizer simply paraphrases the input sequence trying to reduce the overall number of sentences composing the text itself.

Generating summaries requires the system to choose relevant facts and relevant entities. To this end we set up a procedure to select from the Discourse Model individuals and sets and their associated facts and then to assign them scores according to their relevance in the current text. This is done by keeping trace of their topichood, as well as the semantic role assigned in each relation. Main Topics are scored the highest, then we score Expected Topics, and finally Secondary Topics. As to semantic roles, we use a hierarchy where Agent comes first.

3.1. Planning and Tactical Component

If we want to characterize the input to the Tactical Component we can paraphrase its contribution as follows:

> *Select the most relevant sequence of relations for the most important entity of the discourse model and order them temporally; then establish coordinate or subordinate dependancies among adjacent relations. Finally recover arguments for each relation.*

Having done that, there are two main problems that require particular attention, and they are, choice of cue words and choice of syntactic structure which in turn is cast into another important task, concept aggregation(Hovy, 1994:366). In other words, we have a set of discourse structures that we need to express more concisely: we need to know how (which syntactic structure to use) and what cue word to use. In order to do this, we need to aggregate concepts which are semantically related.

The Focus mechanism allows the Tactical Component to inspect a set of discourse structures to see whether they contain the same focus value; in addition there is a number of additional issues to be taken into account, such as the complexity of the remainder of the discourse substructure, the overall style of the text and its rhythm. In more detail, Hovy suggests a number of heuristics to govern sentence formation, including:

- Embedding of background information can be realized as an adjective, appositive NP, PP or relative clause in this order of preference;
- Sentences should contain at most one level of embedding which should occur before focus transformation, and in the leftmost nuclear clause with the same focus value;
- Coordination occurs only between clauses headed by the adequate rhetorical relation such as JOIN, SEQUENCE, CONTRAST;
- Sentences should contain no more than three clauses.

We will now briefly turn to cue words which are paramount in the task of signalling both inter and intrasentential changes of meaning and semantic relations. We assume as valid the following list which is drawn from Cohen(84):

I. Connective Taxonomy
   1. Parallel
      first, second, secondly, next, then, finally, last, in the first place, for one thing, for a start, to begin with, to conclude, furthermore, moreover, in addition, above all, and what is more, and, neither... nor, either... or, as well as, rather than, as well, too, likewise, similarly, equally, again, also, further
   2. Summary
      altogether, overall, therefore, thus, all in all, in conclusion, in sum, to conclude, to summarize, I will sum by saying, My conclusion is
   3. Reformulation
      namely, in other words, that is to say, alternately
   4. Detail
      for example, for instance, another instance is, in particular
   5. Inference
      that is, accordingly, consequently, hence, as a consequence, as a result, if so, if not, that implies, I deduce from that, You can conclude from that
   6. Contrast
      otherwise, conversely, on the contrary, in contrast, by comparison, however, nonetheless, though, yet, in any case, at any rate, after all, in spite of that, meanwhile, rather than, I would rather say, The alternative is

II. Attitudinal expressions(expressing degrees of belief of the speaker)
   primarily, principally, especially, chiefly, largely, mainly, mostly, notably, actually, certainly, clearly, definitely, indeed, obviously, plainly, really, surely, for certain, for sure, of course, frankly, honestly, literally, simply, kind of, sort of, more or less, mildly, moderately, partially, slightly, somewhat, in part, in some respects, to some extent, scarcely, hardly, barely, a bit, a little, in the least, in the slightest, almost, nearly, virtually, practically, approximately, briefly, broadly, roughly, admittedly, decidedly, doubtless, possibly, reportedly, amazingly, remarkably, naturally, fortunately, tragically, unfortunately, delightfully, annoyingly, thankfully, correctly, justly

III. Empasis(to indicate and defend a claim)
to be sure, it is true, there is little doubt, I admit, it cannot be denied, the truth is, in fact, in actual fact

IV. Transitions(to re-direct a structure)
let us now turn to, speaking of, that reminds me

3.2. Building up the Temporal Sequence

After choosing the first entity in the entity list we activate the procedure for building up the most adequate sequence of events. For each discourse structure starting from the first one, we collect all the information and push it into a stack. Then we go back to discourse structure and collect the second discourse structure. To decide whether the second one is a relevant event we look at the discourse relation: to this end, we divided up discourse relations into two separate sets, background and foreground relations.

fore_discrels([setting, narration, obligation, inception, result, egression, prohibition, cause, adverse, contrast, purpose]).

back_discrels([evidence, motivation, definition, elaboration, parallel, evaluation, description, permission, hypothesis, condition, circumstance]).

In case the current discourse relation belongs to the background set, we reject it and look for the following discourse structure. If a ds has a relevant discourse relation belonging to the foreground set, we simply check whether the temporal logical relation is semantically adequate. Temporal relations are organized into three separate sets:

SET 1
includerel(contains).
includerel(during).
includerel(finished_by).
SET 2
afterrel(after).
SET 3
beforrel(before).
beforrel(started_by).
When an after relation is found the ds is chosen and pushed onto the stack.

3.3. Extracting Relevant Facts from the DM

We are now able to pick up the relevant fact and its semantic structure from Discourse Model. We extract the relation and its arguments from the list of facts associated to the current first entity. In particular we are interested in highlighting the semantic role of the main entity in the current fact. This will be used to decide whether the Voice to be associated to the generating phase has to be set in the Active or in the Passive mode.

3.4. Establishing Coordination and Subordination

At this point we are ready to establish dependancies between two adjacent dss. Complex or compound sentences are originated from the need to establish some commonality between two events: this may take place whenever we refer to the same topic or to the same main relation or to the spatiotemporal location which is lexically expressed for the first time and is a relevant topic.

For instance in Derr, McKeown, Focus or Topic Hierarchy is used to check whether the same focussed entity is present over a stretch of three sentence structures: in that case a complex sentence is built out of the three. The need for content aggregation, however, is not in itself sufficient to ensure the construction of a well-cohesive and coherent text, at paragraph level. On a very simple level, the sequence of clauses building up a paragraph of text may either be coordinated as in a list, or it may be subordinated, either by an explicit semantic marker like a subordinating conjunction or implicitly by relative clauses, gerundives, participials, and other types of modifiers and closed and open adjuncts and complements. The choice between one such type of structure is determined by many factors, some of which are related to stylistic variations, which in turn require knowledge of interpersonal and situational effects.

In Polanyi & Scha, complex discourse constituent units can be divided into four structurally different types (ibid.415):

a. ***sequences***, which construct a dcu out of arbitrarily many constituents (e.g.: lists, narratives);
b. ***expansions***, consisting of a clause and a subordinate unit which expands on it;
c. ***structures formed by a binary operator***, such as A because B, If A then B;
d. ***adjacency structures***, involving speaker change, such as question/answer pairs and exchanges of greetings.

In what follows, the authors discuss a. and b. in more detail. SEQUENCES are decomposed into three different types: ***lists, narratives and topic chaining***.

In LISTS they assume that tense, mood, modality are kept fixed by conjoining the semantics of one clause to that of the second and so on. Clauses in a list are conjoined by "and".

NARRATIVES are defined as "successive event clauses (that) specify what happens at successive timepoints in the world described by the narrative"(ibid.416). In turn NARRATIVES may be subdivided into the following four types:

1. ***specific past time narratives*** (marked by clauses in the simple past, though clauses in the historical present may also occur;
2. ***generic past time narratives*** (marked by the use of "would" and "used to");
3. ***procedural narratives*** (present tense) and ***simultaneous reporting*** (present tense);
4. ***plans*** (use of "will" and "shall"; present tense also occurs).

Events in any type of narratives may either be durative and describe some circumstance or elaboration; it may be non-durative and describe some activity or some accomplishment; it may be resultative and describe some achievement or result-state. It may also be inchoative, continuative, egressive, etc. as may be inferred from lexical specifications included in Chapter 5. Events in a narrative may overlap thus requiring an adequate subordinator like "while", and an adequate mood like "progressive". In order to plan the appropriate semantic structure, time sequencing must be built within the system and appropriate symbolic identifiers must be included for each event type(see Novak, 1985).

Narratives may include flashbacks, which may be defined as embedded discourse units which present events taking place in a period before the reference time of the main narrative. Tense used in this case is pluperfect.

Finally Topic Chaining simply consists of a series of clauses which are centered around the same topic or focus. As shown previously, this can be done by a Topic Hierarchy mechanism that checks for the presence of the same topic in a stretch of discourse.

Going now back to Expansions, the authors indicate two types: Elaborations and Topic-Dominant Chaining. Elaboration is just an expansion in more detail of a main event introduced by a previous clause. Each clause is elaborated on a number of events internal to the main event. On the contrary the Topic-Dominant Chaining, expands on the main topic by introducing some additional information while keeping Main Topic fixed.

The authors give one example of a story, a discourse unit which is typically made up of an entrance, which sets the topic and establishes main relation with the context; it follows a setting phase which introduces the necessary background material before the actual event sequence; then follows the core, a specific past narrative relating a sequence of events(ibid.418). The story is concluded with an explicit exit clause, connecting the story with more general discourse topics.

3.5. Referring Expressions and Topic Hierarchy

When generating a text, each time a nominal expression has to be generated a decision must be taken as to its linguistic form or description. Describing an entity in a given context requires the system to keep under control all previously used linguistic expressions: in particular, assuming that human entities are individuated at best by means of their names, this will be the first description associated to an human entity. However, on second mention, a decision must be taken as to whether using a pronoun or any other property associated to the same entity. The problem is defined in (Dale, 1991) and it is a problem related to the need of finding a description of the entity that distinguishes it from other potential referents with which it might be confused. Clearly this problems also arises in any generation systems in which there is no one-to-one relationship between entities known to the system and the linguistic forms available for describing them. Take for instance the frame reported above where a single main character is associated with any given proper name, and also with a number of main relation roles, like being a student, a hockey player, a daughter and a friend. Each such relation roles requires a specification of the spatiotemporal location and/or as in the case of "daughter" a specification of some other relative or just the family. But clearly a property like "friend" is in itself deprived of any distinguishing feature, and requires in addition, a complete change of perspective.

A text requires change of point of view which alone can make it readable and natural-sounding. On the one side, we need to state constraints that control changes in the Topic Hierarchy and introduce new properties and new entities, as allowed by the domain. On the other side we need principles like Gricean conversational maxims that give directions as regards informational content of each description introduced for a given referring expression.

Strictly speaking, we should also take care that the lexical form introduced follows criteria related to its status as antecedent (see Granville, 1984). In other words, not only the linguistic description associated to a certain entity must be contextually relevant, informative, but also adequate to the task of recovering its referring content. Granville establishes a hierarchy of recoverability for lexical substitutes which ranks in first position the strongest substitute - or the easiest to recover - and runs as follows:

1. The sole referent head last mentioned within an acceptable distance or the focus of the previous sentence, a pronoun;
2. The last referent within an acceptable distance, by a superordinate substitution;
3. An element that filled the same syntactic role in the previous sentence, and was the Subject, a pronoun;
4. A referent that has been previously mentioned, or a referent that is a member of a previously mentioned set within an acceptable distance, by a definite NP.

4. Tactical Component

It is generally agreed that a suitable input to the realization component must be constituted by some form of semantic representation which may include the actual lexical choice or some abstract conceptual representation of each lexical item for the final realization.

However, there are many differences that can be found between the approaches documented in the literature and ours. In our system, input to the realization has a general argument structure and a number of functional features associated that are used by the grammar to generate the most adequate structural configuration. Top-down semantic, rhetoric and pragmatic decisions are paired with bottom-up lexical requirements imposed by each predicate on the fly, while realizing each lexical item. In particular, argument specification only reflects the order each argument has in canonical predicate argument structure. Syntactic non-canonical realizations, like for instance passive construction, expletive subject insertion, left-dislocation and any other possible grammatically relevant structural decision is left to the phrase structure rule component of the grammar. Consider the need to realize one argument as clitic pronoun, as is required in Romance languages: the semantic structure would carry the information that the second argument of the predicate belongs to TOP type, as for instance in the following representation for Mario, which is realized as the clitic pronoun "lo"/him independently by the grammar. The fact that Mario has been assigned the TOP type in the slot reserved for Definiteness does not depend on syntactic but merely on pragmatic and semantic information. Features for the choice of the adequate pronominal form are partially extracted from the lexical entry associated to Mario, which are Person=3, Gender=Masculine, Animacy=Human,

```
[top, nil, sing, mario] --> lo
```

In addition, Number is set to singular, and Case is equal to Accusative owing to the fact that the argument is the second. The additional information that “lo” should be anteposed to the verbal predicate is not encoded in the semantic structure but is independently imposed by phrase structure rules associated to “transitive verb” syntactic class, and the presence of a TOP argument. On the contrary, by interleaving focus rules with the realization grammar, McKeown & Paris(1989) have the undesirable side-effect of having to check where the Focus argument has been assigned in the case frame slots of the sentence level predicate before entering the correct vp rule. In our grammar, we capture passive structures very simply by means of the feature PASSIVE in slot assigned to VOICE in the input semantic structure. The grammar will look for second argument or third argument according to argument structure and execute a Lexical Redundancy Rule, according to LFG: the argument selected will be set to Subject of the current structural realization and realized first. Then second argument will be passed to VP structure as Adjunct Oblique with the semantic role of Agent. Semantic role will trigger the adequate preposition “by” to be instantiated in front of the NP. Choice of focussed constituent is again present in the linear disposition of arguments: in case Recipient/Beneficiary/Goal should be fronted, it would have been positioned as second argument, for ditransitive verbs only, however. In other words, we perform dative shift in the pragmatic/semantic component before entering the realization phase.

4.1. Presenting Other Systems

Before discussing in more detail our realization component, we shall comment upon the realization component of three systems: LILOG, MUMBLE, and SYNPHONICS.

The first system, LILOG uses a unification formalism to generate output sentences. The final module, the Formulator takes as input a semantic-based representation with no grammatical properties available. Some of these properties are derived from the lexicon, seen that the approach chosen is basically a HPSG-like grammar formalism, which is a lexicalized approach very much like LFG. Lexical information for verb predicates includes Auxiliary, Case and Argument Syntactic Constituency, Thematic Roles associated to each Argument, separable particles if any. In general, the grammar formalism does not affect nor direct the computation of output surface representations. Rather than going into too much detail we shall discuss one example included in the book of system performance the author include with passive voice and a relative clause. The example is the sentence “Das Gebauede, das mit einer geschwungene Fassade versehen ist, entstand als...” (Sect.3.3.1)

```
sent(pred(entstehen,past,active),
   thema(np(‘Gebauede’,sg,det_def,
       mod(
        rel_s(patiens(relpro),
           instrument(mit,np(Fassade,sg,det_indef,
                    mod(attr(geschwungen)))),
           pred(versehen,present,z_passive))))),
   pred(np(...
```

It is important to note that semantic role names are used to trigger the appropriate grammatical process. It is then clear that - even though not explained by the authors - the label “relpro” associated to the role name “patiens” is substituted by the appropriate pronoun “das” in force of a procedure that is included in the grammar unification formalism and has the task to pass down to the “mod(rel_s” role morphological features of the head noun governor of the relative pronoun. On the contrary, the decision to associate the “patiens” role to the relative pronoun is taken in the semantics and in particular in the planning phase. Roles are assigned to concepts by the Planner and then are checked in the lexicon by the Realizer which is responsible for the input semantic-based structure to be passed to the Formulator.

In fact, decisions about pronominalization and modifiers are taken by the realizer only when all the plan has been executed and all elements like entities, attributes, events and qualities have been correctly assigned. As the authors comment, the problem of deciding which construction to choose among all possible realizations is a matter of style, rules of sentence complexity, and coherence which have to be treated by a discourse-grammar in the post-planning phase and are currently under construction.

SYNPHONICS approach aims at reaching psycholinguistic insights into the nature of language production processes. The authors discuss two instances of stimuli: one deriving from the planner, and a second instance which they define as “the effect of the constraints of rapid, incremental utterance production: in particular, it causes the Formulator to integrate a thematically underspecified increment in a prominent structural environment”(ibid., 3). In the second case passive sentence formation is a matter of a constraint by the structural representation of the utterance produced and the grammatical properties of both lexicon and grammar rules. The authors build an HPSG-like grammar and lexicon: however, in the treatment of passive construction they follow a GB-style strategy. The first instance which is defined as a case of “agent backgrounding”, sees the Conceptualizer deliver a situation type whose agent role remains unspecified or has as yet not been specified. The choice of the corresponding Lemma linguistic form - whether infinitive (verb-like) or participle(adjectival-like) - is thus determined by the lack of first argument. Rather than activating a lexical redundancy rule of Subject Demotion and Object Promotion, the authors comment that the same result is achieved by tracing the effect to linguistic properties of the passive participle and the passive auxiliary within the GB framework. In particular, the participle is not a proper governor for the theme internal argument which is thus forced to move to subject position leaving an NP-trace behind. This is what they call an ergativization of the verb(ibid.,7).

We comment now on MUMBLE, mainly presented by D.McDonald: in this case differences can be found in the use of what they call realization classes whose content is then carried over to TAG driven syntactic structural choices. TAG formalism itself is different from any other grammatical formalism in that it has an incremental policy in the structure building process which is peculiar to that theory, even though it may be partly traced back to X-bar theory. It is syntactically based and has a link to subcategorization through lexical syntactic classes like transitive, ditransitive, sentential complement, intransitive, light verbs, adjectival small clause and other main lexically driven constructions. Other syntactic constructions are specified, like ergative, passives etc. The problem with generation in TAG is due to the lack of a semantic or functional link from planning to specification phases and syntactic choice.

The structure-building process is started by the individuation of an initial tree which is successively iteratively expanded by means of constraints and the interaction with lexically driven structural types. Each node has a procedure attached to it which leads to the process of phrase structure execution. As a matter of fact our grammar unifies constituents and checks for their grammaticality on the basis of lexical information in a similar way, even though no procedure is actually activated: rather, phrase structure rules have constraints threaded through which allow for the interleaving of lexical and structural information. In addition, Prolog allows for simple matching by means of variable unification. It is not clear to us how constraints are represented in MUMBLE seen that some flexibility is required in order to generate more than one possible output structure for a single conceptual choice. XTAG has a single VP structure corresponding both to a single lexical subcategorization class and to an extended number of structural possibilities for the same verb class already expressed in terms of elementary trees available for adjunction. This means that the same verb class may choose among an extended number of structural types: in other words the choice should be determined by the planner, or better by the "message level" which alone determines choices in the specification language. However these choices are redundant since realization functions specify a class of choices which define the set of initial trees (1987, 212). Now consider the case of deciding when to specify the presence of a gap in adjunct infinitival purpose and rational clauses(1987): as the authors note, decisions about the information an utterance is to convey have to be made before decisions about syntactic form or serial order (ibid.,210). Since information to be conveyed relates to arguments of predicates we only need to specify the way in which a certain argument must be realized. In our model, this is divided up into ten semantic types affecting the way in which a certain head noun will be realized and by selecting its referentiality.

We now comment in much more detail the way in which the problem of lexicalizing the subject of the Purpose Clause(PC) is solved in Huettner, Vaughan & McDonald. Gapping of the subject is optional and not obligatory as in Rational Clauses and is dependent on a number of conditions to be checked in the argument structure of the matrix clause. The example discussed at length in the paper leaves out crucial passages from the message level, to the specification level and finally from the specification level to the realization level. However, the point we want to make regards the realization level which is responsible for the actual calls to syntactic constituency and morphological and lexical realization of the output utterance. In Figure 2 (pag.212) the realization specification created by the schema of the specification language of the message level, where the adjunct with the function purpose-of is declaratively specified; in addition, an adhoc indication that an argument must be present as an obligatory trace is also specified, as follows:

```
: specification adjunct
: attachment-function 'purpose-of)
(locate-argument-&-force-to-a-trace
object :containing-rspec adjunct) ))
```

When the event-bundle related to the adjunct clause is specified, the required information that the PC's subject corresponds to Helga, the matrix subject is spelled out, but there is no indication whatsoever from previous discussion, how this would be realized. Further on in the paper, Figure 6 presents a structural representation of the generation process where the infinitival PC appears with a "for-subject" already assigned to Helga and arguments are morphologically realized as the tree is traversed. The comment of the authors is as follows:

"the optional subject gap of the adjunct is considered: since Helga is available as an explicit argument of the matrix clause, the subject is realized as a trace and the "for" is suppressed"(ibid.,213). The need for such a move was previously presented as a surface-level rule and dubbed: "gap if the subject is mentioned in the matrix or is arbitrary (and non-emphatic)"(ibid.211). Even though the authors comment on the fact that such an implementation is not actually working but is only available on their "stand-alone" interface and the details are all wrought out by hand rather than produced automatically by the system(ibid.212), we are very skeptical on the possibility that such a result could ever be achieved by the system the author presents. Decision on how to realize the morphologically unexpressed subject of infinitival PCs are very hard to get as the authors themselves have to admit(ibid.210). The descriptive analysis best suited for the generation of PC, the one couched in terms of thematic roles is preferred since it allows for a single description of the antecedent of the obligatory gap: but in the actual specification language and in the realization specification there is no indication of thematic roles. In addition, TAG formalism does not consider the possibility of addressing thematic roles as attributes of syntactic nodes. We report here below the algorithm the authors suggest as possible solution to the problem of subject gapping in PCs:

"A possible algorithm for locating gaps in PC would be as follows (assuming that arguments of the matrix verb are still accessible from within the adjunct and are annotated with their thematic roles):

1. Gap the first argument in the PC which is an occurrence of the matrix Theme.

2.a. If the PC subject matches the matrix Goal, gap it; or

b. If there is no matrix Goal and the PC subject matches the matrix Source or Location, gap it; or

c. If there is no matrix Source or Location either, and the PC subject is given as "unspecified", gap it.

While for our purposes such an algorithm is an improvement over a structural description, it is still unnecessarily complicated. For instance, there is no need to search the matrix clause for its theme since we already know trivially which argument to obligatorily gap when generating -- the one that the purpose clause was chosen to express the purpose of."(ibid.210)

We also included the authors' comments which seem to solve the problem in a very simplified and straightforward way: information about the object gapping is specified explicitely in the message level plan. However no information whatsoever is added as to the subject argument of the PC clause which has to be gapped by means of decisions taken after matrix has already been lexically realised. We do not see how this gapping could be realized unless wrought out manually by an adhoc specification. It is funny to see that the authors criticize Derr and McKeown's approach because they lack in generality. However we may comment that McDonald's approach lacks in perspicuity and granularity even though this is what the author assumes to be the most important feature a natural language generation system must have, together with modularity(1989,41).

Tag formalism has been commented by many authors who also use it but in a different manner from the one proposed by MUMBLE. In particular, since TAG does not address the question of which syntactic structure of a given logical form is most appropriate in a certain context, this aspect must be addressed by some other component(see McCoy et al., 48). As we saw, MUMBLE generates from an L-Spec(Linguistic Specification) which captures the content of what is to be generated along with the goals and rhetorical force. This is transformed into an elementary TAG tree by a dictionary-like lookup operation. The translation process allows fine-grained decisions to be made. Syntactic structure is built from the inside out starting from an initial tree - i.e. a minimal non-recursive structure, where an auxiliary tree is the minimal recursive structure - and other initial or auxiliary trees are adjoined or substituted into the initial structure. No tree deletion nor backtracking can be performed: once a TAG tree is chosen to realize the initial fragment, that structure is traversed left to right and grammar routines are run to ensure grammaticality. In addition, wherever new information can be added in the resulting surface structure, L-Spec is consulted to see if it contains any item to be realized at that position. As McCoy et al. note (ibid.,49), L-Spec does not correspond to what is usually regarded a logical form representation, since each piece must be broken down and available for correspondance with TAG requirements, but also referenced to each other logical form piece in the overall structure. The need to generate from elementary tree would break the ties existing between governing predicate and its arguments in case the argument is a proposition or an indirect question as the authors note (ibid.). In other words, there is no principled way to characterize the realization process since syntactic and functional aspects are encoded procedurally into the same instruction - the L-Spec - which is executed blindly by TAG. At the same time, each L-Spec contains more information than just logical form and it is not clear what theory is behind this. Since TAG is syntax-driven, functional information is simply coded into L-Spec and no control is passed over to TAG. The authors introduce a functional systemic input representation to be then passed to TAG for syntactic generation: this allows for a clear and clean separation between the two aspects of sentence generation. In following the description of the system realized we found it too complex, this is perhaps due to the need to keep the two systems, the systemic functional one and the syntactic one based on TAG, separate.

In case of active assertions the surface structure realizer has no problems in building the corresponding structure. However problems arise when a derived structure should be realized, as in passive, interrogative, left dislocated or other non canonical syntactic structure. For instance in (Wendholt, 1990), sentence structure is built by iteratively evaluating each feature of the template structure produced by the planner. The result is a set of terms made up of a governing main predicate and its arguments which are instantiated as roles each one containing its constituency. Semantic roles include typical case labels like theme, instrument, agens, goal, patiens, but also more domain dependent labels such as time, poss, mod, attr, pred, app, coord, dir_app, lokal. Nested semantic labels are mixed up with syntactic labels like np, rel_s, sub_s, inf. Nps have a variable structure according to whether a modifier is present - four arguments - or not, with three arguments defining Head, Number, Definiteness. On the contrary, in McDonald & Pustejovsky(1987), the linguistic component uses the structure of the realization specification it is given, plus the syntactic surface structure of the text in progress which it extends incrementally as the specification is realized, to directly control its actions, interpreting them as though they were sequential computer programs(ibid., 96).

An interesting illustration of generation is offered by Rambow O. and T.Korelsky(1992) in their paper. As the authors comment, there is a certain amount of disagreement about where the line between text and sentence planning has to be drawn. In functionally based systems, the two are mixed up together in the planning phase; on the contrary McKeown shifts sentence planning in the realization phase. We take text planning to mean strictly what the authors also mean, "content selection and organization". This has links with pragmatic aspects like knowledge of the world and knowledge of stylistic requirements related to genre which can be made more or less specific according to goals of generation processes. On the contrary, sentence planning represents the real semantic representation process that mediates between pragmatic needs and surface linguistic realization. This is where referring properties of each NP must be determined; this is also where propositions are combined into complex sentences. It applies both to coordinate and subordinate constructions, and to embedded structures like restrictive or non-restrictive relative clauses, appositives and other adjunct and complement sentential level constructions. Semantic properties of sentence planning processes are determined by discourse level pragmatic factors, which as before are partly stylistic or rhetorical and partly content related, determined by the need to highlight some portion or fragment of the overall generation content, or simply to include it in the current sentence. The sentence planner has a number of strategies to make decisions about sentence structure consistent: for instance, to combine two consecutive Deep-Syntactic Representations(DSyntR), they should either have the same main verb at clause level, or have the same "actants". One strategy is the adjectival attachment strategy that turns a copulative construction which predicates some property of one actant already present in a previous DSyntR.

4.2. One Example

As commented above, input to our Tactical Component is as follows:

Voice: active/passive
Tense: any tense
Mood: any mood including imperative, interrogative etc.
Modality any modality
Main Relation: the main clause relation
Main Relation:Modification Adverbial Phrase
Subordinate Clause
Coordinate Clause
Prepositional Phrase
Predicative Adjunct
List of Arguments:
First Argument: Subject argument - Sentential subject
Second Argument: Object, Oblique, Sentential Object
Third Argument: IndirectObject or Oblique
Argument specifications 1.
Semantic Type: a. prop (proper name),
b. def (definite common noun),
c. ndef (indefinite common noun),
d. foc (focussed noun to be fronted by syntactic structures like left dislocation, it-cleft, topicalization, etc.),

e. top (topic noun - to be pronominalized),
f. rel (relative pronoun argument),
g. trace(controllee of syntactic or lexical controller),
i. pro(empty or lexically unexpressed noun),

Cardinality: a number/nil
Number: sing(ular)/pl(ural)
Head: lexical head

alternatively

Head a concept

Argument specifications 2.

Modification Adjectival Phrase,
Prepositional Phrase,
Predicative Adjuncts

The following constitutes the input to the Tactical Component:

Ex.1: Ieri Mario corse a casa / Yesterday Mario ran home

```
Voice=act,
Tense=past,
Mood=indic,
Modality=assert ,
Main_relation=correre,
Main_relation_modifier=[dtemp,ieri],
List_of_arguments=[First_argument=[prop, nil, sing, mario],
                   Second_argument=[meta, casa]
                   ]
```

Ex.2: Maria che ieri lo cercava lo insultò / Maria who yesterday was looking for him, insulted him

```
Voice=act,
Tense=past,
Mood=indic,
Modality=assert ,
Main_relation=insultare,
List_of_arguments=[
    First_argument=[prop, nil, sing, [maria,
    First_argument_modifier=[
        Voice=act,
        Tense=imperf,
        Mood=indic,
        Main_relation=cercare,
        Main_relation_modifier=[dtemp,ieri],
        List_of_arguments=[First_argument=[rel, nil, sing, maria],
                           Second_argument=[top, nil, sing, mario]
                           ]
     Second_argument=[top, nil, sing, mario]
          ]
```

Chapter 7

LINGUISTICALLY-BASED SEMANTIC EVALUATION FOR TEXT ENTAILMENT

1. INTRODUCTION

This chapter is devoted to inferencing and semantic evaluation. It is tightly linked to the socalled RTE Challenge – Recognizing Textual Entailment – which addresses couple of small texts or snippets extracted semi automatically from the web. They are organized into Text-Hypothesis pairs in which the Hypothesis text must be fully entailed by the Text snippet. Thus it requires deep processing embedded though in a partial/shallow version of GETARUN. The organizers of RTE have taken a special stance with respect to semantic inference evaluation which we quote from Dagan, I., et al., p.1:

" Textual entailment recognition is the task of deciding, given two text fragments, whether the meaning of one text is entailed (can be inferred) from another text. This task captures generically a broad range of inferences that are relevant for multiple applications."

As the authors comment in their introductory paper to the Workshop, semantic inference evaluation is viewed from an applied empirical perspective, with an effort at "recognizing meaning-entailing variability at the lexical and syntactic level" [ibid.:2], rather than addressing logical representational issues. As a matter of fact, we believe that any applied semantic task would have to cope also with semantic and logical issues and not just in an empirical way, seen that the algorithm that each participant had to implement, was intended to work on a very large range of linguistic phenomena. In fact, in order to capture the "many-to-many mapping between language expression and meanings" – as the same authors comment [ibid.:1] – the system for RTE evaluation has to address lexical, syntactic, semantic, logical, and sometimes pragmatic aspects (whenever the intended meaning is not linguistically expressed).

As also mentioned in Zaenen, A. et al., when analysed in more detail, the problem of semantic inference evaluation is more complex: for instance, the "intersectivity" issue, as we call it, or what the authors define as the more specific/less specific semantic relation needs to be encoded appropriately if monotonicity has to be detected from syntactic analysis. In addition, in many if not in most cases, the relevant data are not clear-cut relatable to one or the other aspect of linguistic analysis. Lexical issues are mixed up with semantic, syntactic and logical issues in such a way that the implementation of semantic evaluation needs to address them all at the same time.

Even though we build some Logical Form – in the form of flat fully indexed Dependency structures - which might be used for semantic inference and eventually logical proof, as Bos et al., Harabagiu et al., Raina et al. also do, we abandoned this idea. This decision has been supported by empirical data and also on theoretical grounds. We worked on such hypothesis when we used the KL-ONE version available in Prolog and discussed in the following chapter. In fact, our system can produce a Discourse Model in Situation Semantics terms, which could be used to do reasoning and inferencing: we tried to work on such a hypothesis just to discover that the amount of information made available in the model was insufficient and in many cases it suffered too much from parser brittleness, to guarantee an inferential engine or a theorem prover to work properly. So we turned to a less theoretically demanding system setup and decided to use linear semantically Augmented Head Dependent representations which allowed us to work at a propositional level without sacrificing, however, any of the inferential and logical operations we intended to produce on the T/H pairs. There are also elements of uncertainly in FOL representation usually hard to deal with, which on the contrary play an important role in semantic inference: they may be summarized by the following points, which will be discussed below: Modality, Future Tense, Progressive Mood; Lexicalized Negation; Opaque Second Order Operators (Conditionality); Governing Verbs of Doubt, Verbs of Process, Non-Factives; Temporal Inference; Formulaic Expressions; Non-/Anti-intersective Modifiers.

2. System Description

Our system for semantic evaluation is called VENSES (Venice Semantic Evaluation System) and is organized as a pipeline of two subsystems: the first is a reduced version of GETARUNS, our system for Text Understanding; the second is the semantic evaluator which was previously created for Summary and Question evaluation (see Delmonte, 2003b) and has now been thoroughly revised for the new more comprehensive RTE task.

The reduced GETARUNS is composed of the usual sequence of sub-modules common in Information Extraction systems, i.e. a tokenizer, a multiword and NE recognition module, a PoS tagger based on finite state automata; then a multilayered cascaded RTN-based parser which is equipped with an interpretation module that uses subcategorization information and semantic roles processing. The system has a pronominal binding module (see Delmonte & Bianchi 1991) that works at text/hypothesis level separately for lexical personal, possessive and reflexive pronouns, which are substituted by the heads of their antecedents - if available. The output of the system is a flat list of head-dependent structures (HDS) with Grammatical Relations (GRs) and Semantic Roles (SRs) labels (for similar approaches see Lin D. et al.; Punyakanok et al.). Notable additions to the usual formalism is the presence of a distinguished Negation relation; we also mark modals and progressive mood.

The evaluation system uses a cost model with rewards/penalties for T/H pairs where text entailment is interpreted in terms of semantic similarity: the closer the T/H pairs are in semantic terms the more probable is their entailment. Rewards in terms of scores are assigned for each "similar" semantic element; penalties on the contrary can be expressed in terms of scores or they can determine a local failure and a consequent FALSE decision – more on scoring below. In Figure 4 below is a presentation of the system:

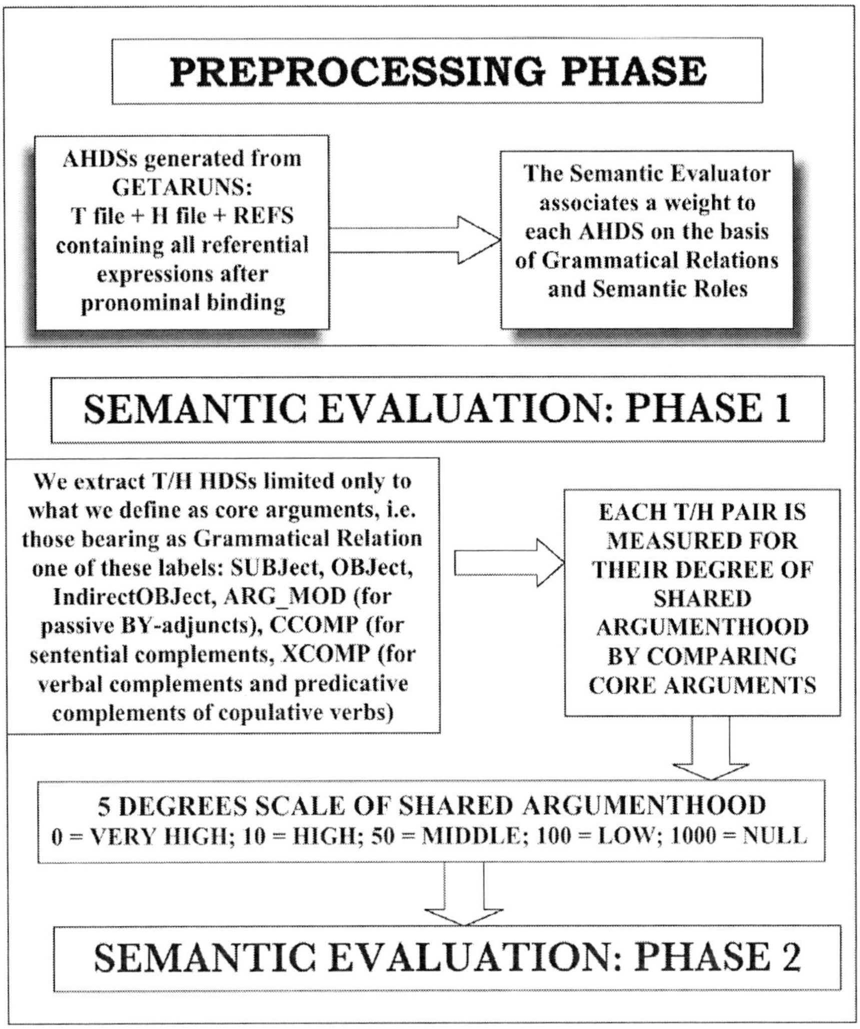

Figure 4. SE Preprocessing and Semantic Evaluation Phase 1.

The evaluation system accesses the output of GETARUNS, i.e. the linguistic representation of the input texts, written on files. It is made up of four main Modules: the first three are a sequence of linguistic rule-based sub-modules; the fourth is a quantitatively based measurement of input structures. The latter is basically a count of heads, dependents, GRs and SRs, scoring only similar elements in the T/H pair. Similarity may range from identical linguistic items, to synonymous or just morphologically derivable. As to GRs and SRs, they are scored higher according to whether they belong to the subset of core relations and roles, i.e. obligatory arguments, or not, that is adjuncts. All modules go through General Consistency checks which are targeted at high level semantic attributes like presence of modality, negation, and opacity operators, the latter ones as expressed either by the presence of discourse markers of conditionality or by a secondary level relation intervening between the main predicate and a governing higher predicate belonging to the class of non factual verbs. Two other general consistency checks regard temporal and spatial location modifiers which must be identical or entailed in one another, if present.

Linguistic rule-based sub-modules are organized into a sequence of rules going from those containing axiomatic-like paraphrase HDSs which are ranked higher, to rules stating conditions for similarity according to the scale of argumentality which are ranked lower. All rules address HDSs, GRs and Srs together with predicates in the form of lemmata or multiwords. All modules strive for True assessments: however, the Quantitative sub-module can output True or False according to general consistency and scoring. Modifying the scoring function may thus vary the final result dramatically: it may contribute more True decisions if relaxed, so it needs fine tuning. More experimentation has been carried out on a much bigger data set – the training data of the MSR made available by Microsoft on their website http://research.microsoft.com/research/nlp/ msr_paraphrase.htm, (see also Dolan et al.) - to achieve a more general definition of this function, and will be discussed below.

The remainder of this paper is organized as follows: in section 2 we present our parser and its performance results. In section 3 we discuss the task of Semantic Inference evaluation, we give a linguistically-based definition of the task and present a set of semantic items heuristically related to T/H pairs taken from the RTE dataset. Also, in the same section we briefly comment on previous work. In section 4 we present the implementation of the Semantic Evaluator(SE). In section 5 we present results and a discussion of most common mistakes made by the SE.

2.1. The Shallow Getaruns

The shallow version of the system uses what can be defined as the Shallow/Robust Processing Hypothesis. The system has now to be positioned in relation to other shallow or partial systems: we will briefly comment on LaSIE the Information Extraction system implemented at Sheffield as has been presented in [25]. In section 2: Background and context, the authors come to the conclusions that IR systems can be ranked up along a line which has at the two extremes, two typologies: on the one side there are systems which produce semantic representations which are fragments of the target template for just those sentences that yield template relevant information, and then merge them using ad hoc heuristics to produce the final template; at the other extreme there are systems that use abductive theorem provers and axiomatizations of the domain to compute the least cost explanation of the first order logic expressions derived from every sentence in the input, and then generate the template from the resulting underlying logical model [25:150]. LaSIE is somewhere in the middle being defined as a system that has an approach to syntactic analysis described as fragmentary parsing: a bottom-up chart parser applying in sequence two simple unification-based grammars (one for proper names, one for phrases) to yield a set of partial parses, from which a 'best' is selected and then semantically interpreted to yield a predicate-argument like representation. Semantic information is subsequently used to extend these partial analyses.

As in LaSIE we use a cascade of finite-state transducers to produce our syntactic analysis. However, as will be commented in detail below, we then go through a grammatical functional labeling of each syntactic constituent before passing the output of constituent analysis to the semantics in order to convert semantically interpretable phrases to canonical predicate-argument forms. As to the higher discourse level processing, the aim of LaSIE is similar to ours, i.e. that of building a single meaning representation for a text called discourse model, from which the information required to fill any IE task specific template may be derived. And we do this by using the semantic information derived from WordNet and other similar knowledge bases, to build up a database of facts represented in terms of situation semantics, as shown in detail in previous sections of this paper. Discourse level information is used to help the module for anaphora resolution do its job properly. The main problems we are facing when comparing the shallow approach to the complete version of the system, are to be referred to difficulties in relating arguments and adjuncts to their governing predicate on the one side; on the semantic side, since no specific domain knowledge has been encoded to do all inferences usually required in the understanding process of any text, some of the meaning relations are simply missing.

2.2. Incremental Shallow-to-Deep Parsing

Shallow or partial parsing produces minimal and incomplete syntactic structures, often in an incremental descriptive schema. In order to repeat some if not all of the features successfully analysed by full GETARUNS, we need to extend shallow parsing to deeper language analysis, while preserving robustness. In order to tackle deeper linguistic aspects we assume the following are essential requisites to fulfil:

- structural information must be extended in order to recover clause-level structure safely;
- lexical information should be tapped in order to help differentiate arguments from adjuncts; i.e. the lexicon should contain full subcategorization frames for most if not all verb, adjective, noun predicates that require them;
- grammatical functions should also be mapped onto the syntactic representation in order to take advantage of fundamental distinctions these descriptions afford: predicative vs. non-predicative functions are distinguished thus allowed a correct semantic mapping to take place.

As in most shallow parsers, we use a sequence or cascade of transducers: however, in our approach, since we intend to recover sentence level structure, the process goes from partial parses to full parses. Sentence and then clause level is crucially responsible for the right assignment of arguments and adjuncts to a governing predicate head. This is clearly paramount in our scheme which aims at recovering predicate-argument structures, besides performing a compositional semantic translation of each semantically headed constituent. The parser is organized into eleven layers as described below:

- Tokenizer produces input sentence which is a list of tokens obtained from the input text by sentence splitting;
- Tokenizer produces input sentence which is a list of tokens obtained from the input text by sentence splitting;

- Tagger associates lexical categories to words from dictionary lookup or from morphological analysis;
- Tag disambiguation with finite-state automata and the aid of lexical information;
- Head-based Chunk building phase;
- Recursive argument/adjunct (A/A) constituent building procedure as a list of syntactic-semantic structures with tentative GFs labels, interspersed with punctuation marks;
- Clause builder that takes as input the A/A vector and tries to split it into separate clauses;
- Recursive clause-level interpretation procedure, that filters displaced or discontinuous constituents;
- Complex sentence organizer which outputs DAG structures;
- Logical Form with syntactic indices and Semantic Roles;
- Transducer from DAGs to AHDSs by recursive calls;
- Pronominal Binding at clause level.

So the first parser receives the input sentence split by previous processors, which is recursively/iteratively turned into a set of non-sentential level syntactic constituents - some of which can incorporate a PP headed by "of". Other operations solved at constituent level are those of collecting under the same constituent structure head level coordinate structures separated by "and/or". Non-sentential level constituents, can be interspersed by heads beginning subordinate clause markers, like subordinating conjunctions, or parentheticals - by punctuation, indirect interrogative clauses - by interrogative pronouns. The final output is a list of headed syntactic constituents which comprise the usual set of semantically translatable constituents, i.e., ADJP, ADVP, NP, PP, VC (Verb Cluster). In addition to that, sentence level markers interspersed in the output are the following:

- FINT, interrogative clause marker;
- DIRSP, direct speech clause marker;
- FP, parenthetical clause marker;
- FC, coordinate clause marker;
- FS, subordinate clause marker;
- F2, relative clause marker.

The task of the following transducer is that of collapsing into the corresponding clause the clause material following the marker up to some delimiting indicator that can be safely taken as not belonging to the current clause level. In particular we assume that at each sentence level only one VCluster can appear: we define the VC as IBAR indicating that there must be a finite or tensed verb included in it. VClusters containing non-tensed verbal elements are all defined separately,

- SV2, for infinitive VCs;
- SV5, for gerundive VCs;
- SV3, for participial VCs.

The second transducer has also two additional tasks: it must take care of ambiguity related to punctuation markers such as COMMA, or DASH, which can either be taken as beginners of a parenthetical or indicators of a list, or simply as separators between main clause and subordinate/coordinate clause. It has also the task of deciding whether conjunctions indicated by FC or by FS are actually starting a clause structure or rather an elliptical structure.

The third pass is intended to produce an improvement on the sentence-level full parse, by transducing each constituent label into a corresponding grammatical function label. The rules are the following, and are taken from the inventory LFG theory and follow its rules and principles. In order to account for the ambiguous labelling of NPs, we use a logical flag associated to IBAR: it is set to false at the beginning of the parser; when the first NP is met and ibar(false) has success, it will be turned into SUBJ. When the IBAR is taken the flag is set to true so that the following NP will be turned into OBJ. We also compute another important feature of IBARs: their passivity. So whenever a passive IBAR is taken, we do not expect a following NP to belong to that clause level, but rather to the following one. Grammatical functional labels are then the following:

- ADJPs are turned into ACOMP;
- ADVPs are turned into ADJ;
- NPs are turned into SUBJ, in case the ibar flag is set to false; and into OBJ in case the ibar flag is set to true;
- PPs are turned into OBL;
- SV2, SV5, SV7, are all turned into VCOMP.
- Some of these functional labels may undergo further changes when subcategorization is looked up in the lexicon: in particular,
- OBJs may become NCOMP;
- OBLs may become PCOMP;
- ADJs may become ADVCOMP.

Finally the fourth pass has the task of splitting complex sentences into simplex ones, or clauses. This may require recovering IBAR and complement structures following a relative clause or a subordinate clause functioning as noun complement, and rejoining it to its subject while preserving control information. This level as the previous ones may lead to failures, which is recovered by simply considering all functions as belonging to the same clause and using IBARs as filters, by means of subcategorization.

The output of the four transducers is passed to the algorithm that takes care of the creation of predicate-argument structures which has the additional task of taking into due account interclausal relations. To do that, semantic indices of governing predicates are used to assert dependencies between two adjacent clauses. This may also apply to a main clause and a clause-like adjunct like a gerundive or a participial.

Our parser has been presented in detail lately in a number of papers (Delmonte, 2002; 2004b) and will also be discussed at length in Book 1 by the same publisher (due to appear late 2007), and has achieved 90% recall on the Greval Corpus and 89% recall on the XEROX-700 corpus, this latter test limited only to SUBJ/OBJ GRs. Sentence and then clause level parsing are crucial to the right assignment of Arguments and Adjuncts (hence A-As) to a governing predicate head. This is paramount in our scheme which aims at recovering predicate-argument structures, besides performing a compositional semantic translation of each semantically headed constituent.

We would like to define our parser "mildly bottom-up" because the structure building process cycles on a subroutine that collects constituents until it decides that what it has parsed might be analysed as Argument or Adjunct. This proceeds until a finite verb is reached and the parse is continued with the additional help of Verb Guidance by subcategorization information. Punctuation marks are also collected during the process and are used to organize the list of arguments and adjuncts into tentative clauses.

The clause builder looks for two elements in the input list: the presence of the verb-complex and punctuation marks, starting from the idea that clauses must contain a finite verb complex: dangling constituents will be adjoined to their left adjacent clause, by the clause interpreter after failure while trying to interpret each clause separately. The clause-level interpretation procedure interprets clauses on the basis of lexical properties of the governing verb: verbless clauses or fragments are dealt with by adding a default BE dummy predicate.

The final processor takes as input fully interpreted clauses which may be coordinate, subordinate, or main clauses. These are adjoined together according to their respective position. Care is taken to account for Reported Speech complex sentences which require the Parenthetical Clause to become Main governing clause. Specialized procedures are used to deal with non-declarative non-canonical structures like Questions, Imperatives, sentences with Reported Direct speech, Clausal Subject sentences and extraposed That-clause fronted sentences (see Delmonte, 2002). Fragments are computed at the end as a default strategy.

2.3. Parsing and Robust Techniques

As far as parsing is concerned, we purport the view that the implementation of a sound parsing algorithm must go hand in hand with sound grammar construction. Extra grammaticalities can be better coped with within a solid linguistic framework rather than without it. Our parser is a rule-based deterministic parser in the sense that it uses lookahead to reduce backtracking. It also implements Finite State Automata in the task of tag disambiguation, and produces multiwords whenever lexical information allows it. In our parser we use a number of parsing strategies and graceful recovery procedures which follow a strictly parameterized approach to their definition and implementation. Recovery procedures are also used to cope with elliptical structures and uncommon orthographic and punctuation patterns.

The grammar is equipped with a lexicon containing a list of fully specified inflected word forms where each entry is followed by its lemma and a list of morphological features, organized in the form of attribute-value pairs. However, morphological analysis for English has also been implemented and used for OutOfVocabulary words. The system uses a core fully specified lexicon, which contains approximately 10,000 most frequent entries of English, where every predicate – be it verb, noun, or adjective – is annotated for Syntactic Category, Aspectual Category, Semantic Category (see Delmonte, 1990 – and also Book 1); then the list of subcategorized arguments follows (if any exist), each argument being specified by Syntactic Constituency, Grammatical Function, Semantic Role and a list of Semantic Features from a set of 75, the same that we used to relabel WordNet . In addition to that, there are all lexical forms provided by a fully revised version of COMLEX. In order to take into account phrasal and adverbial verbal compound forms, we also use lexical entries made available by UPenn and TAG encoding. Their grammatical verbal syntactic codes have then been adapted to our formalism and is used to generate an approximate subcategorization scheme with an approximate aspectual and semantic class associated to it. Semantic inherent features for OOV words, be they nouns, verbs, adjectives or adverbs, are provided by a fully revised version of WordNet – 270,000 lexical entries - in which we used 75 semantic classes similar to those provided by CoreLex. These are all consulted at runtime. We use these features to induce semantic similarity for two entities whenever at least 2 identical features are matched in their feature list.

Another important element of analysis is constituted by Semantic Roles: we have reformatted all publicly available inventories, such as FrameNet, VerbNet and PropBank, and use them in that order, seen that FrameNet has more specific labels than the other two lexica. However, we also produced our own fully specified lexicon which is accessed before VerbNet.

Our training corpus for the complete system is made up 200,000 words and is organized by a number of texts taken from different genres, portions of the UPenn WSJ corpus, test-suits for grammatical relations, narrative texts, and sentences taken from COMLEX manual.

We don't have space here to describe the Pronominal Binding module which accesses Referential Heads at clause level and establishes possible antecedent-pronoun candidate lists which are then weighted and the best one chosen (but see Delmonte & Bianchi, 1991). As for the 1367 T/H pairs of the RTE Challenge, the parser has spotted 85 pronominal expressions which have received an antecedent: we checked the bindings and the result is 82% accuracy.

As an example of an ADHS we report here below Snippets 78 (All examples are from the corpus released for the RTE Challenge available at: http://www.pascal-network.org/Challenges/RTE, and have the same identifier):

T. Clinton's new book is not big seller here.
H. Clinton's book is a big seller.

Whose structure is computed respectively as follows:

```
T.
be(adj-locative, here).
seller(ncmod, big).
book(ncmod-specif, 'Clinton-s_').
be(xcomp-prop, seller).
be(subj-theme_bound, book).
be(neg, not).
H.
seller(ncmod, big).
book(ncmod-specif, 'Clinton-s_').
be(xcomp-prop, seller).
be(subj-theme_bound, book).
```

The presence of the negation operator in the T portion of the snippet will prevent the evaluator from assessing to TRUE even though the relevant HD structures are identical.

3. The Task of Semantic Inference Evaluation

Even though at the bottom of any computation, semantic evaluation - in any case of non equality of the linguistic descriptions involved - needs lexical chains of some kind to be produced or attempted, we consider it less relevant than an appropriate setup for semantic inference. Here below we assess the contribution of a number of different linguistic scenarios – which will be further commented below – that we tried to set apart as can be derived from our SE. In Table 1. we can see their productivity in terms of number of T/H pairs inferred as TRUE, disregarding for the moment the fact that some of these might be false positives.

Table 4. Ratio of TRUE classified snippets by Rule type accessed by the SE

Rule Type / Datasets	Test set	Training set	Test + Train
Quantitative evaluation	66 20.5%	52 21.7%	118 21%
Paraphrase evaluation	31 9.62%	23 9.58%	54 9.61%
Syntactic + Semantic eval.	128 39.7%	99 41.2%	227 40.39%
Lexical chains evaluation	75 23.3%	51 21.2%	126 22.42%
Hybrid for short snippets	22 6.8%	15 6.2%	37 6.58%
total no. snippets	322 100%	240 100%	562 100%

All rule types will be commented in detail below. What we wanted to highlight at this point, is the minimal impact of the Rule set used for Paraphrase evaluation, where we actually use the lemmas to be matched together in axiomatic-like structures: in other words, it is only in these cases that the actual linguistic expressions play a determining role in the task to derive a semantic inference. The number of axioms we built on the basis of Development and Test sets is 47: considering the number of T/H pairs evaluated to True, the mapping is almost one rule to each pair. On the contrary, the great majority of rules applied by the SE come from the combination of Syntactic and Semantic Inference, where Lexical Inference also plays a role.

We also want to point out that our system produced antecedents for pronominal expressions at snippet level, however we haven't been able to find many examples in which such information would have been useful to the RTE task – they are all discussed below. We are not here referring to all those cases defined as Control in LFG theory, where basically the unexpressed subject of an untensed proposition (infinitival, participial, gerundive) either lexically, syntactically or structurally controlled is bound to some argument of the governing predicate.

We have also been working on the MSR training dataset, made available by Microsoft, which has 4076 T/H pairs. We noticed however that it has a major flaw: the annotators judged True pairs in which anaphoric binding applied between T and H. Under the entailment perspective, we think this impossible and a bad mistake, considering the fact that snippets are just small portions of text taken randomly and not in the appropriate context – same text, sequentially with the antecedent preceding the pronoun – to allow such an inference. However, under the "Paraphrase" perspective, i.e. under the additional constraints that the two snippets are taken from a cluster with the same content, it is certainly correct: there are some 250 such cases. Results obtained by our system – which we will not report in this paper - are close to the ones obtained under RTE (accuracy is 59.46%), with the proviso however that the proportion of FALSE to TRUE pairs was 1/3, and accuracy for TRUE is 63%.

3.1. Defining the task of the Semantic Evaluator (SE)

As the examples discussed here below will make clear, the task of the SE is in no way definable on a purely theoretical semantic basis (but see Zaenen et al.). One such particularly revealing case is the one constituted by the socalled (Non/Anti)-Intersective modifiers dealt with in current semantic and linguistic literature. It is a fact that presence of an intersective attribute in the Text and its omission in the Hypothesis hampers the entailment in theoretical terms, but not always in the application-oriented scenario of RTE. A typical case is shown in the following examples,

i. John bought a red car.
ii. John bought a car.
   where example i. is more informative than example ii. due to the presence of the adjective "red". In addition, "car" and "red" can be interpreted compositionally so that ii. is entailed by i. Consider the next pairs:
iii. John was presented to an alleged great Italian scientist.
iv. John was presented to a great Italian scientist.
v. John was presented to a great scientist.
vi. John was presented to a scientist.

In iii. we inserted a "non-intersective" adjective "alleged", which causes the referential expression headed by "scientist" to become non extensional - the same applies to "anti-intersective" modifiers like "fake". In this case the two sentences cannot be interpreted compositionally and are not entailed; also sentence v. is not entailed in iv. in our context, by virtue of the presence of a geographical/intersective modifier in iv.; on the contrary vi. is entailed in v. "great" being a subjective modifier, but theoretically it belongs to "relative intersective" class which is not compositional.

To cope with similar problems, all modifiers that imply non-entailment have been listed separately and constitute a checklist against which modifier heads are checked when attempting to assess the entailment of two snippets.

3.1.1. Lexical Inference for Reasoning and Paraphrase

Differently from what happened in the RTE Challenge 1, the 2nd year's Challenge was characterized by the presence of T/H pairs which require two particularly hard NLP processes to set up:

- reasoning
- paraphrases (reformulation)

Setting up rules for Paraphrase evaluation, requires the system to actually use the lemmas to be matched together in axiomatic-like structures: in other words, in these cases the actual linguistic expressions play a determining role in the task to derive a semantic inference. The number of axioms we found in the Development and Test sets constitutes almost one third of all T/H pairs. And of course, in order for these rules to be applied by the SE it is important to be able to address a combination of Syntactic and Semantic Inference, where Lexical Inference also plays a role. We will present here below examples taken from the Test Dataset of RTE2. In the entailed example 58 below, "be sentenced to life in prison" should match with IMPRISON the governing predicate of the Hypothesis:

T/H pair n. 58
T: Across the Atlantic, on July 13, a radical Islamic cleric named Ali Al-Timimi was sentenced to life in prison, in Virginia, for soliciting treason.
H: Ali Al-Timimi is imprisoned in Virginia.

Now consider the following entailed pair, 468, where KILL, the governing predicate of the Hypothesis, should match with the nominal expression "the death toll"

T/H pair n. 468
T: The death toll of a fire that roared through a packed Buenos Aires nightclub climbed on Friday to at least 175, with more than 700 injured as young revellers stampeded to reach locked exit doors.
H: At least 174 had been killed and more than 410 people injured.
In the example below, n.266, reasoning is required by the need to match "associated with decreased risk" in the T snipped, with PROTECT in the H snipped:

T/H pair n. 266
T: Green tea consumption is associated with decreased risk of breast, pancreatic, colon, oesophageal, and lung cancers in humans.
H: Tea protects from some diseases.

Reasoning again is required in the following pair, where some numerical computation has to be performed on the T snippet in order to match it with the H snippet:

T/H pair n. 389
T: In Rwanda there were on average 8,000 victims per day for about 100 days.
H: There were 800,000 victims of the massacres in Rwanda.

Now consider the following pair, n.48, where none of the words and lemmata contained in the Hypothesis matches directly with those of the Text. In this case, both the SUBJect of the Hypothesis "Shipwreck savaging" and the predicate ATTEMPT have to be fully derived from a reasoning process:

T/H pair n. 48

T: Hundreds of divers and treasure hunters, including the Duke of Argyll, have risked their lives in the dangerous waters of the Isle of Mull trying to discover the reputed 30,000,000 pounds in Gold carried by this vessel--the target of the most enduring treasure hunt in British history.

H: Shipwreck salvaging was attempted.

Three examples now which are not entailed. The first one is based on non intersectivity:

T/H pair n. 260

T: These folk art traditions have been preserved for hundreds of years.

H: Indigenous folk art is preserved.

The presence of "indigenous" in the H snippet is computed as a case of additional information which is not contained in the T sentence: thus entailment does not hold.

In the example below, 403, the entailment is falsified by the presence in the T snippet of a nominal governing predicate: HAVE POTENTIAL which dummifies the presence of such predicates as DESTROY and DAMAGE, possible synonyms for HOLE in the H snippet:

T/H pair n. 403

T: In the mid-1970s, scientists first noticed that chlorine produced in the atmosphere from human-made CFCs and similar chemicals had the potential to destroy ozone and damage the ozone layer.

H: The ozone hole was first noticed in the mid-1970s.

In the following example, the system has to suspend lexical semantic inferencing and to privilege the propositional semantic role of a nominal governor, the word "failure". This is due to the presence of a factive nominal governor, which has to be computed for its semantic import, that of introducing a negative mark for its governed predicate. In other words, FAILURE of the INVASION implies that the invasion did not TAKE_PLACE as the H states.

T/H pair n. 552

T: The failure of the Bay of Pigs invasion in 1961 seriously embarrassed the Kennedy administration.

H: The Bay of Pigs invasion took place in 1961.

T.

embarrass(cl1, adj-mod, seriously-sn7).
kennedy_administration(sn3, det, the).
failure(sn1, ncmod-specif, of, invasion-sn5).
invasion(sn5, ncmod-specif, pigs).
failure(sn1, ncmod-specif, of, bay-sn4).
bay(sn4, det, the).
failure(sn1, det, the).
embarrass(cl1, obj-theme, kennedy_administration-sn3).
embarrass(cl1, ncmod-theme, in, 1961-sn2).

embarrass(cl1, subj-agent, failure-sn1).
H.
bay(sn1, det, the).
take_place(cl2, ncmod-theme, in, 1961-sn3).
take_place(cl2, subj-agent, invasion-sn2).
take_place(cl2, subj-agent, bay-sn1).

RTE LINGUISTIC RULE – Definition 1

A linguistically based approximation to a sound definition of the task at hand may be represented by the Rule below:

Two text fragments approximate the same meaning - are semantically equivalent - whenever they are:

a. linguistically coherent
b. semantically consistent
c. propositionally compatible

In order to make the definition above more concrete, we created a set of Syntactic-Semantic Classes, both theoretically and empirically derived from the RTE examples dataset. They are divided up into two subsets because the actions carried out by our Semantic Evaluator address conditions necessary for True T/H pairs separately from those for False T/H pairs. We would like to comment extensively each semantic item with an example from RTE dataset: however this would make the paper too lengthy. So we decided to limit our analysis to an abbreviated comment of relevant linguistic elements (see also Zaenen et al.). All snippets are individuated by their original number and the texts are included in an Appendix at the end of the paper. All these cases are positively dealt with by our SE.

3.1.1.1. Syntactic-Semantic Classes for Linguistic Coherence

i. Conditions for TRUE
Same Main Heads; Same Main Dependents; Identity of GRs; Identity of SRs; Morphologically derived Heads

ii. Examples
Snippets 238 TRUE (Same SUBJect, Assassination/Assassinate, Same Temporal Adjunct)
T/H pair 238
Following the assassination attempt in 1981, Reagan said he felt God had spared him for a purpose, and he intended to devote the rest of his life in dedication to his God and to that purpose.
Regan was almost assassinated in 1981.

Snippets 693 TRUE (Invasion/Invade, Swedish/Swedes, Entailed Temporal Adjunct)
T/H pair 693

This growth proved short-lived, for a Swedish invasion (1655-56) devastated the flourishing city of Warsaw.
Warsaw was invaded by the Swedes in 1655, and the city was devastated.

Snippets 947 TRUE (murder/kill, police commander/police officer)
T/H pair 947
The extraditables today claimed responsibility for the murder of Antioquia police commander colonel Waldemar Franklin Quintero, which occurred this morning in Medellin.
police officer killed.

ii. Conditions for FALSE
Opposite GRs/SRs; Non-identical GRs/SRs; Argument/Adjunct Swap; Missing Argument; Missing Main Predicate; Modifier/Attribute Swap

ii. Examples
Snippets 152 FALSE (Same SUBJect swapped, same verb predicate)
T/H pair 152
Twenty-five of the dead were members of the law enforcement agencies and the rest of the 67 were civilians.
25 of the dead were civilians.

Snippets 602 FALSE (Same verb predicate, same Patient SUBJect/OBJect, missing omitted Agent/SUBJect)
T/H pair 602
Historians estimate that 800,000 Chechens were stuffed into rail cars and deported to Kazakhstan and Siberia, and 240,000 of them died en route.
Stalin deported 800,000 Chechens.

3.1.1.2. Syntactic-Semantic Classes for Semantic Consistency

i. Conditions for TRUE
Synonyms with adequate GRs / SRs; Entailment of Main Predicates with adequate GRs/SRs; Definitional Paraphrase; Formulaic Expressions; Pronominal Binding

i. Examples
Snippets 466 TRUE (Same SUBJect, presence of formulaic expression "would like to acknowledge and thank"/recognize, same OBJect)
T/H pair 466
The Yellowstone Park Foundation recognizes the following organizations for their generous support in helping to protect the wonders and wildlife of Yellowstone National Park.
The Yellowstone Park Foundation would like to acknowledge and thank the following organizations for their generous support.

Snippets 496 TRUE (Same SUBJect, Same main predicate BE, paraphrase indirectly

derivable from definitions in WordNet)
T/H pair 496
Like Jews and Christians, Muslims believe there is only one God.
Muslims are monotheistic.

Snippets 648 TRUE (Same SUBJect, appositive nominal head “widow” in text entails “wife” in hypothesis)
T/H pair 648
Yoko Ono, widow of murdered Beatles star John Lennon, has plastered the small German town of Langenhagen with backsides.
Yoko Ono was John Lennon's wife.

Snippets 783 TRUE (Same SUBJect, “fire” predicate/”send letter dismissal” complex predicate, same OBJect/ToOBJect)
T/H pair 783
Sharon sent dismissal letters to Benny Elon and Avigdor Lieberman, who oppose his withdrawal plan, on Friday.
On Friday,Sharon fired Benny Elon and Avigdor Lieberman.

Snippets 876 TRUE (Same SUBJect, Kill and Die are treated as antonyms but they also share a part of same meaning – Die is implied in the action of Kill, the SUBJects have different SRs, same temporal location)
T/H pair 876
Officials said Michael Hamilton was killed when gunmen opened fire and exchanged shots with Saudi security forces yesterday
Michael Hamilton died yesterday.

Snippets 912 TRUE (Same/entailed SUBJect, “hurl obscenity” complex predicate/”curse” predicate, same IndirectOBJect)
T/H pair 912
Vice President Dick Cheney on Tuesday hurled an obscenity on the Senate floor to punctuate an angry exchange with Vermont Sen. Patrick Leahy as all senators gathered for their annual photo.
Cheney cursed at Sen. Patrick Leahy.

Snippet 933 TRUE (Same SUBJect, Synonym Main Predicate: same GRs with same SRs)
T/H pair 933
Crude Oil Prices Slump.
Oil prices drop.

Snippets 1121 TRUE (Pronominal SUBJect “it” bound as controller for Relevant Verb Predicate BUY/ACQUIRE, same OBJect) *see also Snippets 74*; *Snippets 201 below.*
T/H pair 1121
Continuing its buying spree, IBM said Wednesday that it plans to acquire Alphablox, a Mountain View, Calif.-based analytics software company.
IBM plans to buy Alphablox.

Snippets 1639 TRUE (Synonym Main Predicate more/less specific, same SUBJect-OBJect arguments with different GRs vs same SRs)
T/H pair 1639
Lennon was murdered by Mark David Chapman outside the Dakota on Dec. 8, 1980.
Mark David Chapman killed Lennon.

ii. Conditions for FALSE
Antonymity; Non-coincidence of Referential Attributes; Propositional/Full Paraphrase; Opposite Entailment (Non)-Intersective Modifiers; Inexistent Relevant Semantic Relations

ii. Examples
Snippets 12 FALSE (Same SUBJect, opposite meaning of governed verb keep_from/release, lexical inference for OBJect form/document)
T/H pair 12
Oracle had fought to keep the forms from being released.
Oracle released a confidential document.

Snippets 46 FALSE (PP adjunct nominal head morphologically derived/main verb Hypothesis – loss/lose, reverted GRs-SRs)
T/H pair 46
The Yankees split Hollywood with something to feel OK about after last night's 5-4 loss to the Dodgers.
Dodgers lose first game ever at Fenway.

Snippets 67 FALSE (Same SUBJect, opposite meaning of main verb come_down/rise)
T/H pair 67
Total coal stocks with the thermal power stations came down to 9.6 million tonnes on March 3, 2003 from 11 million tonnes on October 1, 2002.
Coal stocks rise.

Snippets 148 FALSE (Same SUBJect, opposite meaning of main verb rise/drop)
T/H pair 148
The Philippine Stock Exchange Composite Index rose 0.1 percent to 1573.65.
The Philippine Stock Exchange Composite Index dropped.

Snippets 220 FALSE (Same main phrasal verb predicate – begin legal action, reverted GRs/SRs)
T/H pair 220
Canadian wireless technology licensing company Wi-LAN has begun legal action against Cisco, alleging the networking giant's Linksys and Aironet products are making use of its intellectual property without permission.
Linksys and Aironet begin legal action against a Canadian company.

Snippets 2049 FALSE (Same SUBJect, same verb complement, non synonym, non entailed main verb predicate – order/demand – non identical SRs)

T/H pair 2049
Five other soldiers have been ordered to face courts-martial.
Five other soldiers have been demanded to face courts-martial.

Snippets 2064 FALSE (Same clause, Intersective modifier in Text – Western, geographical adjective/omitted non entailed modifier due to superlative relation)
T/H pair 2064
The Osaka World Trade Center is the tallest building in Western Japan.
The Osaka World Trade Center is the tallest building in Japan.

Snippets 2084 FALSE (Same clause, Different non entailed nominal predicate – "Israel" predicate nominal postmodifier)
T/H pair 2084
Microsoft Israel was founded in 1989 and became one of the first Microsoft branches outside the USA.
Microsoft was established in 1989.

Snippets 2120 FALSE (SUBJect non entailed – less specific, different cardinality, spatial location specified for main verb FREE in Text not it Hypothesis)
T/H pair 2120
Six hostages in Iraq were freed.
The four Jordanian hostages, kidnapped about a week ago, were freed.

Snippets 2141 FALSE (SUBJect negated in Text, main verb negated in Text)
T/H pair 2141
No Weapons of Mass Destruction Found in Iraq Yet.
Weapons of Mass Destruction Found in Iraq.

Inexistent Relevant Semantic Relations: *Snippets 619* FALSE; *Snippets 6120* FALSE; *Snippets 700* FALSE; *Snippets 677* FALSE*; Snippets 712* FALSE
T/H pair 619
Fiat's Gianni Agnelli, owner of Juventus, was quoted by Italian newspapers as saying that when Baggio came off the field after the Mexico game, "He looked like a wet rabbit".
Giovanni Agnelli is the president of Fiat.
T/H pair 620
PERSPECTIVE ON BOSNIA; A BALKANS PEACE THAT CANNOT LAST.
Bosnia is located in the former Yugoslavia.
T/H pair 677
The Dutch, who ruled Indonesia until 1949, called the city of Jakarta Batavia.
Formerly (until 1949) Batavia, Jakarta is largest city and capital of Indonesia.
T/H pair 700
There are many Baroque churches of the Counter-Reformation period, including the Jesuit Church next to the cathedral and the Church of the Holy Cross, which contains Chopin's heart.
Sigismund made Warsaw the capital of Poland in 1611.

T/H pair 712
To the south of Castle Hill rises the higher Gellert Hill (771 feet), a steep limestone escarpment overlooking the Danube, which provides a panoramic view of the whole city.
To the south is Gellert Hill, which features the 19th-century Citadel.

3.1.1.3. Syntactic-Semantic Classes for Propositional Compatibility

i. Conditions for TRUE
Modality, Future Tense, Progressive Mood; Negation, Lexicalized Negation; Light Verbs (Copulative, SpatioTemporal locating, etc.); Governing Verbs of Doubt; Governing Verbs of Process; Opaque Second Order Operators; Factuality and Counterfactuality; Temporal Inference & Operators
ii. Examples
Snippets 74 TRUE (Same SUBJect – by virtue of pronominal binding, his/foreign ministry; and lexical inference country/South Korea -, continue/Negated Modal Verb won't + change governing main verbal head SEND)
T/H pair 74
South Korea's deputy foreign minister says his country won't change its plan to send three-thousand soldiers to Iraq, despite the kidnapping of a South Korean man there.
South Korea continues to send troops.

Snippets 172 TRUE (Same SUBJect, verbal head Suspect governing light verb BE/Modal May governing Cause, Same OBJects – More/Less Specific)
T/H pair 172
The terrorist is suspected of being behind several deadly kidnappings and dozens of suicide attacks in Iraq.
The terrorist may have caused suicide attacks and kidnappings.

Snippets 294 TRUE (Same SUBJect,Take_place/Last, three-day/three day)
T/H pair 294
The three-day G8 summit will take place in Scotland.
The G8 summit will last three days.
Snippets 1014 TRUE (Same SUBJect, More/less specific Heads, Lexicalized Negation Paraphrase Verb+It+Predicate Adjective /Modal Verb + negation)
T/H pair 1014
The thick atmosphere of Titan makes it difficult for even the largest telescopes on Earth to see anything clearly.
Telescopes on Earth cannot see Titan clearly.

Snippets 1164 TRUE (Same SUBJect, Tell/Lexically inferred verbal head Announce, Negated morphologically derived Noun OBJect Cooperation/Negated main verbal head)
T/H pair 1164
Ramadan told reporters at the opening ceremony of the Baghdad International Exposition, "No cooperation and no inspection or monitoring by the American

Zionist espionage commission (the Special Commission for disarming Iraq's banned weapons - UNSCOM) before Iraq's demands are met.".
Ramadan announced that Iraq will not cooperate with the inspectors.

Snippets 1168 TRUE (Same SUBJect, lexically inferrable main predicate tell/say, Negated Modal verb cannot + Operator unless, Same governing verb LIFT, Synonymous OBJect noun heads blockade/embargo)
T/H pair 1168
Ramadan told reporters in Baghdad that "Iraq cannot deal positively with whoever represents the Security Council, unless there was a clear stance on the issue of lifting the blockade.
Ramadan said that Iraq would cooperate when the UN considers lifting the embargo.

Snippets 1197 TRUE (Similar Adjunct with synonymous main verb Focus/Concentrate, main IndirectOBJect noun head matched to Adverbial Modifier + main verb, Future Tense / Modal Verb)
T/H pair 1197
Contact with the press will be restricted to "perodic meetings", as promised by all three parties, in order to "focus their energies" on the most important issues.
The delegations may only speak periodically to the press, in order to concentrate on the issues.

Snippets 1214 TRUE (Same SUBJect, Same main verb Head, Temporal Inference and Modal Verbs (will + by the end of year 2001/should + before 2002)
T/H pair 1214
It is planned that by the end of the year 2001, France will have minted 7.6 billion Euro coins weighing 30 thousand tons or approximately four times the equivalent weight of the Eiffel Tower.
According to plans, France should have minted 7.6 billion Euro coins before 2002 .

Snippets 1261 TRUE (Operators but-until + negation on main verb/if, Light verb HOLD/propose, Nominal head AGREEMENT morphologically derived from verbal head AGREE)
T/H pair 1261
Zeroual proposed February 25 as elections date, but this date will not become final until after the agreement between all of the political partners, according to what was reported by the First Secretary of the Socialist Forces Front, Ahmed Djeddai.
The election will be held on the 25th of February if all of the political partners agree.

Snippets 1265 TRUE (Same SUBJect, main verbal head Prepare is synonymous with Make in hypothesis, Progressive Mood / Future Tense)
T/H pair 1265
Egyptian television is preparing to film a series that highlights the unity and cohesion of Moslems and Copts as the single fabric of the Egyptian society, exemplifying in particular the story of former United Nations Secretary-General Boutros Ghali.
Egyptian television will make a series about Moslems, Copts and Boutros Boutros Ghali.

Snippets 1284 TRUE (Lexical Transformation noun Reduction/verb Reduce in Hypothesis; verb Reduce negated in Text but governed by Expect)

T/H pair 1284

Economic experts were surprised by this coordinated reduction of interest rates; they were expecting, before the meetings of officials in the German Central Bank and French Central Bank today, that the two main central banks in the Euro countries would not reduce interest rates this week.

Two main banks reduced their interest rates.

ii. Conditions for FALSE

Negation; Modality; Conditionality; Opacity; Doubt Verbs

ii. Examples

Snippets 60 FALSE (Operator IF with conditional clause, non entailed main verb predicate try/continue)

T/H pair 60

If a Mexican approaches the border, he's assumed to be trying to illegally cross.

Mexicans continue to illegally cross border.

Snippets 73 FALSE (opaque nominal predicate governor – discussion, same inferrable clause – allow/grant, same governed TO_OBJect/main OBJect)

T/H pair 73

There are discussions in California and Arizona to allow illegal aliens to have driver's licenses.

California driver's licenses granted to illegal immigrants.

Snippets 77 FALSE (opaque governing predicate talk_about, same clause – Dow_Jones be_down)

T/H pair 77

The media always talk about the Dow being up or down a certain number of points.

Dow Jones is down.

Snippets 98 FALSE (SUBJect non inferrable by Knowledge of the world – Arafat/prime minister, same governed verb predicate, same IndirectOBJect)

T/H pair 98

Sharon warns Arafat could be targeted for assassination.

prime minister targeted for assassination.

Snippets 171 FALSE (Same/entailed SUBJect, verbal head Suspect governing Same verb/nominal predicate of BE, Same/entailed OBJects – More/Less Specific)

T/H pair 171

The terrorist is suspected of being behind several deadly kidnappings and dozens of suicide attacks in Iraq.

Terrorist kidnaps dozens of Iraqis.

Snippets 227 FALSE (Same SUBJect, lexically inferrable main verb predicate say/decide, negated/quantified governed clause SUBJect, deontic/can modality on governed clause verb predicate, same OBJect)

T/H pair 227

A closely divided U.S. Supreme Court said on Thursday its 2002 ruling that juries and not judges must impose a death sentence applies only to future cases, a decision that may affect more than 100 death row inmates.

The Supreme Court decided that only judges can impose the death sentence.

Snippets 516 FALSE (Modal + governing verb/Same verb predicate , same OBJect)

T/H pair 516

If this challenge interests you, you might enjoy reading "Punished by Rewards" by Alfie Kohn.

I read "Punished by Rewards" by Alfie Kohn.

4. Implementing the Semantic Evaluator (SE)

As said above, the SE is organized into two main group of modules: a quantitatively based module, and a sequence of linguistic rules where quantitive scoring is also taken into account when needed, to increase confidence in the decision process. The two modules must then undergo General Consistency Checks which ascertain the presence of possible mismatches at semantic level. In particular, these checks take care of the following semantic items:

- presence of spatiotemporal locations relative to the same governing predicate, or a similar one as has been computed from previous modules;
- presence of opacity operators like discourse markers for conditionality having scope over the governing predicate under analysis;
- presence of quantifiers and other referentiality related determiners attached to the same nominal head in the T/H pair under analysis and chosen as relevant one by previous computation;
- presence of antonyms in the T/H pair at the level of governing predicates;
- presence of predicates belonging to the class of "doubt" expressing verbs, governing the relevant predicate shared by the T/H pair.

In some cases the General Consistency Checks have to be suspended: in particular whenever both T/H pairs contain opacity operators and negation, as for instance in Snippets no. 1014 reported above, and other similar examples.

4.1. The Linguistic Rule-Based Modules

These Modules are organized as a sequence of sub-modules which start from exceptional cases down to default cases.

Exceptional cases of Semantic Inference are those constituted by Paraphrase and Reformulation rules where axiomatic structures are addressed; then Lexical Inference follows in snippets where the linguistic elements checked should be identical, synonymous, morphologically derivable or sharing a congruent number of semantic features; Syntactic and Semantic inference rules follow in which different structures are transformed and checked on the basis of GRs and SRs first, then lexical chains are attempted; finally Hybrid (partially heuristic) rules are tried in which both structures and lexical items are matched.

Each rule operates at propositional level within each clause to find matches: however, head-dependent representations are just an unordered and set of terms where the hierarchical organization of syntactic structures needs to be reconstructed. Since predicate-argument structures have to be addressed separately from predicate-adjuncts ones, before entering the semantic evaluator, we assign scores to GRs and SRs and then sort AHDSs accordingly. In this way, the core arguments are always in the front of the list containing all current structures, as for instance in Snippet 46 reported here below,

T - The Yankees split Hollywood with something to feel OK about after last night's 5-4 loss to the Dodgers.
H - Dodgers lose first game ever at Fenway.

TEXT
1000-loss(ncmod-specif, '5/4').
1000-loss(ncmod-specif, 'night-s_').
1000-loss(ncmod-specif, to, dodger).
400-feel(ncmod-temporal, after, loss).
200-feel(obj-theme, ok).
250-split(xcomp-prop, feel).
100-feel(subj-agent, 'Hollywood').
20-split(iobj-comitative, with, something).
10-split(obj-source, hollywood).
0-split(subj-theme, 'Yankee').

HYPOTHESIS
1500-lose(adj-mod, ever).
1000-lose(ncmod-location, at, 'Fenway').
50-lose(xcomp-agent, game).
0-lose(subj-theme_aff, dodger).

We also address main clause first always by means of scoring, seen that SUBJects and OBJects of secondary clauses are weighted differently.

The level of main clause is then switched to that of dependent clause when needed. Dependent clauses may be very important to determine the outcome of an inference: they may be tensed (head label CCOMP) or untensed (head label XCOMP). The governing head predicate is responsible for the factitivity of the dependent. To this aim, important elements checked at propositional level are opacity, modality, and negation. Opacity is determined by type of governing predicates, basically those belonging to the class of nonfactive predicates.

Modality is revealed by the presence of modal verbs at this level of computation. Modality could also be instantiated at sentence level by adverbials, and be verified by General Consistency Checks. Finally, negation may be expressed locally as an adjunct of the verb, but also as a negative conjunction and negative adverbial – see examples above. It may also be present in the determiner of the nominal head and checked separately when comparing referring expressions considered in the inference. Negation may also be incorporated lexically in the verb in the class of the so-called "doubt" verbs.

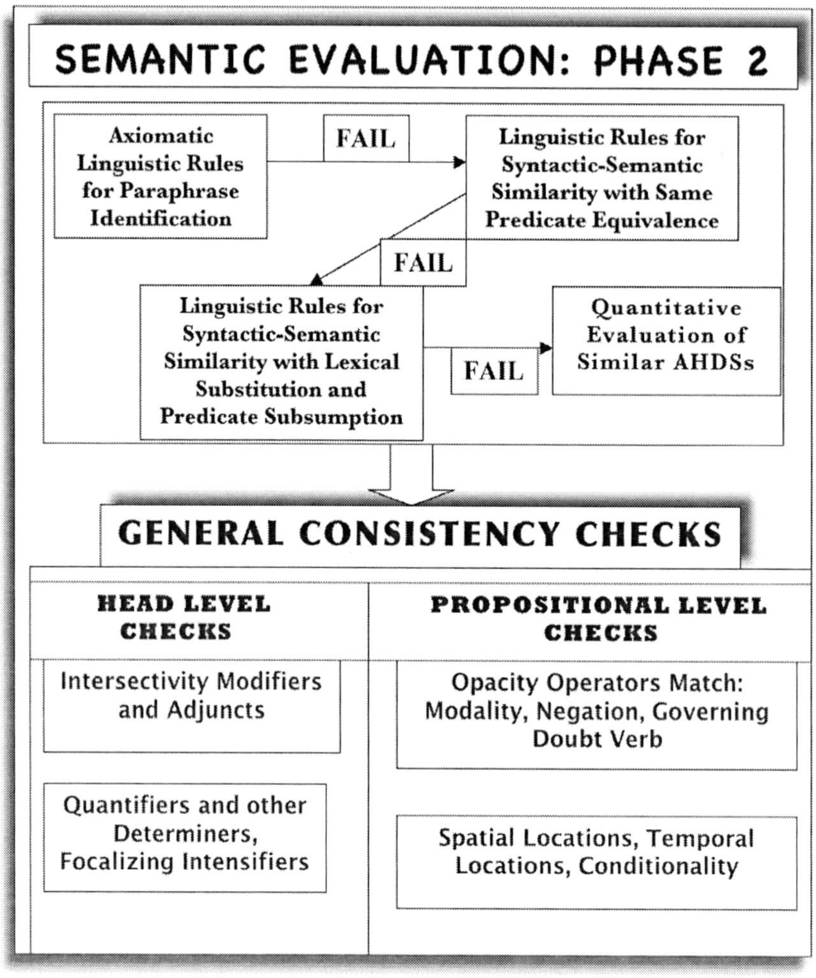

Figure 5. SE Semantic Evaluation and General Consistency Checks - Phase 2.

4.1.1. The Paraphrase Rule Sub-Module

This sub-module addresses definition-like H sentences, or simple paraphrases of the meaning expressed by the main predicate of the T text. Generally speaking, every time one such rule is fired, the T/H pair contains a conceptually complex lexical predicate and its paraphrase in conceptually simple components.

Examples of such cases are constituted by pairs like the following:

interview --> conduct an interview
pressurise --> apply pressure
treat --> receive treatment (provide)
fire → send letter of dismissal

where both a. and b. were actually present in WordNet while c. did not figure with the same predicates but rather with the one in brackets; d. was totally absent.

Definitions and paraphrases are looked up at first in the glosses made available by WordNet. In case of failure a list of some 50 manually made up axiomatic rules are accessed – built on the basis of the training dataset. Each such rule addresses main predicates in the T/H pair, together with the presence of semantically relevant dependent if needed, and whenever the concept expressed by the lexically complex predicate requires it. Together with the predicates, the rules select relevant GRs and SRs when needed. In addition, more restrictions are introduced on additional arguments or adjuncts. As is the case with all the rules, penalties are explored in terms of semantic operators of the main predicate like negation, modality and opacity inducing verbs which must either be absent or be identical in the T/H pair. Below we report one of the axiomatic-like rules (The SE is written in SWI Prolog and runs under Unix or any other compatible system),

```
complex_induct(Text,apply,_,pressure,obj-_),
complex_induct(Text,pressure,_,Ent,ncmod-_),
nonvar(Ent),
(complex_induct(Hypo,pressurize,Ent,_,obj-_);
complex_induct(Hypo,pressurise,Ent,_,obj-_)),
 assess_penalty([apply,pressurise],Hypo,Text,Scores),
 Scores=[],
!.
```

where Text contains all AHDSs for Text snippet, Hypo contains all AHDSs for Hypothesis snippet; "complex_induct" is a recursive call that looks into the list of AHDSs and tries to instantiate the appropriate structure with the constants indicated above: i.e., APPLY as head predicate, with PRESSURE as dependant, with the GR "obj". In the second call, the head predicate must be PRESSURE and the GR ncmod. "Ent" should not be empty and will have to be instantiated in the same linguistic expression in the following calls, applied this time to the Hypothesis list of AHDSs, where the main head predicate should be PRESSURIZE and its spelling variant PRESSURISE. The two main predicates are checked for propositional level penalties, if any: Scores should be empty otherwise a fail will ensue.

4.1.2 The Syntactic-Semantic Rule Sub-Module

The syntactic-semantic rule sub-module is organized into a sequence of subcalls where the T/H pairs are checked for semantic similarity starting from sameness of main predicates to semantic approximate match.

The first subcall requires the presence of same HDs as main predicates with core arguments, i.e. the ones which have been computed as subject, object, indirect object, arg_mod (passive "by" agent adjunct), xcomp. Nonconflicting SRs are checked in all subcalls: i.e. subject-agent are allowed to match with arg_mod-agent and subject-theme_affected with object-theme_affected but not viceversa. These matches take care of what are usually referred to as lexical alternations for verb sucategorization frames, and lexical rules in LFG terms which encompass such syntactic phenomena as passive, intransitivization, ergativization, dative shift, etc. Here below we report one example of such rules,

```
        same_pred(Hypo,Text,Pred,Score1),
        best_role1(Hypo,Text,Role),
        evaluate_opaques(Pred, Hypo,Text),
        assess_penalty(Pred, Hypo,Text,Score), Score=[],
        check_veridicity(Pred, Hypo,Text,Head),
        same_mainhead(Hypo,Text,Score2),
        same_role(Role,First,Score3),
        same_head(Rte,First,Score4),
    evaluate_scoring(Score1,Score2,Score3,Score4,Weight),
        !.
```

where "same_pred" looks for identical governing head predicate which is then further checked for best role, again by cycling in the lists of AHDSs for Text and Hypothesis. From this point onward, the SE checks at propositional level for the presence of possible penalty issuing main governing predicates with the two calls "evaluate_opaques" and "access_penalty". The following calls on the contrary check predicate-argument structures for the soundness of Semantic Roles and Grammatical Relations. Scores are then produced which are summed up and computed as Weight. This is then finally evaluated at higher level together with high level General Consistency Checks.

The second subcall requires the presence of semantically similar HDs as a combination of main head and main dependent and at least another identical HD structure within the core argument subset. Other subcalls included in this group check nominalization derivational relations intervening between main predicate of T and H, which in one case is checked with edit distance measures. A certain number of additional rules checks for semantic similarity, which can range from synonymous, down to morphologically derived.

The third subcall takes as input a list of "light-verbs" in semantic terms, i.e. verbs including "be", "have", "appear", and other similar copulative and locational verbs – like "live", "hold", "take_place", "participate", etc. - which are used to either make a definition, assert a property of the subject, individuate a location of the subject etc. These verbs are matched against main predicates and core arguments of the T portion, which must be identical to H. Quantitative measures are added to confirm the choice. Notable exceptions are sentences containing "be_born" predication which require specific constructions on the other member of the T/H pair.

The fourth subcall takes as input at least one identical main predicate HD non argument structure and one additional core argument or adjunct structure. Quantitative measures are added to confirm the choice.

The fifth subcall looks for different main predicates with core arguments which however must be non antonyms, non negative polarity and be synonyms. In addition, there must be at least another important identical non argument HD structure shared. Quantitative measures are added to confirm the choice. One such case is represented by Snippets 1639 reported in the Appendix.

These cases must be treated appropriately to distinguish them from what happens in real opposite meaning snippets where the SE considers SRs which must also be opposite, as in snippets 933; or cases in which the snippet is rescued due to the presence of same SRs, see Snippets 876, where DIE and KILL have entailed meaning; but when KILL is used in the passive, the SRs attached to their SUBJects will be identical.

4.2. The Quantitative Module

In this module all Heads, Dependents, GRs and SRs are collected for each member of the T/H pair and then they are passed to a scoring function that takes care of identical or similar members by assigning a certain score to every hit. Penalties correspond to high scores, while rewards correspond to low scores. A threshold is then set at a certain value which should encode the presence of a comparatively high number of identical/similar linguistic items. As said above, higher scores are assigned to core GRs and there is a scale also for SRs where Agent has higher score.

As with previous subcalls, at the end of the computation semantic consistency and integrity is checked by collecting and comparing semantic operators, as well as performing a search of possible governing "doubt" verbs.

Generally speaking, we also treat short utterances differently from long ones. A stricter check is performed whenever an utterance has 3 or less HD structures, the reason being that in these structures some of the above mentioned subcalls would fail due to insufficient information available. (This could be related to Application Domain, in particular QA having always shorter Hypotheses than others).

5. Results and Discussion

The RTE task is a hard task: this may be partly due to the way in which it has been formulated – half of the snippets are TRUE, the other half are FALSE. It is usually the case that 10-15% of mistakes are ascribable to the parser or any other analysis tool – at least this is what we expect from our parser, or other off-the-shelf parsers freely available from the web; another 5-10% mistakes will certainly come from insufficient semantic information – and this is what we measured on our results. Whenever a system makes 20% errors this is doubled to 40% due to corpus setup, and the final result will become 60% overall Recall.

As far as the Test set is concerned, our system correctly classified 285/400 False annotated snippets, and 194/400 True annotated snippets. As a result, the system misclassified 321 pairs out of 800 examples. The majority of mistakes – 193, i.e. 60.1% - were false negatives, which are T/H pairs which the system classified as false but were annotated as true. The number of false positives is 128, i.e. 39.9%, which the system wrongly classified as true. If we compute the internal consistency of classification of the algorithm, we come up with the following data: 128 false positives over an overall number of 322 pairs classified as true by the system corresponds to 60.3% overall accuracy for true snippets; 193 false negatives over a total number of 478 pairs classified as false by the system corresponds to 59.5% overall accuracy for false snippets.

Table 5. Results for training and test-set

Test-set Results		Training-set Results	
cws:	0.6306	cws:	0.6459
accuracy:	0.5950	accuracy:	0.6032
precision:	0.6180	precision:	0.6250
recall:	0.4975	recall:	0.5124
f:	0.5512	f:	0.5631
QA cws:0.5295	acc:0.5692	QA cws:0.6360	acc:0.5556
PP cws:0.8563	acc:0.8200	PP cws:0.6249	acc:0.6585
IE cws:0.6534	acc:0.5833	IE cws:0.6119	acc:0.6000
CD cws:0.7139	acc:0.6667	CD cws:0.7416	acc:0.6633
IR cws:0.7163	acc:0.6556	IR cws:0.6795	acc:0.6286
RC cws:0.5796	acc:0.5357	RC cws:0.5529	acc:0.5243
MT cws:0.4693	acc:0.4750	MT cws:0.6359	acc:0.6111

As can be seen from Table 5 above, the system has produced different result in each Application domain, so we will now look with more details at accuracy data for each of the seven application fields:

- IR cws:0.7163 accuracy:0.6556
- CD cws:0.7139 accuracy:0.6667
- PP cws:0.8563 accuracy:0.8200

These three fields are by far those obtaining the best scoring by our system. In particular the Paraphrase Acquisition dataset fares higher simply because we acquired a good number of paraphrases from a number of sources including WordNet Definitions and turned them into appropriate “axiom-like” rules as described above. As to Comparable Documents and Information Retrieval, both syntax and semantics play a role in selecting the required synonyms and antonyms, within the appropriate predicate-argument structure as defined by GRs and SRs. The second set of data fares somewhat worse:

- IE cws:0.6534 accuracy:0.5833
- QA cws:0.5295 accuracy:0.5692
- RC cws:0.5796 accuracy:0.5357

In all these cases, results are better than chance overall but they are not up to the expected results partly because of semantic inadequacies in the thesaurus, as RC may suggest. But also partly because of the lack of suitable syntactic transformation rules for syntactic alternations, in particular all those cases involving modifiers treated as arguments in one of the T/H pair. Finally the worst result obtained by the system,

- MT cws:0.4693 accuracy:0.4750

is represented by the MT data subset. The strange thing is that the Development set diverges only in this case from the Test set, by reaching a much higher result

- MT cws:0.6359 accuracy:0.6111

The other divergent case is represented by the PP results which fare lower than the ones obtained for the Test set,

- PP cws:0.6249 accuracy:0.6585

On a closer look, reasons for these differences are not due to system performance but to differences in distribution of the two application settings in Test and Development datasets, which are almost reversed: in the Test set MT pairs are almost the double of the PP pairs; the opposite applies to the Development set. In fact, if looked at from this perspective the results become absolutely comparable. These are the total figures in the two datasets:

TEST SET
MT – 120 T/H pairs = 15%
PP – 50 T/H pairs = 6.25%
DEVELOPMENT SET
MT – 54 T/H pairs = 9.5%
PP – 82 T/H pairs = 14.5%

In other words, the system performs slightly over chance in the MT application field - summing up the accuracy data and dividing by 2 we get 50.4%. In the PP field the results fare around 74% accuracy, still higher than other fields but no so much as 82% of the test set.

We looked into our mistakes to evaluate the impact of the parser on final Recall and we found out that: 10 snippets out of 100 TRUE ones have a wrong parse which can be regarded the main cause of the mistake. In other words only 10% of wrong results can be ascribed to bad parses. The remaining 10% is due to insufficient semantic information. In turn, this may be classified as follows:

80% is due to lack of paraphrases and definitions;
10% is due to wrong SemanticRole assignment;
10% is due to lack of synonym/antonym relations.

When we started working on the training corpus, verb predicates synsets made available by WordNet have been augmented by the information contained in Grady Ward's MOBY Thesaurus (http://www.dcs.shef.ac.uk/research/ilash/Moby/). Additional information has been derived from a manually reorganized version of Roget's Thesaurus, again limited though to verb predicates. In particular, antonymity is lacking in WordNet where the choice has been that of listing only contradictory items (male/female). However antonymity has two more types to be taken into account: scalar antonyms where the two items don't need to be one or the other and can be between the two extremes of a particular scale (hot/cold); then relational opposites which are pairs that don't represent extremes of some scale (stop/go).

We also felt we needed information related to negative polarity verb predicates which we derived from Harvard Dictionary derived from Harvard IV-4 e Laswell's dictionary on the Dynamics of Culture (http://www.wjh.harvard.edu/). The paraphrase and definition list for verb predicates taken from WordNet and transformed into HD structures was also updated in order to cover some missing cases. For instance, we had to implement a new paraphrase for the verb FIRE which is paraphrased as "send dismissal letter to" in Snippets 783. The list of HDSs will be accessed by the Evaluator in the appropriate Module.

6. Related Work

Our approach to textual entailment can be compared to other similar approaches based on deep parsing, in particular see Bos et al., Raina et al., which however, eventually derive a logical form to undertake semantic processing by means of a theorem prover. As a matter of fact, we also produce a logical form of each snippet, where syntactic indices generated by the parser are accompanied by semantic role labels, and levels of dependency or modification are encoded in embedding. However, since unification could only be applied whenever lexical substitutions or lexical paraphrases for semantically similar predicates have been accomplished, we assume our system to be a better tool for achieving the same goal. In this sense, we follow closely what Punyakanok et al, Braz et al. also do in their system, apart again from the theorem prover. Also Lin et al. can be regarded another example of a system using dependency trees to do semantic similarity measures. We believe our structures to be a much better approximation of what other systems can produce: in particular in Punyakanok et al, Braz et al., only syntactic constituency is being produced and no further semantic processing is carried out, apart from semantic role assignment directly at word level. The same applies more or less to Bos et al., Raina et al., seen that these approaches rely on the output of a constituency only syntactic parser. Only superficially relevant relations will be encoded by these system: all lexically unexpressed relations will be omitted. So not only SUBJects of untensed clauses, but also long distance dependency syntactically controlled arguments will not appear. On the contrary this is fully expressed in our representation which can thus be regarded syntactic-semantic in the intended sense. As to the use of a theorem prover, we rather prefer a more flexible rule-based semantic approach, as discussed above; in addition, Equality and Subsumption can be expressed very effectively by the paradigm of variable and constraints instantiation in Prolog, once the appropriate information is available. So in a nutshell, the real problem is getting the appropriate representation: we think that dependency structure are to be regarded equivalent to any other flat or hierarchical logical structure.

Another different case is constituted by Lin et al. which computes syntactic constituency on the basis of a chomskian approach and then a mapping into Grammatical Relations is produced by the system. When we look at results reported by Bos et al., we see that the best accuracy scores are obtained by the Hybrid Task and the domains with better score are CD and IR; the same applies to Raina et al. where best scores are obtained by CD, PP, and IR. This is very much in line with our results and reflects some bias involved in the deep parsing approach.

If we consider probabilistic Bag Of Words (BOWs) approaches - see for instance Punyakanok et al., Glickman et al. Corley et al. – the picture changes dramatically. In this cases, semantic similarity is derived from term cooccurence frequency measures, usually taken from a big corpus or the web itself. The main criticism we can raise to these approaches is that semantic elements contained in a sentence very often coincide with stopwords such as negation, auxiliaries, modals, prepositions. All these are function words which shouldn't be erased, because they are used to express relations (grammatical, semantic, discourse), which these systems attempt to capture by the usual cooccurence paradigm contained in such measures as Inverse Document Frequency (idf) or the Mutual Information. Even though we think that such approaches are needed in a real life application setting, they are nonetheless in themselves insufficient to determine with enough confidence whether what is being measured is actually semantic similarity at propositional level – i.e. the two snippets are saying the same thing – or just an instance with good approximation of parallel texts. If we look at results reported in Glickman et al., we see a remarkably high accuracy in two domains, CD and MT. The same appears to be the case in Punyakanok where MT, QA and CD receive a very high accuracy score – over 80%; Corley et al. doesn't report separate evaluations for each domain, so we are left with a single overall score. Best systems seem to be Glickman et al., and Corley et al.: both fare around 59% accuracy. In all the three papers, error analysis is omitted: we take this to be a fundamental step in assessing the validity of their approach and look forward to see it in future papers. However, this seems to be a weakness of BOWs approaches.

7. CONCLUSIONS

We have presented an approach based on linguistic rules where representations are intended to convey all possible syntactic and semantic knowledge in a linear dependency-based compact but consistent format. Limitations of this approach are basically due to parsing errors and insufficient semantic/world knowledge, so we don't expect to go over 62/64% accuracy in future experiments with a similar dataset as the one provided by RTE. While deep parsing accuracy cannot reasonably be expected to improve easily beyond the 85% threshold, we hope to achieve better results with augmented thesauri and other semantic similarity repositories available on the web. Another possibility would be that of assuming a probabilistically based BOWs approach on the same issue, in order to recover missing information for term cooccurence, especially in such thorny cases as paraphrase and definition related semantic similarities. Approaches attested in the literature seem to be quite successful and could thus be integrated with the linguistically-based stance of our system. We are currently experimenting with a version of LinkGrammar (LG) ported under SWI Prolog, where we have implemented our semantically and discourse oriented labelling modules which provide information as to semantic roles, pronominal binding and other relevant logical operators and discourse markers. We intend to produce an evaluation based on the augmented LG output in order to ascertain whether it compares positively with our system.

Chapter 8

REASONING FROM DISCOURSE MODEL FOR QUESTION ANSWERING AND TEXT PARAPHRASING

1. INTRODUCTION

In this final chapter we explore the possibility to do Reasoning for Paraphrasing and Question/Answering from the Discourse Model produced by the system together with knowledge encoded in the lexicon and in the associated computational lexicon of Conceptual Representations. Differently from existing systems for Question/Answering in which all knowledge and constraints needed to cope within a given domain is carefully manually grafted into the system, in our case only what the system actually computes from linguistic descriptions will be made available to the KL-ONE-like Knowledge Representation language. In addition, there will be no specific domain-related constraints nor overall planning strategy, seen that we only intend to concern ourselves with a more limited task: that of building sensible questions and/or answers without any internal dialogue structure.

The language we use is a specific implementation called BACK - Berlin Advanced Computational Knowledge Representation System. We are currently using Version 5.2 released in September 1993. Functionality of the system as reported in the Readme file are as follows:

- reasoning based on terminological logics (KL-ONE)
- supporting inheritance,
- consistency checking,
- cycle detection,
- classification,
- completion of partial descriptions,
- role inferences,
- abox revision,
- extended query answering.

Main system components are: TBox (KB scheme), ABox (KB assertions), IBox (extensional implications). System interfaces: uniform access language.

In order to go from the Discourse Model to the reasoning modules we need to introduce an important component of our computational lexicon, Conceptual Representations. World knowledge however has also a dynamic important component which is represented in our case by the intersection of aspectual semantics and temporal reasoning as has been carried out in the DM.

We shall now give an overview of KL-ONE, as described in Brachman & Schmolze(1985), a system for knowledge representation which we used in a previous version of our system(see Delmonte, 1990). KL-ONE has an "epistemological level" to cope with such elements as "description, attribute, concept, role, inheritance, and instantiation", in order to form descriptions of the objects of the domain, as well as an inference mechanism for deriving the consequences of the use of descriptions in particular contexts. On the contrary, in our system an individual is described with an Initial Description which is a statement of existence. As we have extensively shown, Coreference is not achieved in the model itself, but in two steps: at first the discourse module checks whether pronominal or nominal expressions corefer to topics of discourse, these in turn are identified by a unique identifier in the model and this is then used to activate coreference. Equality is simply given by Prolog language. Predication on the contrary is assumed to hold between all properties and attributes associated to a given individual in the model: the ISA relation is assumed unless a more specific one can be found. Subsumption holds between members of a set and inheritance as a whole is activated every time is needed: particularly at the end of the computation, all properties and attributes belonging to a given individual or set are subsumed under the same identifier, and in case it is a set, are propagated to its members.

Other important component of the ontology of KL-ONE are Roles, Restriction and Differentiation, which are naturally incorporated in our framework, being either the instantiation of a new individual, or an attribute. However, note that only actual roles appear in the description, the ones being extracted dynamically from the text. We take Restrictions in KL-ONE to be simply necessary information, in case they characterize a set with a given cardinality - a plural NP is restricted in case we know the number or the identity of its components. As to Cases, as semantic roles are usually called in Knowledge Representation literature, they are instantiated by the predicate, or they are absent from the description. In this case, the relevant information would be encoded at the level of lexical form rather than in the Knowledge Base. The same applies to RoleSet Restrictions. On the contrary RoleSet Differentiation should be encoded in the Knowledge Base since we would like to know in advance that the President of a Company can be coreferred by the common noun Officer. However we think it a misconception altogether the way in which RoleSet Restrictions - what has been defined as bridges in previous chapters – and Case are encoded in KL-ONE: as also the authors note, we might not know in advance whether a special restriction may be attached to a CC-Recipient or a To-Recipient of a CC-Message Concept, until we analyse the text. These are taken to be necessary but not sufficient conditions, so that a Recipient can also be a To-Recipient, and "the details of the Role-defining mechanism have not yet been worked out satisfactorily"(ibid.,186).

The same applies to the definition of the conditions for determining the referent of an Individual Concept. As to Generic Concepts, the equivalent of a general term, the authors also note that potentially many individuals in any possible world can be described by it. Each Generic Concept for animal, mammal, human, female human, woman etc. is a description that can be used to describe many individuals. However there is no indication of how in a real text these descriptions can be used efficiently. In our system some such questions are tackled in particular, when in Chapter V, we discuss the role of quantifiers in discourse. As the model description has shown, universal quantifiers can be encoded as IDs with a restriction in terms of Generic Concept, the semantic feature [+human] or any other feature made available by the semantic role being assigned to it by the linguistic analysis. However, when to use these IDs to draw inferences in a text is a matter of discourse theory rather than Knowledge Representation Theory. As discussed in Chapter V, there are certain text typologies which allow the use of quantifier to describe entities in the world and to draw inferences on the basis of quantified expressions or plural definite NPs, or still singular definite NPs in generic statements though. More to the point are the "default properties" discussed further on in this chapter.

We will not go into a discussion of Structural Description whose technical details the authors themselves define as "a bit messy", nor shall we go into a criticism of the Example in the Appendix.

As we already showed in previous chapters, we believe that intensional descriptions of objects of a domain may be necessary in a given application in order to encode commonsense knowledge and other types of apriori knowledge of a domain(see Lang,1991): in a framework like ours in which every entity is simply asserted in the data base as it pops up from the text, intensional entities may have to be distinguished from existing, extensional ones, in the way we have discussed below.

What we really want to stress here is the fact that our Knowledge Representation Model of the Text is not manually added or hand-coded into the system but derived automatically by means of fully general procedures which apply to any Discourse Model as long as it is consistent and fully instantiated. As will be clear from the description below, partial semantic interpretation is insufficient to allow for the full set of question/answering we surmise should be possible in the normal case. However, queries on properties and relations of entities should always be made possible even from partial interpretation.

2. From Conceptual Representations to Inferential Rules

In Question-Answering systems it is usually the plan that allows the system to smoothly carrying on the communicative exchange with the user. The Knowledge Representation of the domain includes either a frame-like description of every action or else a specification of precondition and postconditions with respect to roles and objects involved in the event described by a given predicate. We do not intend to carry out dialogues which would require us to build a plan and take care of any changes in the knowledge base introduced by actions and events happening as a result of the communicative exchange. However, the overall architecture of these systems is important in that it allows us to better understand how static and dynamic knowledge interact in the generation of dialogues in communicative exchanges.

We saw in a previous section how conceptual representations can be used to introduce constraints on spatiotemporal locations of entities; we have also seen that the Discourse Model provides us with the output of the Temporal Reasoning algorithm which allows us together with the spatial location inferential module to determine when and where entities, their relations and properties are situated. Rather than hand-coding the knowledge specific to a given example as shown above, the task we have to face now is a more general mapping from the DM, its ontology and the KL-ONE environment where consistency checking is performed.

As a first step we need to establish a set of semantic fields with certain properties so that actions and events have fixed effects on its objects and participants. Semantic fields are just a superset of the fields already presented in the section on CRs.

```
fields :- semanticfield :< anything,
     spatial :< semanticfield,
     perceptive :< semanticfield,
     existential :< semanticfield,
     possessional :< semanticfield,
     circumstantial :< semanticfield.
```

Then we need to define the set of primary functions associated to CRs in more detail and in the language specification used in our implementation of KL-ONE. The primary functions we introduced above are the following ones: GO, BE, STAY, CAUSE, LET, ORIENT, IDENT and might all be preceded by negation NOT and we shall only take into account the first four functions:

```
definePrimitives:-primitive :<anything,
       defineGo,defineStay,defineBe,defineCause.

defineGo:- fromgo:<anything,
      togo:<anything,
      themego:<anything,
      pathgo:<oneof([to,toward,via]),
primgo:< primitive
       and all(from,fromgo) and all(to,togo) and all(path,pathgo)
       and all(semanticfieldGo, semanticfield)
       and all(theme,themego).

defineStay:- themestay :< anything,
statestay :< anything,
      pathstay :< oneof([in,at]),
      primstay :<primitive
       and all(state, statestay) and all(path,pathstay)
       and all(semanticfieldstay, semanticfield)
       and all(theme, themestay).

defineBe:- themebe :< anything,
     placebe :< anything,
     pathbe :< oneof([in]),
     primbe :<primitive
      and all(places,placebe) and all(path,pathbe)
      and all(semanticfieldbe, semanticfield)
```

```
        and all(themeNonAgent,themebe).

defineCause:- themeCause :< anything,
     primCause :< primitive and all(theme,themeCause)
          and all(primitiveIntroduced,primitive).
```

Now we can build recursively all instances of objects for relations specified by verbs, as follows:

```
generate :-
fact(_,isa,[arg:K,arg:ev],1,A,B),
    fact(K,Pred,[Agent:X,Locat:Y],1,A,B),
    associate_primary_function_and_roles(K, Pred, Agent:X, Locat:Y).
```

Mapping from the Discourse Model to Knowledge Database is filtered from Conceptual Representations by means of verbal linguistic description and its semantic roles. All roles present in the surface sentence should be mapped into the corresponding CR in order for the conceptual mapping to be consistent. In addition, other semantic roles might be present in the corresponding CR which need not be lexically expressed but are conceptual components of the semantic frame associated to the "going" event. These roles will have to be instantiated in the knowledge DataBase-mapping.

```
associate_primary_function_and_roles(K, go, Agent:X,Locat:Y):-
    role_saturation(go, Agent, Locat, SuperFunct, PrimFunct, ExtraRoles),
db_mapping(SuperFunct, PrimFunct, [X, ExtraRoles,Y], K).
```

These calls are very important because they attains the lexicon to knowledge mapping by means of CRs. All semantic roles coming from the surface sentence level realization should be present in the lexical CR entry and should be fully saturated. As we saw above, more than one meaning may be associated to the lexical head of the verb predicate; however only one of those meanings needs to be selected. In addition, the CR should provide the mapping procedure with further unrealized roles and with the labels of Super Functions like CAUSE and Primary Functions like GO: these latter functions will trigger the appropriate mapping rule in KL-ONE.

```
role_saturation(go, agent, locat, CAUSE, GO, [source]):-
go[CAUSE(<agent>(GOexten(FROM<source>(TO<locat>)))
{(en,tn),(e1,t1)}],!.
```

In addition to two realized and saturated roles, the CR contains an unrealized role which is mapped as a variable or nil in case no information is available in the Model. Remember that only semantic Ids are mapped here into the KRDB.

```
db_mapping(MainPrimitive,PrimaryFunction,[Agent|ArgumentRoles],SemanticIndex) :-
R::MainPrimitive and theme:Agent and primitiveIntroduced:Primitive,
introduce_specific_primitive(PrimaryFunction, [Agent |ArgumentRoles], Primitive),
    linkverb(SemanticIndex,R),!.
```

```
introduce_specific_primitive(primgo, [Agent,From,To], Primitive):-
Primitive=(S:: primgo and theme:Agent and from:From and to:To
        and semanticfieldgo:spatial ),!.
linkverb(A,B) :- A::anything and prim:B.
```

2.1. Definition of Sets, General Class, Social Roles and Time Intervals

We can now come to the assertion of default properties and Generic Concepts, but also of other items of the interpretation process like polarity values, time location labels, prepositions used in the mapping and finally constant values like proper names.

At first, very general roles and properties are declared, like for instance the set of proper names or the set of prepositions:

```
set :- proper_names  := aset([john,mary]),
   masfem            := aset([male,female]),
   pol               := 0..1,
   special           := aset([in,on,under,near]).

generic_class :- general :< anything.

int :- time :< general,
       tloc  :< tempo.
```

We then define attributes to be associated to individuals which we recover from the DM and divide up accordingly into three main general group: PERSONS, OBJECTS and PLACES.

```
persons :- man    :< general,
has_name   :< domain(man) and range(proper_names),
sex      :< domain(man) and range(masfem),
get_persons.
objects :- thing  :< general,
get_objects.
places :- place   :< general,
get_places.
get_objects:-
fact(_,inst_of,[ind:Y,class:thing],1,_,_),
    fact(_, isa, [ind:Y, class:Class], 1, _, _),
    fact(_, in, [arg:Y, locativo:Loc], 1, _, _),
Class :< thing
and all(locat,place) and all(spec,special)
and all(location,place) and all(partOf,thing),!.
get_objects:-
fact(_,inst_of,[ind:Y,class:thing],1,_,_),
    fact(_, isa, [ind:Y, class:Class], 1, _, _),
```

```
Class  :< thing and all(location,place).
get_places:-
   fact(_, isa, [arg:Y, arg:Class], 1, _, Y),
    Class :< place.
get_persons:-
fact(_,inst_of,[ind:Y,class:social_role],1,_,_),
   fact(_, isa, [ind:Y, class:Class], 1, _, _),
   fact(_,role,[Class,X,Y],1,_,_),
Class  :< man and all(work_in,X).
```

Subsidiary properties and relations associated to entities in the DM are associated automatically in case they are actually present: a location of an entity, a role of an individual as defined by the semantic inherent feature "social_role" is further defined as related to a certain spatial location, when available, thus instantiating a partial frame structure.

Aspectual information is used to individuate the appropriate internal constituency of the event (see also Delmonte, 1997 and above), and also to drive the semantics, which together with the information coming from arguments and adjuncts will be able to trigger the adequate knowledge representation. In particular, as shown in Passonneau 1988, we need to process reference to entities and events in the discourse model, in order to know what predicates are asserted to hold over what entities and when.

EVENTS, STATES and PROCESSES are special objects which possess a polarity, a reference time and an agent that causes something: it may be a process as in the case of BEGIN, or an event of going to a place as for GO, or still a theme_unaff (a non affected theme that stays in a given location).

```
events :- ev    :< general
and all(time,tense) and all(polarity,pol),
specify_event_predicates.
states :- st   :< general
and all(time,tense) and all(polarity,pol),
specify_state_predicates.
processes :- pr    :< general
and all(time,tense) and all(polarity,pol),
specify_process_predicates.
specify_event_predicates:-
fact(_,isa,[arg:X,arg:ev],1,A,B),
fact(X,Pred,[Agent:_,locat:_],1,B,_),
Pred :< ev
and all(agent,man) and all(location,place)
  and all(prim,primCause) .
specify_state_predicates:-
fact(_,isa,[arg:X,arg:st],1,A,_),
fact(X,Pred,Arguments,1,B,_),
Pred :< st
and all(theme_nonaff,thing) and all(prim,primbe).
specify_process_predicates:
```

```
fact(_,isa,[arg:X,arg:pr],1,A,_),
fact(X,Pred,[Agent:_,theme_aff:_],1,B,_),
Pred :< pr
and all(Agent,man) and all(theme_aff,thing)
and all(prim,primCause),!.
```

From general entities we then declare instances as they have been collected in the DM with their semantic ids, for example for all instances of man we use,

```
facts :- fact(_,inst_of,[ind:Y,class:man],1,_,_),
    Y :: man.
```

For all instances of individuals belonging to the class of social_roles,

```
facts :- fact(_,inst_of,[ind:Y,class:social_role],1,_,_),
   fact(_, isa, [ind:Y, class:Class], 1, _, _),
    Y :: Class.
```

Names and roles are associated to a specific relation:

```
facts :- fact(_,name,[X,Y],1,_,_),
    Y :: has_name:X.
facts :- fact(_,role,[Class,X,Y],1,_,_),
    Y :: works_in:X.
```

The same applies for ids associated to spatiotemporal locations, both for entities and relations like events, processes or states,

```
facts :- fact(_,isa,[ind:X,class:Y],1,A,Z),
    X :: Y and time:A and location:Z.
facts :- fact(_,isa,[arg:X,arg:ev],1,A,B),
    X :: ev and time:A and location:B.
```

Then we associate to a relation id all its semantic properties, from semantic roles to spatiotemporal relations, as for instance with predicates like GO,

```
facts :- fact(X,Pred,[agent:Z,locat:A],1,B,_),
X :: Pred and agent:Z and location:A and time:B.
```

2.2. Internal Knowledge DATABASE of Classes and Instances

The internal representation of the mapping produced so far from the DM into the KRDB is organized into two separate DBs: one containing all classes characterized by the prefix b5st_class_db, and the other containing all instances of the Model, characterized by the prefix b5st_instance_db. Here below we list a small excerpt from both DBs.

i. Db of Classes

```
b5st_class_db(proper_names, (a, 0), 16, proper_names:=aset([john, mary])).
```

```
b5st_class_db(masfem, (a, 0), 24, masfem:=aset([male, female])).
b5st_class_db(pol, (n, 0), 25, pol:=0..1).
b5st_class_db(special, (a, 0), 30, special:=aset([in, on, under, near])).
b5st_class_db(prim(general), (c, 0), 31, internal).
b5st_class_db(general, (c, 0), 32, general:<anything).
b5st_class_db(prim(social_role), (c, 0), 37, internal).
b5st_class_db(social_role, (c, 0), 38, social_role:<general).
b5st_class_db(prim(man), (c, 0), 39, internal).
b5st_class_db(man, (c, 0), 40, man:<general).
b5st_class_db(prim(has_name), (r, 0), 41, internal).
b5st_class_db(has_name, (r, 0), 42, ha_nome:<domain(man)and range(proper_names)).
b5st_class_db(prim(sex), (r, 0), 43, internal).
b5st_class_db(sex, (r, 0), 44, sex:<domain(man)and range(masfem)).
b5st_class_db(prim(waiter), (c, 0), 45, internal).
b5st_class_db(prim(works_in), (r, 0), 46, internal).
b5st_class_db(works_in, (r, 0), 47, works_in:<domain(anything)and range(anything)).
b5st_class_db(prim(restaurant), (c, 0), 49, forward).
b5st_class_db(restaurant, (c, 0), 50, restaurant:<anything).
b5st_class_db(waiter, (c, 0), 51, waiter:<man and all(works_in, restaurant)).
prop:<domain(anything)and range(anything)).
b5st_class_db(prim(agente), (r, 0), 113, internal).
b5st_class_db(agente, (r, 0), 114, agente:<domain(anything)and range(anything)).
b5st_class_db(prim(prim), (r, 0), 118, internal).
b5st_class_db(prim, (r, 0), 119, prim:<domain(anything)and range(anything)).
b5st_class_db(prim(st), (c, 0), 126, internal).
b5st_class_db(st, (c, 0), 127, st:<general and all(time, tempo)).
b5st_class_db(prim(tema_nonaff), (r, 0), 131, internal).
b5st_class_db(tema_nonaff, (r, 0), 132, tema_nonaff:<domain(anything)and
    range(anything)).
b5st_class_db(prim(have), (c, 0), 135, internal).
b5st_class_db(prim(tema_aff), (r, 0), 136, internal).
b5st_class_db(tema_aff, (r, 0), 137, tema_aff:<domain(anything)and range(anything)).
b5st_class_db(have, (c, 0), 139, have:<st and all(agente, man)and all(tema_aff, thing)).
b5st_class_db(prim(there_in), (c, 0), 140, internal).
b5st_class_db(prim(goal), (r, 0), 141, internal).
b5st_class_db(goal, (r, 0), 142, goal:<domain(anything)and range(anything)).
b5st_class_db(there_in, (c, 0), 144, there_in:<st and all(location, place)and all(goal,
    general)).
b5st_class_db(prim(pr), (c, 0), 145, internal).
b5st_class_db(pr, (c, 0), 146, pr:<general and all(time, tempo)).
b5st_class_db(prim(begin), (c, 0), 147, internal).
b5st_class_db(begin, (c, 0), 148, begin:<ev and all(agente, man)and all(prop, pr)).
```

ii. Db of Instances

```
b5st_instance_db(mary, (a, 0), 14, no_definition).
b5st_instance_db(john, (a, 0), 15, no_definition).
```

```
b5st_instance_db(restaurant, (c, 0), 159, ([], [])).
b5st_instance_db(id3, (c, 0), 155, ([man, has_name:john], [])).
b5st_instance_db(id10, (c, 0), 158, ([waiter, lavora_in:id2, locazione:id2, time:id1], [])).
b5st_instance_db(tes(f5_r01), (c, 0), 162, ([], [])).
b5st_instance_db(tes(f3_free_a1), (c, 0), 164, ([], [])).
b5st_instance_db(tes(f2_free_aq), (c, 0), 166, ([], [])).
b5st_instance_db(tes(finf1_free_a1), (c, 0), 168, ([], [])).
b5st_instance_db(tes(f4_free_r02), (c, 0), 175, ([], [])).
b5st_instance_db(id18, (c, 0), 178, ([book, location:id2, time:id14], [])).
b5st_instance_db(id21, (c, 0), 165, ([begin, ev, agente:id3, location:id2, prop:id19,
    time:tes(f3_free_a1)], [])).
b5st_instance_db(poss, (c, 0), 179, ([have, agente:id3, tema_aff:id18, time:id14], [])).
b5st_instance_db(id6, (c, 0), 157, ([table, thing, locaz:id7, location:id2, spec:in,
    time:id1], [])).
b5st_instance_db(id7, (c, 0), 156, ([corner, thing, location:id2, partOf:id2, time:id1], [])).
b5st_instance_db(go_id4, (c, 0), 284, ([primgo, semanticfieldgo:spatial, from:nil,
    tema:id3, to:id2], [])).
b5st_instance_db(cause_id4, (c, 0), 285, ([primCause, primitiveIntroduced:go_id4,
    tema:id3], [])).
b5st_instance_db(id4, (c, 0), 163, ([anything, ev, go, agente:id3, location:id2,
    prim:cause_id4, time:tes(f5_r01)], [])).
```

3. Linguistic Knowledge and Reasoning for Error Diagnosis and Feedback Generation

In the knowledge representation we establish a semantic relation that holds between a sentence and an interval in the spirit of interval semantics. We specify what property of an interval is entailed by the input sentence and then compositionally we construct a representation of the event from the intervals and their associated properties. The Discourse Model provides us with the output of the Temporal Reasoning algorithm which allows us together with the spatial location inferential module to determine when and where entities, their relations and properties are situated. Rather than hand-coding the knowledge specific to a given example as shown above, the task we have to face now is a more general mapping from the DM, its ontology and the reasoning module where consistency checking is performed.

As said above, we present a QA module which is not intended to be used on any domain with open questions. The domain in our case coincides with the text the system has just analysed and transformed into a DM. As before we will be using the short text from the psychological atmosphere texts. Here below are some of the queries that can be addressed to the system. The typology of questions includes spatiotemporal locations in addition to the usual identity questions and the activity ones. Here below is the Discourse Model, the list of Entities of the World and their Properties used by the Question/Answering module to create questions and answers and then the list of Discourse Structures used by the system to generate adequate answers.

The interesting part of the program is obviously the possibility of recovery from failure in case of wrong inferences. According to the type of query, failure may be recovered and an appropriate feedback generated. Students are presented with four questions generated at random from the set of available question reported above. After choosing the question by pushing on one of four buttons,

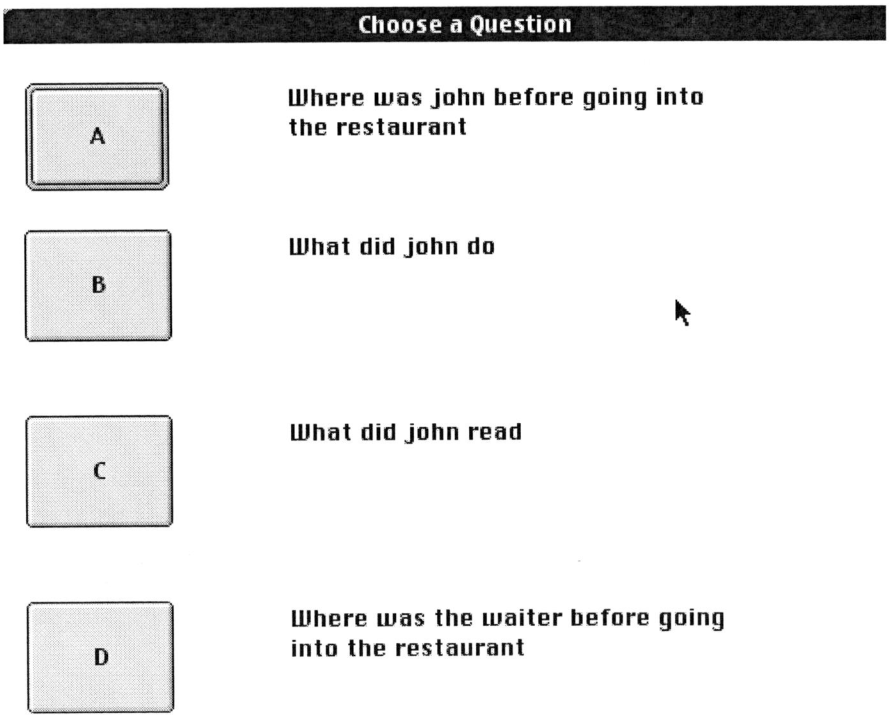

Figure 6. Four randomly chosen questions from the set of automatically generated questions.

The student is then presented with the set of possible answers automatically generated by the system. This time the student has to write the number of what he thinks might be an appropriate answer to the question he chose.

Theoretically, there may be two possible general cases:- right-wrong answers and consistent-inconsistent questions. But then also answers may either be consistent or inconsistent independently of their appropriateness. So the full list of possibilities is as follows:

a. the student chooses both a consistent question and a right and consistent answer;
b. the student chooses a consistent question and a wrong answer;
c. the student chooses a consistent question and a right but inconsistent answer;
d. the student chooses an inconsistent question and a right but inconsistent answer;
e. the student chooses an inconsistent question and a wrong and inconsistent answer;
f. the student chooses a consistent question but there is no inferrable available answer from the context.

However, the problem is how to give cooperative responses in case of semantic inconsistency. Mistakes may be made either because the student did not fully understand the semantic relations explicitely stated in the text, or else because the implicitely stated relations have not been grasped. So in the latter case, the mistake can be due to false or wrong presuppositions, violation of some pragmatic constraint related to the "restaurant" scenery, or some misconceptions. Here below is a listing of student-system interaction where Cooperative Assessment is shown:

A. ANSWER IS RIGHT

CASE 1. Right Question and Right Answer
Your question was the following : What has John begun
Your answer was the following : john has begun to read

COOPERATIVE ASSESSMENT
Your answer was right:
Your question was right and also semantically consistent
Your answer was right and also semantically consistent

CASE 2. - No information available in the text
Your question was the following : Where was the waiter before he was taking the order in the restaurant
Your answer was the following : We don_t know from text

COOPERATIVE ASSESSMENT
Your answer was right:
Your question was right and also semantically consistent
Your answer was right and also semantically consistent

CASE 3. - Pragmatically Inconsistent Question and Right Answer
Your question was the following : Did the restaurant read the book
Your answer was the following : The restaurant did not read the book

COOPERATIVE ASSESSMENT
Your answer was right:
Your question was pragmatically inconsistent
Your answer was right but pragmatically inconsistent

CASE 4. - Semantically Inconsistent Question and Right Answer
Your question was the following : Did the waiter read the book
Your answer was the following : The waiter did not read the book

COOPERATIVE ASSESSMENT
Your answer was right:
Your question was semantically inconsistent
Your answer was right but semantically inconsistent

B. ANSWER IS WRONG

CASE 5. - Semantically Consistent but Syntactically Wrong
Your question was the following : What did the waiter do
Your answer was the following : The waiter was taking the order

COOPERATIVE ASSESSMENT
Your answer was wrong:
Your question was wrong but semantically consistent
Your answer was syntactically wrong but semantically consistent

CASE 6. - Answer Wrong but Semantically Consistent
Your question was the following : What did john possess
Your answer was the following : I do not know what john possesses

COOPERATIVE ASSESSMENT
Your answer was right
Your question was wrong but semantically consistent
Your answer was wrong but semantically consistent

Recovery strategies have been set up by backretrieving information related to the wrong answer and then generate a message which is made up of two parts: an explanation of the error in a first sentence and the right answer in the second sentence.

Here below we show the list of all entities and the discourse structures generated by GETARUNS for the text in the Appendix which we already commented in Chapt. II above.

List of All Entities of the World Ranked by Relevance Score

```
entity(ind,id3,30,facts([
fact(infon5, inst_of, [ind:id3, class:man], 1, univ, univ),
fact(infon6, name, [john, id3], 1, univ, univ),
fact(id5, go, [agente:id3, locat:id4], 1, tes(f1_r01), id2),
fact(id8, sit, [actor:id3, locat:id7], 1, tes(f3_id8), id2),
fact(id14, take_order, [agente:id13, goal:id3], 1, tes(f1_r03), id2),
fact(infon64, poss, [john, id3, id19], 1, id1, id2),
fact(id20, read, [agente:id3, actor:id19], 1, tes(finf1_r05), id2),
fact(id22, begin, [actor:id3, prop:id20], 1, tes(f3_r05), id2)])).
entity(ind,id13,6,facts([
fact(infon40, inst_of, [ind:id13, class:social_role], 1, univ, univ),
fact(infon41, isa, [ind:id13, class:waiter], 1, id1, id2),
fact(infon42, role, [waiter, id2, id13], 1, id1, id2),
fact(id14, take_order, [agente:id13, goal:id3], 1, tes(f1_r03), id2)])).
entity(set,id16,5,facts([
fact(infon54, inst_of, [ind:id16, class:coll], 1, univ, univ),
fact(infon55, isa, [ind:id16, class:atmosphere], 1, id1, id2),
fact(infon57, [friendly, warm], [arg:id16], 1, id1, id2)])).
```

```
entity(ind,id4,2,facts([
fact(infon8, isa, [ind:id4, class:restaurant], 1, id1, id2),
fact(infon9, inst_of, [ind:id4, class:luogo], 1, univ, univ),
fact(id5, go, [agente:id3, locat:id4], 1, tes(f1_r01), id2),
fact(infon29, part_of, [restaurant, id10, id4], 1, id1, id2)])).
entity(ind,id7,1,facts([
in(infon22, id7, id2),
fact(infon20, inst_of, [ind:id7, class:thing], 1, univ, univ),
fact(infon21, isa, [ind:id7, class:table], 1, id1, id2),
fact(id8, sit, [actor:id3, locat:id7], 1, tes(f3_id8), id2),
fact(infon31, corner, [nil:id7], 1, id1, id2),
fact(id11, there_be, [tema_nonaff:id7, prop:infon31], 1, tes(f2_r02), id2),
fact(*, role, [waiter, id7, id13], 1, id1, id2)])).
entity(ind,id2,0,facts([
fact(infon42, role, [waiter, id2, id13], 1, id1, id2),
fact(infon3, main_sloc, [arg:restaurant], 1, _, _)])).
entity(ind,id19,0,facts([
fact(infon64, poss, [john, id3, id19], 1, id1, id2),
fact(infon66, inst_of, [ind:id19, class:thing], 1, univ, univ),
fact(infon67, isa, [ind:id19, class:book], 1, id1, id2),
fact(id20, read, [agente:id3, actor:id19], 1, tes(finf1_r05), id2)])).
entity(ind,id10,0,facts([
fact(infon27, inst_of, [ind:id10, class:thing], 1, univ, univ),
fact(infon28, isa, [ind:id10, class:corner], 1, id1, id2),
fact(infon29, part_of, [restaurant, id10, id4], 1, id1, id2)])).
```

List of Discourse Structures of the Texts

```
discourse_structures([
ds(to(1-1), 5-5, [main:id3:john, secondary:id16:atmosphere], begin([id3:john, id20:read],
    1, id2), after(tes(f3_r05), tes(f1_r01)), inception, 4-[5]),
ds(down(3-3), 4-4, [main:id3:john], be([infon57:[friendly, warm]], 1, id2),
    during(tes(f1_r04), tes(f1_r01)), explanation, 3-[4]),
ds(level(2-2), 3-3, [expected:id13:waiter, secondary:id3:john], take([id13:waiter,
    id3:exist], pol:1, id2), after(tes(f1_r03), tes(f1_r01)), narration, 2-[3]),
ds(down(1-1), 2-2, [main:id3:john], there_be([id7:table, infon31:corner], 1, id2),
    during(tes(f2_r02), tes(f1_r01)), explanation, 1-[2]),
ds(new(1-1), 1-1, [expected:id3:john], go([id3:john, id4:restaurant], 1, id2),
    undef(tes(f1_r01), tes(f1_r01)), narration, 1-[1])]).
```

Answers Generated

1. john has begun to read
2. john
3. john went into the restaurant
4. john ordered

5. the waiter took the order
6. there was a john in a restaurant
7. there was the book in the restaurant
8. there was the corner in the restaurant
9. there was the table in the restaurant
10. 10 there was the waiter in the restaurant
11. the waiter took the order
12. john reads
13. the book reads
14. john ordered something
15. john begins
16. john is reading
17. john is sitting
18. the table was there in restaurant
19. the waiter takes_order
20. john sat at the table
21. john was begining to read
22. john possesses a book in restaurant
23. the atmosphere was friendly and warm in restaurant
24. I do not know what john possesses
25. the atmosphere does not read
26. the corner does not read
27. the restaurant does not read
28. the table does not read
29. the waiter does not read
30. the atmosphere did not go into the restaurant
31. the book did not go into the restaurant
32. the corner did not go into the restaurant
33. the restaurant did not go into the restaurant
34. the table did not go into the restaurant
35. the waiter did not go into the restaurant
36. john was in the restaurant
37. the atmosphere did not read the book
38. the book did not read the book
39. the corner did not read the book
40. the restaurant did not read the book
41. the table did not read the book
42. the waiter did not read the book
43. We don_t know from text

Questions Generated

Who has taken the order?
Who was reading?
Did the corner read the book?
Did the waiter read the book?

Did the atmosphere read the book?
Did the restaurant read the book?
Did the table read the book?
Where was john sitting?
What has John begun?
Who has begun doing something?
How was the atmosphere?
Who went into the restaurant?
Who has ordered?
Who has taken the order?
Who was sitting at the table?
What was there in the restaurant?
Did the corner go into the restaurant?
Did the waiter go into the restaurant?
Did the atmosphere go into the restaurant?
Did the book go into the restaurant?
Did the table go into the restaurant?
What did john order?
What did john possess?
What did the waiter do?
What did the book do?
What did john do?
What did the table do?
Where was john after he was going into the restaurant?
Where was john while he was going into the restaurant?
Where was john before he was going into the restaurant?
Where was the waiter before going into the restaurant?
Where was the waiter after he was going into the restaurant?

4. Question Answering from a General Text

Question/Answering and Summarization are by far the best benchmark for any system that aims at showing how good the semantic mapping has been. We will show how GETARUNS computes the DM by presenting the output of the system for the "Maple Syrup" text made available by Mitre for the ANLP2000 Workshop(see Hirschman et al). Here below is the original text which is followed by the DM only relatively to the linguistic material needed to answer the five questions, though.

How Maple Syrup is Made
Maple syrup comes from sugar maple trees. At one time, maple syrup was used to make sugar. This is why the tree is called a "sugar" maple tree. Sugar maple trees make sap. Farmers collect the sap. The best time to collect sap is in February and March. The nights must be cold and the days warm. The farmer drills a few small holes in each tree. He puts a spout in each hole. Then he hangs a bucket on the end of each spout. The bucket has a cover to keep rain and snow out. The sap drips into the bucket. About 10 gallons of sap come from each hole.

4.1. Discourse Model for the Text Organized Sentence by Sentence

1. How Maple Syrup is Made
   ind(infon1, id1)
   fact(infon2, inst_of, [ind:id1, class:manner], 1, univ, univ)
   fact(infon3, isa, [ind:id1, class:way], 1, univ, univ)
   class(infon4, id2)
   fact(infon5, inst_of, [ind:id2, class:[edible, substance], 1, univ, univ)
   fact(infon6, isa, [ind:id2, class:maple_syrup], 1, univ, univ)
   fact(infon9, isa, [arg:id3, arg:exist], 1, univ, univ)
   fact(id4, make, [agent:id3, theme_aff:id2], 1, tes(f2_es1), univ)
   fact(infon10, isa, [arg:id4, arg:ev], 1, tes(f2_es1), univ)
   fact(infon11, isa, [arg:id5, arg:tloc], 1, tes(f2_es1), univ)
   fact(infon12, pres, [arg:id5], 1, tes(f2_es1), univ)
   during(tes(f1_es7), tes(f1_es6))
   includes(tr(f3_es1), univ)

2. Maple syrup comes from sugar maple trees
   loc(infon24, id8, [arg:main_sloc, arg:tree])
   fact(infon26, sugar_maple, [ind:id10], 1, univ, id8)
   set(infon28, id10)
   card(infon29, id10, 5)
   fact(infon30, inst_of, [ind:id10, class:plant_life], 1, univ, univ)
   fact(infon31, isa, [ind:id10, class:tree], 1, univ, id8)
   fact(infon32, maple, [nil:id10], 1, univ, id8)
   fact(id11, come, [actor:id2, locat:id10], 1, tes(f1_es2), id8)
   fact(infon35, isa, [arg:id11, arg:ev], 1, tes(f1_es2), id8)
   fact(infon36, isa, [arg:id12, arg:tloc], 1, tes(f1_es2), id8)
   fact(infon37, pres, [arg:id12], 1, tes(f1_es2), id8)
   during(tes(f1_es2), tes(f1_es7))
   includes(tr(f1_es2), univ)

3. At one time, maple syrup was used to make sugar
   class(infon42, id13)
   fact(infon43, inst_of, [ind:id13, class:substance], 1, univ, univ)

fact(infon44, isa, [ind:id13, class:sugar], 1, univ, id8)
fact(id14, make, [agent:id2, theme_aff:id13], 1, tes(finf1_es3), id8)
fact(infon47, isa, [arg:id14, arg:ev], 1, tes(finf1_es3), id8)
fact(infon48, isa, [arg:id15, arg:tloc], 1, tes(finf1_es3), id8)
fact(infon49, pres, [arg:id15], 1, tes(finf1_es3), id8)
fact(id16, use, [theme_aff:id2, result:id14], 1, tes(f2_es3), id8)
fact(infon51, isa, [arg:id16, arg:pr], 1, tes(f2_es3), id8)
fact(infon52, isa, [arg:id17, arg:tloc], 1, tes(f2_es3), id8)
fact(infon53, trap_pross, [arg:id17], 1, tes(f2_es3), id8)
fact(infon55, at_one_time, [arg:id16], 1, tes(f2_es3), id8)
before(tes(f2_es3), nil)
includes(tr(f2_es3), univ)

4. This is why the tree is called a "sugar" maple tree
ent(infon61, id18)
fact(infon62, prop, [arg:id18, disc_set:[id16:use:[theme_aff:id9, result:id14]]], 1, univ, id8)
ind(infon63, id19)
fact(infon64, tree, [nil:id19], 1, univ, id8)
fact(infon65, inst_of, [ind:id19, class:plant_life], 1, univ, univ)
fact(infon66, isa, [ind:id19, class:tree], 1, univ, id8)
in(infon67, id19, id10)
ind(infon68, id20)
fact(infon69, inst_of, [ind:id20, class:thing], 1, univ, univ)
fact(infon70, isa, [ind:id20, class:reason], 1, univ, id8)
fact(infon72, reason, [nil:id18], 1, univ, id8)
fact(id21, be, [prop:infon72], 1, tes(f15_es4), id8)
fact(id22, call, [actor:id19, theme:id10, prop:infon72], 1, tes(f15_es4), id8)
fact(infon73, isa, [arg:id22, arg:st], 1, tes(f15_es4), id8)
fact(infon74, isa, [arg:id23, arg:tloc], 1, tes(f15_es4), id8)
fact(infon75, pres, [arg:id23], 1, tes(f15_es4), id8)
during(tes(f15_es4), tes(f2_es3))
includes(tr(f15_es4), univ)

5. Sugar maple trees make sap
class(infon85, id24)
fact(infon86, inst_of, [ind:id24, class:substance], 1, univ, univ)
fact(infon87, isa, [ind:id24, class:sap], 1, univ, id8)
fact(id26, make, [agent:id10, theme_aff:id24], 1, tes(f1_es5), id8)
fact(infon92, isa, [arg:id26, arg:ev], 1, tes(f1_es5), id8)
fact(infon93, isa, [arg:id27, arg:tloc], 1, tes(f1_es5), id8)
fact(infon94, pres, [arg:id27], 1, tes(f1_es5), id8)
during(tes(f1_es5), tes(f15_es4))
includes(tr(f1_es5), univ)

6. Farmers collect the sap
   class(infon100, id28)
   fact(infon101, inst_of, [ind:id28, class:man], 1, univ, univ)
   fact(infon102, isa, [ind:id28, class:farmer], 1, univ, id8)
   fact(id29, collect, [agent:id28, theme_aff:id24], 1, tes(f1_es6), id8)
   fact(infon105, isa, [arg:id29, arg:ev], 1, tes(f1_es6), id8)
   fact(infon106, isa, [arg:id30, arg:tloc], 1, tes(f1_es6), id8)
   fact(infon107, pres, [arg:id30], 1, tes(f1_es6), id8)
   during(tes(f1_es6), tes(f1_es5))
   includes(tr(f1_es6), univ)

7. The best time to collect sap is in February and March
   ind(infon112, id31)
   fact(infon113, inst_of, [ind:id31, class:substance], 1, univ, univ)
   fact(infon114, isa, [ind:id31, class:sap], 1, univ, id8)
   in(infon115, id31, id24)
   ind(infon116, id32)
   fact(infon117, best, [ind:id32], 1, univ, id8)
   fact(infon118, inst_of, [ind:id32, class:time], 1, univ, univ)
   fact(infon119, isa, [ind:id32, class:time], 1, univ, id8)
   set(infon120, id33)
   card(infon121, 2)
   fact(infon122, inst_of, [ind:id33, class:time], 1, univ, univ)
   fact(infon123, isa, [ind:id33, class:[march, February]], 1, univ, id8)
   fact(id35, collect, [agent:id28, theme_aff:id31], 1, tes(finf1_es7), id8)
   fact(infon126, isa, [arg:id35, arg:ev], 1, tes(finf1_es7), id8)
   fact(infon127, isa, [arg:id36, arg:tloc], 1, tes(finf1_es7), id8)
   fact(infon128, nil, [arg:id36], 1, tes(finf1_es7), id8)
   fact(infon130, [march, February], [arg:id32], 1, univ, id8)
   fact(id37, be, [prop:id35, prop:infon130], 1, tes(f1_es7), id8)
   fact(infon131, isa, [arg:id37, arg:st], 1, tes(f1_es7), id8)
   fact(infon132, isa, [arg:id38, arg:tloc], 1, tes(f1_es7), id8)
   fact(infon133, pres, [arg:id38], 1, tes(f1_es7), id8)
   during(tes(f1_es7), tes(f1_es6))
   includes(tr(f1_es7), univ)

8. The nights must be cold and the days warm
   ind(infon139, id39)
   fact(infon140, cold, [nil:id39], 1, univ, id8)
   fact(infon141, inst_of, [ind:id39, class:time], 1, univ, univ)
   fact(infon142, isa, [ind:id39, class:night], 1, univ, id8)
   in(infon143, id39, id32)
   ind(infon144, id40)
   fact(infon145, warm, [nil:id40], 1, univ, id8)
   fact(infon146, inst_of, [ind:id40, class:time], 1, univ, univ)
   fact(infon147, isa, [ind:id40, class:day], 1, univ, id8)

```
in(infon148, id40, id32)
fact(id41, be, [theme_bound:id32], 1, tes(f1_es8), id8)
fact(infon150, isa, [arg:id41, arg:st], 1, tes(f1_es8), id8)
fact(infon151, isa, [arg:id42, arg:tloc], 1, tes(f1_es8), id8)
fact(infon152, nil, [arg:id42], 1, tes(f1_es8), id8)
fact(id43, be, [theme_bound:id32], 1, tes(f3_es8), id8)
fact(infon155, isa, [arg:id43, arg:st], 1, tes(f3_es8), id8)
fact(infon156, isa, [arg:id44, arg:tloc], 1, tes(f3_es8), id8)
fact(infon157, nil, [arg:id44], 1, tes(f3_es8), id8)
during(tes(f1_es8), tes(f3_es8))
includes(tr(f4_es8), univ)
```

9. The farmer drills a few small holes in each tree

```
fact(infon164, small, [ind:id45], 1, univ, id8)
fact(infon165, inst_of, [ind:id45, class:place], 1, univ, univ)
fact(infon166, isa, [ind:id45, class:holes], 1, univ, univ)
fact(id47, drill, [agent:id28, theme_aff:id45], 1, tes(f1_es9), id8)
fact(infon170, isa, [arg:id47, arg:ev], 1, tes(f1_es9), id8)
fact(infon171, isa, [arg:id48, arg:tloc], 1, tes(f1_es9), id8)
fact(infon172, pres, [arg:id48], 1, tes(f1_es9), id8)
fact(infon173, in, [arg:id45, locat:id10], 1, tes(f1_es9), id8)
during(tes(f1_es9), tes(f1_es8))
includes(tr(f1_es9), univ)
```

10. He puts a spout in each hole

```
class(infon178, id49)
fact(infon179, inst_of, [ind:id49, class:thing], 1, univ, univ)
fact(infon180, isa, [ind:id49, class:spout], 1, univ, id8)
class(infon181, id50)
fact(infon182, inst_of, [ind:id50, class:place], 1, univ, univ)
fact(infon183, isa, [ind:id50, class:hole], 1, univ, univ)
in(infon184, id50, id45)
fact(id51, put, [agent:id28, theme_aff:id49, locat:id50], 1, tes(f1_es10), id8)
fact(infon187, isa, [arg:id51, arg:ev], 1, tes(f1_es10), id8)
fact(infon188, isa, [arg:id52, arg:tloc], 1, tes(f1_es10), id8)
fact(infon189, pres, [arg:id52], 1, tes(f1_es10), id8)
during(tes(f1_es10), tes(f1_es9))
includes(tr(f1_es10), univ)
```

11. Then he hangs a bucket on the end of each spout

```
class(infon196, id54)
fact(infon197, inst_of, [ind:id54, class:thing], 1, univ, univ)
fact(infon198, isa, [ind:id54, class:bucket], 1, id53, id8)
fact(infon201, isa, [arg:id55, arg:end], 1, id53, id8)
fact(infon202, isa, [arg:id56, arg:spout], 1, id53, id8)
fact(infon203, of, [arg:id55, specif:id56], 1, id53, id8)
```

fact(id57, hang, [agent:id28, theme_aff:id54], 1, tes(f1_es11), id8)
fact(infon205, isa, [arg:id57, arg:ev], 1, tes(f1_es11), id8)
fact(infon206, isa, [arg:id58, arg:tloc], 1, tes(f1_es11), id8)
fact(infon207, pres, [arg:id58], 1, tes(f1_es11), id8)
fact(infon209, then, [arg:id57], 1, tes(f1_es11), id8)
during(tes(f1_es11), tes(f1_es10))
includes(tr(f1_es11), id53)

12. The bucket has a cover to keep rain and snow out
class(infon218, id59)
fact(infon219, inst_of, [ind:id59, class:thing], 1, univ, univ)
fact(infon220, isa, [ind:id59, class:cover], 1, id53, id8)
fact(infon222, cover, [nil:id54], 1, id53, id8)
fact(id60, have, [actor:id54, prop:infon222], 1, tes(f1_es12), id8)
fact(infon223, isa, [arg:id60, arg:st], 1, tes(f1_es12), id8)
fact(infon224, isa, [arg:id61, arg:tloc], 1, tes(f1_es12), id8)
fact(infon225, pres, [arg:id61], 1, tes(f1_es12), id8)
fact(infon227, isa, [arg:id62, arg:rain], 1, tes(f1_es12), id8)
fact(infon228, isa, [arg:id63, arg:snow], 1, tes(f1_es12), id8)
fact(id65, keep_out, [agent:id54, theme_aff:id64], 1, tes(finf1_es12), id8)
fact(infon229, isa, [arg:id65, arg:pr], 1, tes(finf1_es12), id8)
fact(infon230, isa, [arg:id66, arg:tloc], 1, tes(finf1_es12), id8)
fact(infon231, pres, [arg:id66], 1, tes(finf1_es12), id8)
fact(infon233, coincide, [arg:id60, prop:id65], 1, tes(f1_es12), id8)
during(tes(f1_es12), tes(f1_es11))
includes(tr(f1_es12), id53)

13. The sap drips into the bucket
fact(id67, drip, [agent:id31], 1, tes(f1_es13), id8)
fact(infon247, isa, [arg:id67, arg:ev], 1, tes(f1_es13), id8)
fact(infon248, isa, [arg:id68, arg:tloc], 1, tes(f1_es13), id8)
fact(infon249, pres, [arg:id68], 1, tes(f1_es13), id8)
fact(infon252, into, [arg:id67, nil:id31, loc_direct:id54], 1, tes(f1_es13), id8)
during(tes(f1_es13), tes(f1_es12))
includes(tr(f1_es13), id53)

14. About 10 gallons of sap come from each hole
set(infon259, id69)
card(infon260, id69, 10)
fact(infon261, inst_of, [ind:id69, class:substance], 1, univ, univ)
fact(infon262, isa, [ind:id69, class:sap], 1, id53, id8)
in(infon263, id69, id24)
class(infon264, id70)
fact(infon265, inst_of, [ind:id70, class:place], 1, univ, univ)
fact(infon266, isa, [ind:id70, class:hole], 1, id53, id8)
in(infon267, id70, id50)

fact(id71, come, [agent:id69, theme_aff:id70], 1, tes(f1_es14), id8)
fact(infon271, isa, [arg:id71, arg:ev], 1, tes(f1_es14), id8)
fact(infon272, isa, [arg:id72, arg:tloc], 1, tes(f1_es14), id8)
fact(infon273, pres, [arg:id72], 1, tes(f1_es14), id8)
during(tes(f1_es14), tes(f1_es13))
includes(tr(f1_es14), id53)

4.2.Question-Answering from the Discourse Model

Coming now to Question-Answering, the system accesses the DM at first looking for relations, then for entities : entities are searched according to the form of the focussed element in the User DataBase of Question-Facts as shown below with the QDM for the first question, « Who collects maple sap? »:

User Question-Facts Discourse Model

q_loc(infon3, id1, [arg:main_tloc, arg:tr(f1_free_a)])
q_ent(infon4, id2)
q_fact(infon5, isa, [ind:id2, class:who], 1, id1, univ)
q_fact(infon6, inst_of, [ind:id2, class:man], 1, univ, univ)
q_class(infon7, id3)
q_fact(infon8, inst_of, [ind:id3, class:coll], 1, univ, univ)
q_fact(infon9, isa, [ind:id3, class:sap], 1, id1, univ)
q_fact(infon10, focus, [arg:id2], 1, id1, univ)
q_fact(id4, collect, [agent:id2, theme_aff:id3], 1, tes(f1_free_a), univ)
q_fact(infon13, isa, [arg:id4, arg:pr], 1, tes(f1_free_a), univ)
q_fact(infon14, isa, [arg:id5, arg:tloc], 1, tes(f1_free_a), univ)
q_fact(infon15, pres, [arg:id5], 1, tes(f1_free_a), univ)

The system replies correctly to all the questions reported here below. As to question 4, at first the system takes « come from » to be answered exhaustively by sentence 14 ; however, seen that « hole » is not computed with a « location » semantic role, it searches the DM for a better answer which is the relation linguistically expressed in sentence 9, where « holes » are drilled « in each tree ». The « tree » is the Main Location of the whole story and « hole » in sentence 9 is inferentially linked to « hole » in sentence 14, by a chain of inferential inclusions. In fact, come_from does not figure in WordNet even though it does in our dictionary of synonyms. As to the fifth question, the system replies correctly.

2. What does the farmer hang from a spout? (A bucket)
3. When is sap collected? (February and March)
4. Where does the maple sap come from? (Sugar maple trees)
5. Why is the bucket covered? (to keep rain and snow out)

As far as anaphora resolution is concerned, the Higher Module computes the appropriate antecedent for the big Pro of the arbitrary SUBject of the infinitive in sentence n. 7, where the collecting action would have been left without an agent. This resolution of anaphora is triggered by the parser decision to treat the big Pro as an arbitrary pronominal and this information is stored at lexical level in the subcategorization frame for the name « time ».

With question n.4 the text only makes available information related to « maple syrup ». Since we start looking for relation, and the « come from » relation has a different linguistic description as SUBJect argument, what we do is to try and see whether there is some inferential link between « sap » and « syrup ». This is not the case seen that WordNet does not link the two concepts explicitly. However both are classified as « substance » thus allowing the required inference to be fired – both are also taken as synonyms in our dictionary. The final question does not constitute a problem seen that the predicate «cover» has become a semantic relation and is no longer a noun or a verb. Also worth noting is the fact that the question is not a real passive, but a quasi-passive or an ergative construction, so no agent should be searched for.

We implemented also another possible and interesting « Why » question:

6. Why is the tree called sugar maple tree?

The answer computed by the system is *"because maple syrup was used to make sugar"*. This answer can be recovered seen that the corresponding sentence has received an appropriate grammatical and semantic analysis. In particular, the discourse deictic pronoun « This » has been bound to the previous main relation « use » and its arguments so that they can be used to answer the « Why » question appropriately. Here below we report the f-structure and the Discourse Model for this question. The interesting point is that, as happens for "why" questions in general – the interrogative pronoun is transformed by the parser into an adjunct whose head is the word REASON. This is then used to search the previous Discourse Model derived for the text analyzed.

```
[why, is, the, tree, called, sugar, maple, tree, ?]

focus:focus_type:interrogative
    index:sn1
    cat:[reason]
    pred:why
    case:[obl]
    tab_ref:[-ref, -pro, -ana, +me]
perform:ask
index:f2
pred:call
lex_form:[np/obj/theme_bound/[inform, legale social], xcomp/prop/[any]]
voice:passive
mood:ind
tense:pres
cat:achiev
subj/theme_bound:indice:sn2
        cat:[abstract, inform, plant, techno]
        pred:tree
        num:sing
```

```
                pers:3
                spec:def:+
                tab_ref:[+ref, -pro, -ana, +class]
    ncomp/prop:indice:sn6
            cat:[ abstract, inform, plant, techno]
            pred:tree
            num:sing
            pers:3
            spec:def:'0'
            subj/nil:index:sn7
                pred:vbl
                controller:sn2
                tab_ref:[+ref, -pro, -ana, -me]
            mods:mod/theme:index:sn4
                    cat:[edible, object, substance]
                    pred:sugar
                    num:sing
                    pers:3
                    tab_ref:[+ref, -pro, -ana, +class]
                mod/tema:index:sn5
                    cat:[plant]
                    pred:maple
                    num:sing
                    pers:3
                    tab_ref:[+ref, -pro, -ana, +class]
            tab_ref:[+ref, -pro, -ana, +class]
    adjs:adj/modal:sem_mark:for
                obj/nil:index:sn3
                    cat:[reason]
                    pred:vbl
                    controller:sn1
                    tab_ref:[+ref, -pro, -ana, -me]
    aspect:achiev
    rel1:[td(f2_q6)=tr(f2_q6)]
    rel2:[included(tr(f2_q6), tes(f2_q6))]
    specific:-
    ref_int:[tr(f2_q6)]
```

So our conclusion is that the heart of a Q/A system should be a strongly restrictive pipeline of linguistically based modules which alone can ensure the adequate information for the knowledge representation and the reasoning processes required to answer natural language queries.

4.3. Evaluating GETARUNS Approach to QA

Totally shallow approaches when compared to ours will always be lacking sufficient information for semantic processing at propositional level: in other words, as happens with our "Partial" modality, there will be no possibility of checking for precision in producing predicate-argument structures.

Most systems would use some Word Matching algorithm that counts the number of words that appear in both the question and the sentence being considered after stripping them of stopwords: usually two words will match if they share the same morphological root after some stemming has taken place. Most QA systems presented in the literature rely on the classification of words into two classes: function and content words. They don't make use of a Discourse Model where input text has been transformed via a rigorous semantic mapping algorithm: they rather access tagged input text in order to sort best match words, phrases or sentences according to some matching scoring function.

It is also common knowledge the fact that only introducing or increasing the amount of linguistic knowledge over crude IR-based systems will contribute substantial improvements. In particular, systems based on simple Named-Entity identification tasks are too rigid to be able to match phrase relations constraints often involved in a natural language query.

First objection is the impossibility to take into account pronominal expressions, their relations and properties as belonging to the antecedent, if no head transformation has taken place during the analysis process.

Second objection is the use of grammatical function labels, like SUBJ/OBJects without an evaluation of their relevance in the utterance structure: higher level or main clause SUBJ/OBJects are more important than other SUBJects. In addition, there is no attempt at semantic role assignment which would come from a basic syntactic/semantic tagging of governing verbs: a distinction into movement verbs, communication verbs, copulative verbs, psychic verbs etc. would suffice to assign semantic roles to main arguments if present.

It is usually the case that QA systems divide the question to be answered into two parts: the Question Target represented by the wh- word and the rest of the sentence; otherwise the words making up the yes/no question and then a match takes place in order to identify most likely answers in relation to the rest/whole of the sentence except for stopwords.

However, it is just the semantic relations that need to be captured and not just the words making up the question that matter. Some system implemented more sophisticated methods (notably Hovy et al.; Litkowski): syntactic-semantic question analysis. This involves a robust syntactic-semantic parser to analyze the question and candidate answers, and a matcher that combines word- and parse-tree-level information to identify answer passages more precisely.

4.4. Answering Generic Question

An important issue in QA is answering generic questions on the "aboutness" of the text, questions which may be answered by producing appropriate headlines or just a title. In our system, given the concomitant work of anaphora resolution modules and the semantic mapping into predicate-argument structures, this can be made as follows. The system collapses all entities and their properties, relations and attributes after the text has been fully analysed by collecting them for each ontological type under each semantic individual. At the same time, each semantic id receives a score for topichood thus allowing a ranking of the entities. Here below we list the most relevant entities of the text reported above:

```
entity(set,id8,30,facts([
card(infon23, id8, 5),
fact(infon24, sugar_maple, [ind:id8], 1, T, P),
fact(infon25, inst_of, [ind:id8, class:plant_life], 1, T, P),
fact(infon26, isa, [ind:id8, class:tree], 1, T, P),
fact(id11, come, [actor:id2, locat:id8], 1, T, P),
fact(id25, make, [agent:id8, theme_aff:id23, patient:id24], 1, T, P)])).

entity(class,id2,115,facts([
fact(infon3, 'Maple', [ind:id2], 1, T, P),
fact(infon4, inst_of, [ind:id2, class:edible_animal], 1, T, P),
fact(infon5, isa, [ind:id2, class:'Syrup'], 1, T, P),
fact(id5, make, [theme_bound:id2, agent:id4], 1, T, P),
fact(id11, come, [actor:id2, locat:id8], 1, T, P),
fact(id14, make, [agent:id2, theme_aff:id13], 1, T, P),
fact(id16, use, [theme_aff:id2, result:id14], 1, T, P)])).

entity(class,id30,77,facts([
fact(infon114, inst_of, [ind:id30, class:man], 1, T, P),
fact(infon115, isa, [ind:id30, class:farmer], 1, T, P),
fact(id39, drill, [agent:id30, theme_aff:id38], 1, T, P),
fact(id42, put, [agent:id30, theme_aff:id41, locat:id38], 1, T, P),
fact(id48, hang, [agent:id30, theme_aff:id44], 1, T, P)])).

entity(ind,id13,10,facts([
in(infon48, id13, id9),
fact(infon46, inst_of, [ind:id13, class:substance], 1, T, P),
fact(infon47, isa, [ind:id13, class:sugar], 1, T, P),
fact(id14, make, [agente:id2, theme_aff:id13], 1, T, P),
fact(*, inst_of, [ind:id13, class:maple], 1, T, P),
fact(*, isa, [ind:id13, class:maple], 1, T, P),
fact(*, isa, [ind:id13, class:sugar_maple], 1, T, P),
fact(*, of, [arg:id10, specif:id13], 1, T, P)])).
```

Where starred facts are inherited by the inclusion relation specified by the “in” semantic predicate. For instance, the fact constituted by a “specifying” relation between “sugar” and “maple” as

```
fact(infon34, of, [arg:id10, specif:id9], 1, univ, univ)
```

becomes a starred fact inherited by id13 in force of the inclusion relation,

```
in(infon48, id13, id9)
```

In this way, an appropriate answer to the question “What is the text about” can be generated directly from the entity list by picking up relations and properties of the most relevant individuals, sets and classes: that's what we have dubbed as "Focalized wh-questions" in the sense that they focus on one single character. One such question is reported below and has been formulated on the Story of the 3 Little Pigs in Italian.

Che cosa è accaduto al lupo? /What happened to the wolf

```
q_ind(infon1, id1)
q_fact(infon2, inst_of, [ind:id1, class:animal_ferocious], 1, univ, univ)
q_fact(infon3, isa, [ind:id1, class:lupo], 1, univ, univ)
q_fact(infon4, isa, [ind:id1, class:lupo], 1, univ, univ)
q_ind(infon5, id2)
q_fact(infon6, isa, [ind:id2, class:thing], 1, univ, univ)
q_fact(infon7, inst_of, [ind:id2, class:thing], 1, univ, univ)
q_fact(infon8, focus, [arg:id2], 1, univ, univ)
q_fact(id3, accadere, [theme_unaff:id2, theme _aff:id1], 1, univ, univ)
q_fact(infon11, isa, [arg:id3, arg:ev], 1, univ, univ)
q_fact(infon12, isa, [arg:id4, arg:tloc], 1, univ, univ)
q_fact(infon13, pass_pross, [arg:id4], 1, univ, univ)
q_fact(infon14, time, [arg:id3, arg:id4], 1, univ, univ)
q_fact(infon18, perf, [arg:id5, ask:id3], 1, univ, univ)
```

The answer is constituted by the list of predicate-argument structures involving the character's related events. It is also made up of a so-called "Focalized Summary" of the story which includes only those sentences in which the character is referred to, directely or indirectly – by means of anaphora resolution. Of course this could be generated from PAS but the result would have been narratively speaking much poorer.

```
###################### FOCALIZED PAS #########################
vivere [actor:lupo, locative:luogo]
proteggere [agent:pPro, experiencer:porcellino, malef:lupo]
apparire [actor:lupo]
pensare [actor:lupo, goal:jimmi]
pensare [actor:lupo, prop:penetrare]
mettersi [actor:lupo, prop:osservare]
avere_calcagna [experiencer:porcellino, actor:lupo]
arrivare [theme_aff:lupo]
riempire [agent:lupo, tema_aff:polmone, matter:aria]
accasciarsi [experiencer:lupo, prop:in]
```

###################### FOCALIZED SUMMARY #####################

C'erano una volta tre fratelli porcellini che vivevano felici nella campagna. Nello stesso luogo però viveva anche un terribile lupo che si nutriva proprio di porcellini grassi e teneri .

Questi allora, per proteggersi dal lupo, decisero di costruirsi ciascuno una casetta.

Ma ecco che improvvisamente il lupo apparve alle loro spalle.

Aiuto , aiuto gridarono i due porcellini e cominciarono a correre più veloci che potevano verso la loro casetta per sfuggire al terribile lupo. Finalmente i porcellini riuscirono a raggiungere la loro casetta e vi si chiusero dentro sbarrando la porta. Dalla finestra cominciarono a deridere il lupo cantando la solita canzoncina: chi ha paura del lupo cattivo. Esso si mise ad osservare attentamente la casetta e notò che non era davvero molto solida. Soffiò con forza un paio di volte e la casetta si sfasciò completamente.

Fecero appena in tempo ad entrare e tirare il chiavistello.

Sicuro di abbattere anche la casetta di mattoni il lupo si riempì i polmoni di aria e cominciò a soffiare con forza alcune volte.

Riconoscenti i due porcellini oziosi promisero al fratello che da quel giorno anche essi avrebbero lavorato sodo.

In case the question were addressing the deeds of the two lazy little pigs, the result would have been as follows:

Che cosa è accaduto ai due porcellini pigri? /What happened to the two lazy little pigs

###################### FOCALIZED PAS ########################

sbrigarsi [agent:porcellino, modal:fretta]
passare [theme_unaff:porcellino, time:giornata]
suonare [experiencer:porcellino]
cantare [experiencer:porcellino, theme_unaff:canzone]
gridare [agent:porcellino, prop:[aiuto, aiuto]]
riuscire [agent:porcellino, prop:raggiungere]
chiudere [agent:porcellino, theme_aff:si]
cominciare [agent:porcellino, prop:deridere]
cantare [experiencer:porcellino, theme_unaff:canzone]
correre [agent:porcellino, loc_direct:casa, prop:perdifiato]
fare [agent:porcellino, patient:exist, prop:entrare]
promettere [actor:porcellino, goal:jimmi, propint:lavorare]

##################### FOCALIZED SUMMARY ####################

C'erano una volta tre fratelli porcellini che vivevano felici nella campagna. Gli altri, Timmy e Tommy, pigri e oziosi se la sbrigarono in fretta costruendo le loro casette con la paglia e con pezzetti di legno.

Ma ecco che improvvisamente il lupo apparve alle loro spalle .

Aiuto, aiuto gridarono i due porcellini e cominciarono a correre più veloci che potevano verso la loro casetta per sfuggire al terribile lupo. Finalmente i porcellini riuscirono a raggiungere la loro casetta e vi si chiusero dentro sbarrando la porta. Dalla finestra cominciarono a deridere il lupo cantando la solita canzoncina: chi ha paura del lupo cattivo. Esso si mise ad osservare attentamente la casetta e notò che non era davvero molto solida.

Fecero appena in tempo ad entrare e tirare il chiavistello .

Sicuro di abbattere anche la casetta di mattoni il lupo si riempì i polmoni di aria e cominciò a soffiare con forza alcune volte .

Riconoscenti i due porcellini oziosi promisero al fratello che da quel giorno anche essi avrebbero lavorato sodo .

5. EVALUATING STUDENTS' SUMMARIES WITH GETARUNS

Evaluating summaries is currently performed by the use of statistically-based tools which lack any linguistic knowledge and are unable to produce grammatical and semantic judgements (Landauer et al., 1997). However, summary evaluation needs precise linguistic information with a much finer-grained coverage than what is being offered by currently available statistically based systems. We assume that the starting point of any interesting application in these fields must necessarily be a good syntactic-semantic parser. The heart of our system GETARUNS is a rule-based top-down parser, which uses an LFG oriented grammar organization. A less constrained version of the parser for the application field of text summarization allows the system to recover gracefully from failures. To this end, the parser is coupled with another concurrent parsing process: a partial or shallow parse is always produced and used to recover from complete failures. As discussed at length above, semantic processing is strongly modularized and distributed amongst a number of different submodules which take care of Spatio-Temporal Reasoning, Discourse Level Anaphora Resolution. Evaluation taps information from the Discourse Model and uses Predicate Argument Structures (PAS) to detect students' understanding of the text to summarize. It also uses the output of the Anaphora Resolution Module to check for most relevant topics in the text which the student should have addressed in his/her summary. The system uses a Topics-Stack while processing the text in order to corefer referential expressions: The Topic-Stack Hierarchy gauges nominal heads as either Main, Secondary or Potential Topic. This grading is used as a score that allows the system to detect the most relevant entities in the text at the end of the computation.

Currently available summary and essay evaluation systems are basically based on statistical and mathematical procedures which are used to assess students linguistic abilities. We are here referring to such tools as LSA-based Summary Street®. Latent Semantic Analysis (Landauer T. et al, 1997) is a statistical theory of meaning which tells the student "…how well your summary covers the information in the original text. It will tell you if your summary is too long for a good summary." It is unable to check for grammaticality issues, neither coherence nor cohesiveness is checked, and what is worse no semantic soundness can be checked. LSA techniques simply allow looking for semantic similarities through comparison of most frequent content words with a knowledge of the surrounding most frequent content words at sentence and paragraph level. LSA does not take into account content words with frequency of occurrence equal/lower than two; nor does it take into account the order in which content words cooccur. It capture text similarity in terms of differences in word choice among different texts. This seems to me to be too poor a way of characterizing meaning: on the contrary, the authors speak of LSA as a tool that "captures a great deal of the similarity of meanings expressed in discourse", and use that as "…the basis for performing automated scoring of essays". Seen that LSA does not take into account word order and discards such important elements as negation items it follows that there is no way to tell whether simple coocurrence indicates similarity of meaning. The experiment commented in the same article is very uncouth. At first glance, Landauer et al. seem to be concerned only with destroying what has gone on in Syntactic Theory and its contribution to the determination of meaning. However in the following paragraph they come up with the opposite statement:

> The fact that LSA can capture as much of meaning as it does without using word order shows that the mere combination of words in passages constrains overall meaning very strongly. How can this be? In addition to the contrary theoretical presumptions mentioned earlier, various intuitive and rational arguments suggest that such representations must fall far short of extracting as much meaning from text as do human readers. For instance, the following two sentences are identical for LSA, but have very different meanings for a human reader: "It was not the sales manager who hit the bottle that day, but the office worker with the serious drinking problem."; "That day the office manager, who was drinking, hit the problem sales worker with a bottle, but it was not serious… Nonetheless, what such examples prove is only that a method that ignores word order cannot always render completely correct comprehension. [ibid:417]

Here it would seem that Landauer et al. recognize that LSA cannot possible capture the same amount of meaning from a text as human beings do, and the conclusions partially confirm this. If LSA is unable to distinguish sentences telling just the opposite of one another, than looking into what has gone on in Syntactic and Semantic Theory might be useful.

Another line of research is represented by the work of J.Burstein et al. who make use of NLP tools without however trying to build any kind of logical form or semantic representation. In their latest work they take advantage of discourse structure as built from syntactic structure. Discourse structure is used to determine whether essays produced by a test-taker contain as their most relevant parts topics which are regarded important for a given prompt. This seems to be a more effective line of research that tackles a specific task: that of assessing whether the essay produced covers most of the important topics and also presents them in a salient manner. This latter aspect can be captured nicely by the traversal of rhetorical structures built on the basis of syntactic structure as the authors comment in their work. So even though this is just one of the aspects to be looked into by a human assessor and does in no way cope with the issue of semantic soundness, semantic coherence and cohesion, it may still be a useful tool in itself.

5.1. Evaluating Summaries with PAS and Topic Relevance Scoring

The context in which the system is used for evaluation is with summary creation exercises in the area of newspaper stories for students of Foreign Languages and Literatures. The student is presented with a short text of approximately 800-1000 words length and is asked to shorten it to no more than 200 words by picking up the most relevant parts of it. He/she is also prompted to use the lexicon present in the text as much as possible. Our evaluation system will tap WordNet and other lexical resources for lexical items not present in the original text, but used by the student to create the summary : it looks for synonyms, hypernyms, hyponyms and other semantic relations in order to understand whether the new lexical item has been introduced with the appropriate meaning relation. In addition, this is done, starting from a complete semantic representation of the text, which constitutes the knowledge representation needed to cope with all semantic relations expressed in the text. Without such a representation, searching WordNet for synonyms would be a nonsensical operation. Systems such as the ones used in « bag-of-words » approaches would be unable to look for the appropriate meaning by simply selecting most frequent content words in context simply because meaning ambiguities must be ameneable to the context, i.e. the PAS in which the concept is expressed.

Coming now to the actual tools used for evaluation, the system produces a list of most relevant entities at the end of the computation, which includes for each entity all the properties asserted in the DM. In the case of the current text, - the Story of the 3 Little Pigs - this is the list generated:

List of Most Important Characters of the Text:

I. due fratelli porcellini, grassi oziosi pigri teneri
II. lupo, terribile
III. fratello jimmi porcellino, grasso tenero
La casa, piccola

The list is organized in order of relevance so that the most relevant character comes first. The system may then generate PAS as an answer to a question related to one specific character – this in case it is working in tutoring and coaching modality. The question – already shown above in section 4.4 - is computed by the system in the same way in which the text has been processed, except that it will not be part of the same DM. As shown above, the system is able to keep under strict control all PAS related to each entity in the text. This is the key to the semantically-driven evaluation phase.

5.2. Evaluating GETARUNS Approach to Essay Evaluation

We have just started experimenting with the system in simulation, using summaries produced by students on paper and comparing the judgements expressed by human tutors with the output of the algorithm: the results are encouraging. As proposed in Burstein (2000:56), we compare test summary with the full text and then evaluate the level of relevance by gauging the number of predicate-argument structures used and their semantic appropriateness. The results are encouraging, but work is needed to produce the didactic cooperative evaluation so that adequate feedback messages can be generated for each type of error or simply lack of coherence/cohesiveness, or still wrong focussing.

6. GETARUNS Approach to WEB-Q/A

Totally shallow approaches when compared to ours will always be lacking sufficient information for semantic processing at propositional level: in other words, as happens with our "Partial" modality, there will be no possibility of checking for precision in producing predicate-argument structures.

Most systems would use some Word Matching algorithm to count the number of words appearing in both question and the sentence being considered after stripping stopwords: usually two words will match if they share the same morphological root after some stemming has taken place. Most QA systems presented in the literature rely on the classification of words into two classes: function and content words. They don't make use of a Discourse Model where input text has been transformed via a rigorous semantic mapping algorithm: they rather access tagged input text in order to sort best matched words, phrases or sentences according to some scoring function. It is an accepted fact that introducing or increasing the amount of linguistic knowledge over crude IR-based systems will contribute substantial improvements. In particular, systems based on simple Named-Entity identification tasks are too rigid to be able to match phrase relations constraints often involved in a natural language query.

We raise a number of objections to these approaches: first objection is the impossibility to take into account pronominal expressions, their relations and properties as belonging to the antecedent, if no head transformation has taken place during the analysis process.

Another objection comes from the treatment of the Question: it is usually the case that QA systems divide the question to be answered into two parts: the Question Target represented by the wh- word and the rest of the sentence; otherwise the words making up the yes/no question are taken in their surface order, and then a match takes place to identify most likely answers in relation to the rest/whole of the sentence except for stopwords.

However, it is just the *semantic relations* that need to be captured and not just the words making up the question that matter. Some systems implemented more sophisticated methods (notably [22;23;24]) using syntactic-semantic question analysis. This involves a robust syntactic-semantic parser to analyze the question and candidate answers, and a matcher that combines word- and parse-tree-level information to identify answer passages more precisely.

6.1. A Prototype Q/A System for the Web

We experimented our approach over the web using 450 factoid questions from TREC. On a first run the base system only used an off-the-shelf tagger in order to recover main verb from the query. In this way we managed to get 67% correct results, i.e. the correct answer was contained in the best five snippets – out of ten - selected by the BOW system on the output of Google API. However, only 30% of the total correct results had the right snippet ranked in position one. To improved on that, we applied GETARUNS (shallow version) on the best five snippets with the intent of improving the automatic ranking of the system and have the best snippet always positioned as first candidate. Here below is a figure showing the main components for the GETARUNS based analysis, where we also included a number of additional modules used to interface the Semantic Web input-output format. The system is also interfaced with Protegé to check the appropriate ontology-encoded relations.

We will present two examples and discuss them in some detail. The questions are the following ones:

Q: Who was elected president of South Africa in 1994?
A: Nelson Mandela
Q: When was Abraham Lincoln born?
A: Lincoln was born February_12_1809

The answers produced by our system are indicated after each question. Now consider the best five snippets as filtered by the BOWs system:

who/WP was/VBD elected/VBN president/NN of/IN south/JJ africa/NN in/IN 1994/CD

Main keywords: president south africa 1994
Verb roots: elect
Google search: elected president south africa 1994

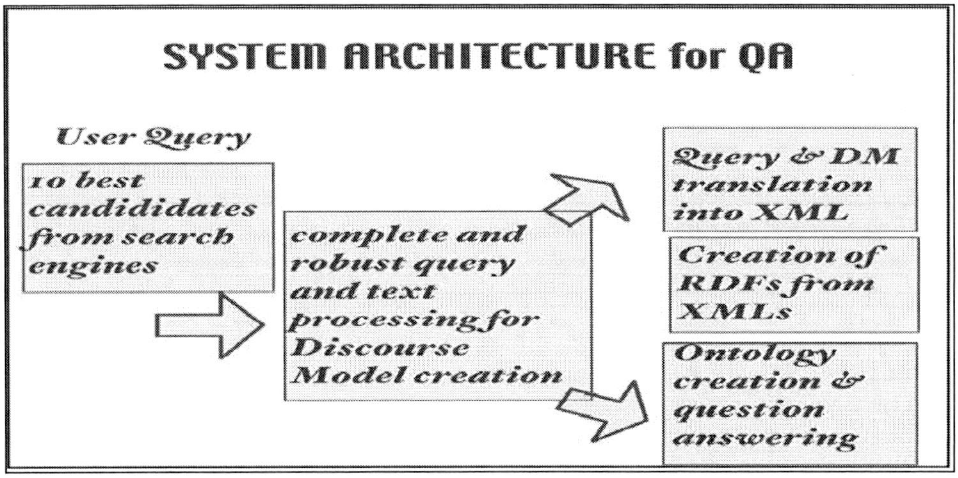

Figure 6. System Architecture for QA on the web.

1. On June 2, 1999, Mbeki, the pragmatic deputy president of South Africa and leader of the African National Congress, was elected president in a landslide, having already assumed many of Mandela's governing responsibilities shortly after Mandela won South Africa's first democratic election in 1994.
2. Washington ? President Bill Clinton announced yesterday a doubling in US assistance South Africa of $600-million (R2 160-million) over three years, and said his wife Hillary would attend Nelson Mandela's inauguration as the country's first black president.
3. Nelson Mandela, President of the African National Congress (ANC), casting the ballot in his country's first all-race elections, in April 1994 at Ohlange High School near Durban, South Africa.
4. Newly-elected President Nelson Mandela addressing the crowd from a balcony of the Town Hall in Pretoria, South Africa on May 10, 1994.
5. The CDF boycotted talks in King William's Town yesterday called by the South African government and the Transitional Executive Council to smooth the way for the peaceful reincorporation of the homeland into South Africa following the resignation of Oupa Gqozo as president.

Notice snippet n.1 where two presidents are present and two dates are reported for each one: however the relation “president” is only indicated for the wrong one, Mbeki and the system rejects it. The answer is collected from snippet no.4 instead. After computing the ADM, the system decides to rerank the snippets and use the contents of snippet 4 for the answer. Now the second question:

when/WRB was/VBD abraham/NN lincoln/NN born/VBN
Main keywords: abraham lincoln

Verb roots: bear

Google search: abraham lincoln born

1. Abraham Lincoln was born in a log cabin in Kentucky to Thomas and Nancy Lincoln.
2. Two months later on February 12, 1809, Abraham Lincoln was born in a one-room log cabin near the Sinking Spring.
3. Abraham Lincoln was born in a log cabin near Hodgenville, Kentucky.
4. Lincoln himself set the date of his birth at feb_ 12, 1809, though some have attempted to disprove that claim .
5. A. Lincoln (February 12, 1809 April 15, 1865) was the 16/th president of the United States of America.

In this case, snippet n.2 is selected by the system as the one containing the required information to answer the question. In both cases, the answer is built from the ADM, so it is not precisely the case that the snippets are selected for the answer: they are nonetheless reranked to make the answer available.

After running Web/QA with GETARUNS, the 450 questions recovered the whole of the original correct result 67% from first snippet.

BIBLIOGRAPHY

Abney, S. (1996), Part-of-Speech Tagging and Partial Parsing, in Ken Church, Steve Young, and Gerrit Bloothooft, eds. *Corpus-Based Methods in Language and Speech,* Kluwer Academic Publishers, Dordrecht.

Adorni G., et al.(1987), Integrating Logic Programming and Structured Knowledge Representation, Journal for the Integrated Study of Artificial Intelligence, Cognitive Science and Applied Epistemology, G.Adorni(ed.), *Cognitive Modelling,* Vol.4, 1, 1987, 7-21.

Alberti G.(1992), *Computing Grammatical Cues for Utterance and Text Understanding,* Unpublished Dissertation, University of Venice.

Allen J.F.(1983b), Maintaining Knowledge about Temporal Intervals, *Communications of the ACM,* 26,11, 832-843.

Allen J.F.(1984), Towards a General Theory of Action and Time, *Artificial Intelligence* 23, 123-154.

Allen J.F.(1994), N*atural Language Understanding,* The Benjaming/Cummings Pub.Co. Redwood City CA.

Appelt D.(1985), *Planning English Sentences,* C.U.P.

Appelt D.(1988), *Planning Natural-Language Referring Expressions.* In D. McDonald and L. Bolc (eds.).

Bach, E. (1982). *Purpose clauses and control.* In Jacobson, P. I. & Pullum, G. K. (eds.), *The nature of syntactic representation.* Dordrecht: Reidel. 35-57.

Balkanski, Cecile T. 1992, Action Relations in Rationale Clauses and Means Clauses, in Proc. COLING-*92*, Nantes, 267-273.

Bara B.G. (2007), *Cognitive Pragmatics: Mental processes of communication,* MIT Press, Boston, MA.

Barwise J.(1985), The Situation in Logic-II: Conditionals and Conditional Information, *Report No. CSLI-85-21.*

Barwise J.(1985), The Situation in Logic-III: Situations, Sets and the Axiom of Foundation, *Report No. CSLI-85-26.*

Barwise J., J.M.Gawron, G.Plotkin, S.Tutiya(eds.)(1991), Situation Theory and its Applications, Vol.2, *CSLI Lecture Notes No.26.*

Berners-Lee, T., Hendler, J., and Lassila, O. The Semantic Web. Scientific American (May 2001)

Bianchi D., R.Delmonte, E.Pianta(1993), Understanding Stories in Different Languages with GETA_RUN, *Proc.EC of the ACL*, Utrecht, 464.

Bianchi D., Rodolfo Delmonte(1999), Reasoning with A Discourse Model and Conceptual Representations, *Proc. VEXTAL,* Unipress, pp. 401-411.

Boguraev B. & C. Kennedy(1997), *Salience-based Content Characterisation of Text Documents,* in I.Mani & M.Maybury(eds.), ibid., 2-9.

Boris Katz, Jimmy J. Lin, Sue Felshin: The START Multimedia Information System: Current Technology and Future Directions, In *Proceedings of the International Workshop on Multimedia Information Systems* (MIS 2002)

Borislav Popov, Atanas Kiryakov, Dimitar Manov, Angel Kirilov, Damyan Ognyanoff, Miroslav Goranov: Towards Semantic Web Information Extraction, Workshop on Human Language Technology for the Semantic Web http://gate.ac.uk/ conferences/iswc2003/ proceedings/popov.pdf (2003)

Bos, J., Clark, S., Steedman, M., Curran, J., Hockenmaier, J.: Wide-coverage semantic representations from a ccg parser. In: *Proc. of the 20th International Conference on Computational Linguistics.* Geneva, Switzerland (2004).

Bosch P.(1993), Lexical Meaning and Conceptual Representation, Bericht Nr. 30, Arbeitspapiere 340 DFG Sonderforschungsbereich, Stuttgart.

Brachman R., Schmolze J.(1985), An Overview of the KL-ONE Knowledge Representation System, *Cognitive Science* 7, 171-216.

Braz, R., Girju, R., Punyakanok, V., Roth, D., Sammons, M.: An Inference Model for Semantic Entailment in Natural Language. In: Proc. of the 1st. PASCAL Recognision Textual Entailment Challenge Workshop, Southampton, U.K., (2005) 29-3.

Bresnan, Joan. 2001. *Lexical-Functional Syntax*. Blackwells.

Brill, E., Lin, J., Banko, M., Dumais, S., & Ng, A. (2002). Data-Intensive Question Answering. In E. M. Voorhees & D. K. Harman (eds.), *The Tenth Text Retrieval Conference (TREC 2001).* 122-131.

Burke T.(1991), *Pierce on Truth and Partiality,* in J.Barwise et al.(eds.), op.cit., 115-146.

Busemann S.(1991), Structure-Driven Generation from Separate Semantic Representation, in Proc.ACL, 113-118.

Burstein, J. and Wolska, M. (2003). Toward Evaluation of Writing Style: Overly Repetitious Word Use in Student Writing. In *Proceedings of the 11th Conference of the EACL.* Budapest,35-42.

Carlson G.(1977), *Reference to Kinds in English,* Ph.D. Dissertation, University of Massachusetts, Amherst.

Carlson, L., Marcu, D., & Okurowski, M. (2002). *RST Discourse Treebank.* Philadelphia, PA:Linguistic Data Consortium.

Chintan Patel, Kaustubh Supekar, and Yugyung Lee, OntoGenie: Extracting Ontology Instances from WWW, Workshop on Human Language Technology for the Semantic Web http://gate.ac.uk/conferences/iswc2003/proceedings/patel.pdf (2003)

Ciravegna, F.: (LP)2, an Adaptive Algorithm for Information Extraction from Web related Texts. In: *Proc. IJCAI-2001 Work.* on Adaptive Text Extraction and Mining (2001)

Clark, H. H., & Clark, E. V. (1977). *Psychology and language: An introduction to psycholinguistics*. New York: Harcourt Brace Jovanovich, Inc.

Cooper R.(1991), *Three Lectures on Situation Theoretic Grammar*, in Situation Theoretic Grammar, op.cit., 1-44.

Cooper R.(1991), *Situation Theoretic Grammar,* 3rd European Summer School in LLI, Universität des Saarlandes, Saarbrücken.

Cooper R.P.(1991), *Persistence and Structural Determination,* in J.Barwise et al.(eds.), op.cit., 295-310.

Corley, C., Mihalcea, R.: Measuring the Semantic Similarity of Texts , in *Proceedings of the ACL 2005 Workshop on "Empirical Modeling of Semantic Equivalence and Entailment",* Ann Arbor, MI. (2005) 13-18.

Dagan, I., Glickman, O., Magnini, B.: The pascal recognising textual entailment challenge. In: *Proceedings of the Recognising Textual Entailment Challenge*, Southampton (UK), (2005) 1-8

Dahlgren K.(1988), *Naive Semantics for Natural Language Understanding,* Kluwer, Boston.

Dahlgren K., J. McDowell(1989), Knowledge Representation for Commonsense Reasoning with Text, *Computational Linguistics,* 15, 3, pp.149-170.

Dale R., Mellish C.S., Zock M.(eds)(1990), *Current Research in Natural Language Generation,* Voll.I-II, AP, London.

Dancygier, B. & Sweetser, E. (2000). Constructions with if, since and because: Causality, epistemic stance, and clause order. In Couper-Kuhlen, E. & Kortmann, B. (eds), *Cause, Condition, Concession, Contrast; Cognitive and Discourse Perspectives.* Berlin/New York: Mouton de Gruyter.

Davidson, D. (1967). The logical form of action sentences. In Rescher, N. (ed.), *The logic of decision and action.* Pittsburgh: University of Pittsburgh Press.

Delmonte R.(1990), Semantic Parsing with an LFG-based Lexicon and Conceptual Representations, *Computers & the Humanities*, 5-6, 461-488.

Delmonte R., D.Bianchi, E.Pianta(1992), GETA_RUN - A General Text Analyzer with Reference Understanding, in *Proc. 3rd Conference on Applied Natural Language Processing, Systems Demonstrations*, Trento, ACL-92, 9-10.

Delmonte, R., Bianchi D.: Binding Pronominals with an LFG Parser. In: *Proceeding of the Second International Workshop on Parsing Technologies,* Cancun (Mexico), ACL. (1991) 59-72

Delmonte R., D.Bianchi(1994), *Computing Discourse Anaphora from Grammatical Representation,* in D.Ross & D.Brink(eds.), Research in Humanities Computing 3, Clarendon Press, Oxford, 179-199.

Delmonte R., 1994: *Inferences and Discourse Structure,* in G.Ferrari(ed), Proc.IV Conference of the Italian Artificial Intelligence Association - AIIA, 11-14.

Delmonte R., Dibattista D.(1995), Switching from Narrative to Legal Genre, *Working Papers in Linguistics,* C.L.I., University of Venice.

Delmonte R.(1995), Lexical Representations: Syntax-Semantics interface and World Knowledge, in *Notiziario AIIA (Associazione Italiana di Intelligenza Artificiale),* Roma, pp.11-16.

Delmonte R.(1997), Lexical Representations, Event Structure and Quantification, *Quaderni Patavini di Linguistica*, 39-94.

Delmonte R. D.Bianchi (1998), Dialogues From Texts: How to Generate Answers from a Discourse Model, *Atti Convegno Nazionale AI*IA,* Padova, 139-143.

Delmonte R.(1999), From Shallow Parsing to Functional Structure, in Atti del Workshop AI*IA - "Elaborazione del Linguaggio e Riconoscimento del Parlato", *IRST Trento,* pp.8-19.

Delmonte R., E.Pianta(1999), Tag Disambiguation in Italian, in *Proc. Treebank Workshop ATALA,* Paris, pp.43-49.

Delmonte R., D.Bianchi(1999), Determining Essential Properties of Linguistic Objects for Unrestricted Text Anaphora Resolution, *Proc. Workshop on Procedures in Discourse,* Pisa, pp.10-24.

Delmonte R. 2000a. Generating from a Discourse Model, *Proc. MT-2000*, BCS, Exeter, pp.25-1/10.

Delmonte R., 2000b. Shallow Parsing And Functional Structure In Italian Corpora, *Proc. LREC*, Athens, pp.113-119.

Delmonte R., 2000c. Parsing with GETARUN, *Proc.TALN2000, 7° conférence annuel sur le TALN*, Lausanne, pp.133-146.

Delmonte R., 2000d. Parsing Preferences and Linguistic Strategies, in *LDV-Forum - Zeitschrift fuer Computerlinguistik und Sprachtechnologie - "Communicating Agents"*, Band 17, 1,2, pp. 56-73.

Delmonte R., D. Bianchi, (2002) From Deep to Partial Understanding with GETARUNS, *Proc. ROMAND 2002*, Università Roma2, Roma, pp.57-71.

Delmonte R.(2002), GETARUN PARSER - A parser equipped with Quantifier Raising and Anaphoric Binding based on LFG, Proc. LFG2002 Conference, Athens, pp.130-153, at http://cslipublications.stanford.edu/hand/miscpubsonline.html.

Delmonte R., 2003a. Getaruns: a hybrid system for summarization and question answering, in *Proc. Workshop "Natural Language Processing for Question Answering"* in EACL, Budapest, pp.21-28.

Delmonte R., 2003b. The Semantic Web Needs Anaphora Resolution, *Proc.Workshop ARQAS, 2003 International Symposium on Reference Resolution and Its Applications to Question Answering and Summarization,* Venice, Ca' Foscari University, pp.25-32.

Delmonte R., 2004a.: Evaluating GETARUNS Parser with GREVAL Test Suite, Proc. ROMAND - *20th International Conference on Computational Linguistics* - COLING, University of Geneva, (2004) 32-41

Delmonte, R., 2004b: Text Understanding with GETARUNS for Q/A and Summarization, *Proc. ACL 2004 - 2nd Workshop on Text Meaning & Interpretation, Barcelona,* Columbia University (2004) 97-104

Delmonte R., Sara Tonelli, Marco Aldo Piccolino Boniforti, Antonella Bristot, Emanuele Pianta, 2005.: VENSES – a Linguistically-Based System for Semantic Evaluation, RTE Challenge Workshop, Southampton, *PASCAL - European Network of Excellence*, 49-52.

Derr M. A., McKeown K.R., 1984.: Using Focus to Generate Complex and Simple Sentences, *Porc. 10th International Conference on Computational Linguistics, COLING,* 319-326.

van Dijk, Teun A., 1979. Pragmatic connectives. Journal of Pragmatics 3, 447-456.

Dolan, W.B., Quirk, C., Brockett, C.: Unsupervised construction of large paraphrase corpora: Exploiting massively parallel news sources. In: *Proceedings of the 20th International Conference on Computational Linguistics*, Geneva, Switzerland. (2004).

Dorr B.,(1993), *Machine Translation*, MIT Press, Cambridge Mass.

Dowty D.(1979), Word Meaning and Montague Grammar, Reidel.

Eikmeyer H.-J., Rieser H.(eds.)(1981), Words, Worlds, and Contexts, de Gruyter, Berlin.

Enç M.(1986), Towards a referential analysis of temporal expressions, *Linguistic and Philosophy* 9.

Faraci, R. (1974). *Aspects of the grammar of in®nitives and for-phrases*. Ph.D. dissertation, MIT.

Fenstad J.E. et al.(1987), *Situations, Language and Logic,* Reidel, Dordrecht.

Fraurud, Keri (1990), Definiteness and the processing of NPs in natural discourse, *Journal of Semantics,* 7, 395-433.

Gazdar G. (1979), *Pragmatics,* Academic Press, New York.

Glickman, O., Dagan, I., Koppel, M.: A Probabilistic Classification Approach for Lexical Textual Entailment, *Twentieth National Conference on Artificial Intelligenc*e (AAAI-05), (2005).

Greimas A.J. (1966), *Structural Semantics: An Attempt at a Method,* University of Nebraska Press, 1983.

Halvorsen P.K. and R.Kaplan(1988), Projections and semantic description, *Proceedings of the International Conference on Fifth Generation Computer System*, Tokyo, 1116-1122.

Halvorsen P.K.(1983), Semantics for Lexical Functional Grammar,*Linguistic Inquiry* 4,567-616.

Halvorsen P.K.(1988), Situation semantics and semantic interpretation in constrained-based grammars, *Proceedings of the International Conference on Fifth Generation Computer System*, Tokyo, 471-478.

Halvorsen P.K. & R.Kaplan(1988), Projections and semantic description, *Proceedings of the International Conference on Fifth Generation Computer System*, Tokyo, 1116-1122.

Harabagiu, S., Pasca, M., Maiorano S.: Open-Domain Question Answering Techniques. Natural Language Engineering 1 (1), CUP. (2003) 1-38.

Hauser, M. D., Chomsky, N., & Fitch, W. T. (2002). The faculty of language: What is it, who has it, and how did it evolve? *Science*, 298, 1569-1579.

Heim I. (1982), *The Semantics of Definite and Indefinite Noun Phrases,* Ph.D. thesis, University of Massachusetts, Amherst.

Hendrix G.(1978), The Representation of Semantic Knowledge, in D.Walker(ed), *op.cit.,* 121-224.

Herzog O., C.-R. Rollinger(1991)(eds), *Text Understanding in LILOG,* Springer Verlag, Berlin.

Higginbotham, J. (1983). The logic of perceptual reports: an extensional alternative to Situation Semantics. *Journal of Philosophy* 80. 100-127.

Higginbotham J.(1985), On Semantics, *Linguistic Inquiry* 16, 4, 547-593.

Higginbotham J.(1989), Elucidations of Meaning, *Linguistics and Philosophy* 12, 4, 465-518.

Hinzen, W. (2006). Mind Design and Minimal Syntax. Oxford: Oxford University Press.

Hinzen, W. (2007a). An Essay on Naming and Truth. Oxford: Oxford University Press.

Hinzen, W. (2007b). 'The successor function + LEX = Human Language?", in K. Grohman (ed.), InterPhases, Oxford University Press, forthcoming.

Hinzen, W. (2007c). Emergence of a systemic semantics through minimal and underspecified code, Talk delivered at the conference "Biolinguitics – Perspective on language evolution and variation", Auditorium S.Margherita, Venezia, June 5th, 2007.

Hirschman, L. Marc Light, Eric Breck, & J. D. Buger. 1999. Deep Read: A reading comprehension system. In *Proc. A CL '99.*University of Maryland.

Hobbs J.R.(1993), I*ntention, Information, and Structure in Discourse:* A First Draft, Artificial Intelligence Center, SRI International.

Hornstein N.(1989), *As Times Goes By: Tense and Universal* , Ms, University of Brandeis.

Hovy E.H.(1988), *Generating Natural Language Under Pragmatic Constraints,* Lawrence Erlbaum Associates, Hillsdale, NJ.

Hovy E.H.(1994), Automated discourse generation using discourse structure relations, in Pereira & Grosz(eds), *Natural Language Processing,* MITPress, 341-385.

Hovy E. & C.Y.Lin (1997), Automated Text Summarization in SUMMARIST, in I.Mani & M.Maybury(eds.), *ibid.,* 18-24.

Hovy, E., U. Hermjakob, & C. Lin. (2002a). The Use of External Knowledge in Factoid QA. In E. M. Voorhees & D. K. Harman (eds.), *The Tenth Text Retrieval Conference (TREC 2001).* 644-652.

Jackendoff R. (1972), Semantic Interpretation in Generative Grammar, The MIT Press, Cambridge, MA.

Jackendoff R.(1976), Towards an Explanatory Semantic Representation, *Linguistic Inquiry* 7, 89-150

Jackendoff R.(1980), Belief Contexts Revisited, *Linguistic Inquiry* 11(2).

Jackendoff R. (1983), Semantics and Cognition, MIT Press, Cambridge Mass.

Jackendoff R. (1985a) Believing and Intending: Two Sides of the Same Coin, *Linguistic Inquiry* 16, 445-460.

Jackendoff R. (1985b), Multiple Subcategorization and theTheta-Criterion: the Case of *Climb*, *Natural Language and Linguistic Theory* 3, 271-296.

Jackendoff R.(1987a), Consciousness and the Computational Mind, The MIT Press, Cambridge Mass.

Jackendoff R.(1987b), The Status of Thematic Relations in Linguistic Theory, *Linguistic Inquiry* 18, 369-411.

Jackendoff, Ray S. 1992. "Parts and boundaries." in Levin and Pinker (1992). 9-46.

Jackendoff R.(1993), The Combinatorial Structure of Thought: The Family of Causative Concepts, in Reuland & Abraham(eds), op.cit., 31-50.

Jackendoff R.(1993b), On the role of Conceptual Structure in Argument Selection: A Reply to Emonds, *Natural Language and Linguistic Theory* 11, 2, 279-312.

Jena http://www.hpl.hp.com/semweb/

Kadmon N.(1990), *Uniqueness, Linguistics and Philosophy* 13, 3, 273-324.

Kahan, J. and Koivunen, M. Annotea: an open RDF infrastructure for shared web annotations, in *Proceedings of WWW10* (May 2001)

Keenan E.(1984), A Boolean Approach to Semantics, in Groenendijk, Janssen, Stockhof(eds), *Truth,Interpretation and Information,* Foris, Dordrecht, 65-98.

Keenan E.(1987), A Semantic Definition of "Indefinite NP", in Reuland and ter Meulen(eds), *op.cit.,* 286-318.

Keenan E., Faltz L.(1985), *Boolean Semantics for Natural Language,* Reidel, Dordrecht.

Kempen G.(ed)(1987), *Natural Language Generation,* Kluwer Academic, Dodrecht.

Klein Dan and Christopher D. Manning: Accurate Unlexicalized Parsing. *ACL, (2003)* 423-430

Landauer, T. K., Laham, D., Rehder, B., & Schreiner, M. E., (1997). How well can passage meaning be derived without using word order? A comparison of Latent Semantic Analysis and humans. In M. G. Shafto & P. Langley (Eds.), *Proceedings of the 19th annual meeting of the Cognitive Science Society* (pp. 412-417). Mahwah, NJ: Erlbaum.

Lang E.(1991), The LILOG Ontology from a Linguistic Point of View, in Herz & Rollinger, op.cit., pp.464-481.

Laresohn P.(1990), Group Action and Spatio-Temporal Proximity, *Linguistics and Philosophy* 13, 2, 179-206.

Lascarides A., Asher N.(1991), Discourse Relations and Defeasible Knowledge, in *Proceedings 29th Annual Meeting of the ACL,* Berkeley, Cal, 55-62.

Lassila, O. and Swick, R. (eds.). Resource Description Framework (RDF) model and syntax specification. Available at http://www.w3.org/ TR/1999/REC-rdf-syntax-19990222.

Levin, Lori, Malka Rappaport and Annie Zaenen. 1983. *Papers on Lexical-Functional Grammar*. Bloomington: Indiana University Linguistics Club.

Levin, Beth and Steven Pinker. 1992. *Lexical and conceptual semantics*. Oxford: Blackwell.

Levin, B., & Rappaport Hovav, M. (1994). A preliminary analysis of causative verbs in English. *Lingua: International Review of General Linguistics,* 92, 35-77.

Levin, Beth and Malka Rappaport Hovav. 1995. Unaccusativity: at the syntax-lexical semantics interface. *Linguistic Inquiry monographs* 26. Cambridge, Mass.: MIT Press.

Lin D.: Dependency-based evaluation of MINIPAR. In *Proceedings of the Workshop on Evaluation of Parsing Systems at LREC 1998*. Granada, Spain, (1998)

Lin, D., Pantel, P.: *DIRTdiscovery of inference rules from text. In: Knowledge Discovery and Data Mining*, (2001) 323–328.

Litkowski, K. C. (2001). Syntactic Clues and Lexical Resources in Question-Answering. In E. M. Voorhees & D. K. Harman (eds.), *The Ninth Text Retrieval Conference (TREC-9).* 157-166.

Litkowski, K. C. (2002). CL Research Experiments in TREC-10 Question-Answering. In E. M. Voorhees & D. K. Harman (eds.), *The Tenth Text Retrieval Conference (TREC 2001).* 122-131.

Litman D.J.(1985), Linguistic Coherence: a Plan-Based Alternative, Proc.ACL, 215-222.

Litman D.J., J.F.Allen(1984), A Plan Recognition Model for Clarification Subdialogues, Coling84, Stanford, 302-311.

Mani I. & M.Maybury(eds.),(1997), Intelligent Scalable Text Summarization, ACL, Madrid.

Mann, W.C. & Thompson, S.A.(1987), Rhetorical Structure Theory: A theory of text organization. Technical Report ISI/RS-87-190, ISI.

Mann, William C., 2005. RST Web Site, http://www.sfu.ca/rst.

Marcu D. 2000. The Rhetorical Parsing of Unrestricted Text: a Surface-based Approach, CL 26:3, pp. 395-448.

Marcu, D. (2000). *The theory and practice of discourse parsing and summarization.* Cambridge, MA: MIT Press.

Marcu D. and A. Echihabi, 2002. An Unsupervised Approach to Recognizing Discourse Relations. In the *Proceedings of the 40th Annual Meeting of the Association for Computational Linguistics* (ACL'02), Philadelphia, PA (2002), pp. 368-375.

Martin W.(1981), Roles, Co-Descriptors, and the Formal Representation of Quantified English Expressions, in *American Journal of Computational Linguistics*, 7, 3, 137-147.

May R.(1985), *Logical Form,* The MIT Press, Cambridge(Mass.).

May R.(1989), Interpreting Logical Form, *Linguistics and Philosophy* 12, 4, 387-436.

McCawley J.(1981), *Everything that Linguistis have Always Wanted to Know about Logic* -* *but were ashamed to ask, The University of Chicago Press,Chicago.

ter Meulen A.(1983), *The representation of time in natural language*, in A. ter Meulen(ed), Studies in Modeltheoretic Semantics, Foris, Dordrecht, 177-192.

McCoy K.F., K.Vijay-Shanker, G.Yang(1992), A Functional Approach to Generation with TAG, *Proc. ACL*, 48-55.

McDonald D.D.(1984), Description Directed Control: Its Implications for Natural Language Generation, in Cercone(ed), *Computational Linguistics,* Pergamon Press, 111-130.

McDonald D.D., Bolc L. (eds.) (1988), N*atural Language Generation Systems,* Springer-Verlag, New York.

McDonald D.D., J.D.Pustejovsky(1987), Tags as a grammatical formalism for generation, *Proc.ACL*, 94-103.

McDonald D.D., M.W.Meteer(1989), FromWater toWine: Generating Natural Language Text from Today's Applications Programs, *Proc.ACL,* 41-48.

McKeown K. (1985), *Text generation,* Cambridge University Press, London.

Meier Einar, "Since you mention it" - A contrastive study of causal subordination in English and Norwegian, *Thesis presented to the Department of British and American studies,* University of Oslo, in partial fulfilment of the Cand. Philol degree Spring term 2001.

Moens M., M.Steedman, *Temporal Ontology and Temporal Reference,* in *Computational Linguistics* cit., 15-28.

Navigli R. and P. Velardi: Learning Domain Ontologies from Document Warehouses and Dedicated Web Sites, *Computational Linguistics, (*30-2), MIT Press, April, (2004)

Novak H.J.(1985), Generating a Coherent Text Describing a Traffic Scene, *Proc.ACL,* 570-575.

Palmer M., D.Dahl, R.Schiffman, L.Hirshman, M.Linebarger, J.Dowding(1986), Discovering Implicit Information, *Proceedings of the ACL,* New York, 10-19.

Palmer M.S., Passoneau R.J., C.Weir, T.Finin(1994), The KERNEL text understanding system, in Pereira & Grosz(eds), *Natural Language Processing,* MITPress, 17-68.

Paris C.L., W.R.Swartout, W.C.Mann(eds)(1991), *Natural Language Generation in Artificial* Intelligence and Computational Linguistics, Kluwer Academic, Dordrecht.

Partee B. (1993), S*emantic Structures and Semantic Properties,* in Reuland & Abraham(eds), op.cit. 7-30.

Pereira F.(1989), A Calculus for Semantic Composition and Scoping, in *Proceedings of the 27th Annual Meeting of ACL,* Vancouver,

Pinker, S. (1989). *Learnability and cognition: The acquisition of argument structure.* Cambridge, MA: The MIT Press.

Poesio M.(1991), Relational Semantics and Scope Ambiguity, in J.Barwise et al.(eds.), *op.cit.*, 469-498.

Polanyi L., Scha R. (1984), A Syntactic Approach to Discourse Semantics, Proceedings of COLING84, ACL.

Polanyi, L. (1996). *The linguistic structure of discourse*. Stanford, CA.

Pollack M., F.Pereira(1988), An Integrated Framework for Semantic and Pragmatic Interpretation, in *Proc. ACL,* Buffalo, 75-86.

Preis J., (2003), Using Grammatical Relations to Compare Parsers, in *Proc., EACL,* Budapest, pp.291-298.

Propp V.(1927), *Morphology of the Folktale*, Trans., Laurence Scott. 2nd ed. Austin: University of Texas Press, 1968.

Punyakanok, V., Roth, D., Yih. W.: Natural language inference via dependency tree mapping: *An application to question answering. Computational Linguistics* (2004)

Pustejovsky J.(1988), The Geometry of Events, *Lexicon Project Working Papers 24,* Center of Cognitive Science, MIT, 19-39.

Pustejovsky J.(1991a), *The syntax of event structure,* Cognition, 41, 47-81.

Pustejovsky J.(1991b), The Generative Lexicon, *Computational Linguistics* 17, 4, 409-441.

Raina, R., Haghighi, A., Cox, C., Finkel, J., Michels, J., Toutanova, K., MacCartney, B., Marneffe, M.C., Manning, C.D., Ng, A. Y.: Robust Textual Inference using Diverse Knowledge Sources. In: *Proc. of the 1st. PASCAL Recognision Textual Entailment* Challenge Workshop, Southampton, U.K., (2005) 57-60.

Rambow O., T.Korelsky(1992), Applied Text Generation, *Proc.3rd Conference on Applied NLP,* 40-47, Trento.

Ravichandran, D. & E. Hovy. (2002). Learning Surface Text Patterns for a Question Answering System. *Proceedings of the 40th ACL.* Philadelphia, PA., 41-7.

Reimer U., U.Hahn, *A Formal Model of Text Summarization Based on Condensation Operators of a Terminological Logic,* in I.Mani & M.Maybury(eds.), ibid., 97-104.

Riloff, E.: *A Case Study in Using Linguistic Phrases for Text Categorization on the WWW.* In: AAAI/ICML Work. Learning for Text Categorization (2001)

Sandstrøm G.(1993), *Narrative Discourse*, Report No.34, DGL-UUM-R.34.

Scha R., B. Bruce, L.Polanyi(1986), Discourse Understanding, *BBN Technical Report No.391,* October 1986.

Schiffrin, Deborah, 2001. *Discourse markers: Language, meaning and context.* In: Schiffrin, D.,

Schwitter R., D. Mollà, R. Fournier & M. Hess, 2000. Answer Extraction: Towards better Evaluations of NLP Systems. *In Proc. Works. Reading Comprehension Tests as Evaluation for Computer-Based Language Understanding Systems*, Seattle, 20-27.

Shieber S.M., F.C.N.Pereira, G. van Noord, R.C.Moore(1990), Semantic-head-driven generation, *Computational Linguistics*, 16:30-42.

Simpson, Jane H. 1983. "Resultatives." In Rappaport, Levin and Zaenen, eds., *Papers in LFG.* Indiana University Linguistic Club.

Sleator, Daniel, and Davy Temperley: "Parsing English with a Link Grammar." *Proceedings of IWPT* '93, (1993)

Smith, C. S. (1970). *Jespersen's 'move and change' class and causative verbs in English.* In M. A. Jazayery, E.C. Palomé, & W. Winter (Eds.), Linguistic and literary studies in honor of Archibald A. Hill. Vol. 2: Descriptive linguistics (pp. 101-109). The Hague: Mouton.

Soricut, R. and Marcu, D.(2003), Sentence level discourse parsing using syntactic and lexical information, *Proceedings of the 2003 Conference of the North American Chapter of the Association for Computational Linguistics on HumanLanguage Technology-Volume 1* pp. 149–156.

Spark Jones K. (1997), *Summarizing: Where are we now? Where should we go?,* in I.Mani & M.Maybury(eds.), ibid., 1.

Talmy G.(1973), Opacity and Reference in language: an Inquiry into the role of modalities, in J.Kimball(ed), *Syntax and Semantics,* 2, Academic Press, New York.

Talmy, Leonard. 1976. Semantic causative types. In Masayoshi Shibatani, editor, *Syntax and Semantics 6: The Grammar of Causative Constructions*. Academic Press, pages 43-116.

Talmy, Leonard. 1988. Force dynamics in language and thought. *Cognitive Science*, 12:49-100.

Talmy, Leonard. 2000. *Toward a Cognitive Semantics* – Vol.1, LCS Series, Chpt. 8, The MIT Press, 471-549.

Talmy, Leonard. 2000. *Toward a Cognitive Semantics* – Vol.2, LCS Series, The MIT Press.

Tannen, D. & Hamilton, H. E. (Eds.), *The Handbook of Discourse Analysis,* Blackwell, Malden, MA, pp. 54-75.

Vander Linden, K.(1993), Rhetorical Relations in Instructional Text Generation, in *Proc.Workshop on "Intentionality and Structure in Discourse Relations",* ACL, Columbus, pp.140-143.

Vander Linden, K.(1994), Generating Precondition Expressions in Instructional Text, in *Proc. 32nd Annual Meeting of the ACL,* N.Mexico.

Vendler, Zeno. 1967. "Verbs and times." in Zeno Vendler. *Linguistics in philosophy.* Ithaca: Cornell University Press. 97-121.

Voorhees E.M. (1999), *Natural Language Processing and Information Retrieval, in* Pazienza M.T.(ed.),(1999), *Information Extraction*, Springer.

Walker M.(1989), *Evaluating Discourse Processing Algorithms, in Proceedings of the 27th Annual Meeting of ACL,* Vancouver, 251-261.

Webber B. L. (1981), *Discourse model synthesis: preliminaries to reference.* In A. Joshi, B. L. Webber and I. Sag (eds.), op.cit..

Webber B. L.(1983), So what can we talk about now?, in Brady M. and Berwick R.(eds), *Computational Models of Discourse,* The MIT Press, 331-372.

Webber B.L.(1988), Tense as Discourse Anaphor, in *Computational Linguistics* - Special Issue on Tense and Aspect - 14, 2, 61-73.

Webber B.L.(1991a), Structure and Ostension in the Interpretation of Discourse Deixis, in *Language and Cognitive Processes* 6 (2), 107-135.

Webber B.L., B.Baldwin(1993), Accomodating Context Change, in *Proc.ACL*, 96-103.

Webber-Nash B.(1977), Anaphora and logical form: on formal meaning representations for natural language, in *Proceedings of 5th IJCAI*, 121-131.

Wolf, Florian & Edward Gibson, Amy Fisher, Meredith Knight, *A procedure for collecting a database of texts annotated with coherence relations,* Technical Manual, December 1, 2003.

Wolff, Phillip, B. Klettke, T. Ventura, G. Song, 2005. Expressing Causation in English and Other Languages, in Woo-Kyoung Ahn et al. (eds.), 2005. Categorization Inside And Outside The Laboratory: Essays In Honor Of Douglas L. Medin, Part I. *Language, culture, categories, and induction,* 29, (20).

Wolff, P., & Song, G. (2003). Models of causation and the semantics of causal verbs. *Cognitive Psychology,* 47, 276-332.

Wolff, P., Song, G., & Driscoll, D. (2002). Models of causation and causal verbs. In M. Andronis, C. Ball, H. Elston, & S. Neuval (Eds.), *Papers from the 37 the Meeting of the Chicago Linguistics Society,* Main Session, Vol. 1, (pp. 607-622). Chicago: Chicago Linguistics Society.

Woods W.(1978), Taxonomic Lattice Structures for Situation Recognition, *American Journal of Computational Linguistics*, 33-41.

WordNet www.cogsci.princeton.edu/~wn/

Zaenen, A., Karttunen, L., Crouch, R.: Local Textual Inference: Can it be Defined or Circumscribed?. In: *Proc. Workshop Empirical Modeling of Semantic Equivalence and Entailment,* ACL05, University of Michigan, Ann Arbor Michigan, (2005) 31-36.

Harvard dictionary: http://www.wjh.harvard.edu/
Moby: http://www.dcs.shef.ac.uk/research/ilash/Moby/

INDEX

A

E

F

G

H

I

J

K

L

M

N

O

P

Q

R

S

T

U

V

W

X

Y